Responses to Traumatized Children

Also by Amer A. Hosin

(ed.) ESSAYS ON ISSUES IN APPLIED DEVELOPMENTAL PSYCHOLOGY AND CHILD PSYCHIATRY

(ed.) TYPICAL OR ATYPICAL DEVELOPMENT: APPLIED PSYCHOLOGY AND CHILD PSYCHIATRY PERSPECTIVES

First published 2007 by
PALGRAVE MACMILLAN
Houndmills, Basingstoke, Hampshire RG21 6XS and
175 Fifth Avenue, New York, N.Y. 10010
Companies and representatives throughout the world

PALGRAVE MACMILLAN is the global academic imprint of the Palgrave
Macmillan division of St. Martin's Press, LLC and of Palgrave Macmillan Ltd.
Macmillan® is a registered trademark in the United States, United Kingdom
and other countries. Palgrave is a registered trademark in the European
Union and other countries.

ISBN 13: 978–1–4039–9680–0   hardback
ISBN 10: 1–4039–9680–6   hardback

This book is printed on paper suitable for recycling and made from fully
managed and sustained forest sources.

A catalogue record for this book is available from the British Library.

Library of Congress Cataloging-in-Publication Data

Responses to traumatized children / edited by Amer A. Hosin
    p. cm.
  Includes bibliographical references and index.
  ISBN 1–4039–9680–6 (cloth)
   1. Psychic trauma in children. 2. Child psychotherapy.

  RJ506.P66R472 2007
  18.92'8914–dc26   2006044687

10   9   8   7   6   5   4   3   2
16   15   14   13   12   11   10   09   08

Printed and bound in Great Britain by
Antony Rowe Ltd, Chippenham and Eastbourne

Responses to Traumatiz
Children

Edited by
Amer A. Hosin

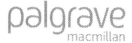

In memory of my eldest brother whose care, passion and sacrifices for me were immeasurable. Indeed, I could neither match nor repay.

To all traumatized children and adult victims of both manmade and natural disasters whose losses, fears, resilience, coping and determination inspired me to produce this volume.

This book is also dedicated to all victims of ethnic cleansing who suffered fear, uncertainty and displacement.

Contents

Foreword

Events that inflict psychological trauma on children are diverse and unfortunately in most cases can lead to catastrophic outcomes. Natural disasters (such as earthquakes, tsunamis and hurricanes) and manmade disasters (such as wars, terrorist attacks and ethnic cleansing) often affect individuals, families, communities and, at times, whole nations. For example, the 2004 south Asian tsunami, hurricane Katrina (2005) in the USA, and the recent earthquake in northern Pakistan and Kashmir took a combined toll of over half a million human lives; the majority of victims were children, women and elderly.

War is the most violent of the manmade disasters and surpasses by far the natural disasters in its impact, lethality and destructive power. It has been estimated that the armed conflicts that have occurred around the world between 1980 and 2005 have resulted in the deaths of 3.5 million children, the disability of 7.8 million individuals, the orphaning of 1.75 million, and made 21 million children homeless (*State of the World's Children*, UNICEF, 2005). Research has shown that wars and natural disasters have a profound impact on children's physical and psychological well-being and the stress produced by such events has the ability to stunt their physical growth and may bring about physiological changes. I met a seven-year-old girl in Bosnia Herzegovina whose hair prematurely turned grey after she was forced to witness the rape, torture and murder of her mother. Most children, exposed to life-threatening events, develop a wide range of symptoms ranging from inability to sleep to palpitations, migraine and stomach aches. Young children may regress to bedwetting, become socially withdrawn and may refuse to attend school.

The psychological reactions to traumatic experiences in children have the potential to arrest their emotional growth and may destroy their hope in the future. Fearfulness, sleep disturbance, nightmares, poor school performance and hyper-arousals are some of the symptoms that haunt traumatized children and impair their capacity to learn and grow in peace and harmony (see Chapters 1 and 2).

The work that we have been doing at the International Center for Psychosocial Trauma at the University of Missouri and in various war zones and disaster areas around the world during the past twelve years or so, led us to conclude that the core reactions to traumatic events tend to be similar across cultures. The majority of the children initially develop psychological symptoms depending on the severity and nature of the trauma, such as direct threat to life, loss of loved ones or witnessing horrific life-threatening events. Children who have witnessed the death of a loved one often suffer depression, suicidal ideation and survivor guilt, which could interfere with the recovery from trauma.

Although references to the impact of traumatic events on human beings have been made as early as in the writings of Homer, Shakespeare and Goethe, the medical literature began to report on many of the above-mentioned symptoms only during the late nineteenth century. Conditions labelled as 'traumatic neurosis', 'shell shock' and 'traumatic sleep disturbance and nightmares' started to appear in the authoritative medical journals and the writings of many medical experts. The medical community became more alarmed about the effects of life-threatening experiences on the survivors in the early 1970s when Vietnam veterans returning from combat duty began reporting symptoms of flashback, intrusive thoughts and nightmares and associated impairment of function and co-existing substance abuse and domestic violence. In 1980, the committee on DSM-III included the diagnosis of Post-Traumatic Stress Disorder (PTSD) in the psychiatric classification. The presence of this condition in children was later accepted in 1987 and was included in the revised edition of *DSM-III-R*. Since these developments, research in the field of trauma psychology has significantly increased. Similarly, the reports on the outcomes of various therapeutic measures are beginning to appear in the scientific literature. However, it is interesting to note that not many training programmes in psychiatry, psychology, counselling, nursing, social work and other allied fields teach the special elements of trauma psychology, making it necessary for clinicians and other professionals interested in working with traumatized individuals to take such a sub-specialty and courses.

Focusing on a more hopeful note, many children are also resilient. That is to say, not all children who are exposed to life-threatening situations suffer from its ill effects. Research has shown (see Chapter 8) that a good majority of children who have been exposed to trauma may bounce back to a normal state after initial adverse reactions due to their resilience. Resilience in children depends on temperament, the quality of attachment during early childhood, a supportive family and a special and positive relationship with an adult. Poverty, early bereavement, physical and sexual abuse, a broken family and multiple traumas, on the other hand, increase the vulnerability of a child to the adverse effects of trauma. Various chapters highlighted in this book will allow the readers to be exposed to the evidence-based outcomes of various techniques utilized by practitioners to overcome trauma in children.

Ideally, the interventions should start with preventive measures aimed at the whole society to make it safe and trauma free. The international and national laws, public policies and public institutions supporting individuals' well-being, human security, equity and participation are crucial for making a society safe and perhaps trauma free.

Overall, this book is divided into two main parts. Part I, 'An Overview of Trauma Psychology', consists of ten chapters, while Part II covers the applied context of trauma psychology through four insightful chapters. The topics covered in Part I include four clinical themes: diagnosis, therapeutic modalities including psychopharmacology and neurobiology of PTSD, and recent understanding of factors influencing resilience and compassion fatigue. The consideration of symptoms of secondary traumatization or compassion fatigue and burnout (highlighted in Chapter 10) is an important addition to the first section. Compassion fatigue and burnout, characterized by physical and emotional fatigue, sleep disturbance, hyper-arousal and feelings of guilt, are often reported by the care providers and relief workers who hear the stories of death, destruction and hopelessness of the survivors. The volunteers who have difficulty setting reasonable limits on their desire to help the survivors are at a higher risk of experiencing 'burnout'. Compassion fatigue is preventable if the care providers or relief workers are trained in recognizing their limits and in taking care of themselves while helping others. Daily debriefing, discussion of success, failure and frustrations with co-workers and finding time for self-care and recreation, despite the surrounding chaos, go very far in combating compassion fatigue.

Part II, entitled 'Applied Context of Trauma Psychology', includes some notably important topics, which are often lacking in other books. These topics include: conflict and reconciliation, special issues facing displaced children and physically and sexually abused children.

Although several books have been published in recent years on trauma psychology, there remains a need for more comprehensive accounts and books that include a more extensive range of coverage, including evidence-based research and the underpinning of theories in this rapidly growing field. This book is an attempt to meet such needs. Additionally, most authors who have contributed to this book have hands-on experience in working with the traumatized children of war zones and disaster areas. Besides their expertise in the field, they bring their personal experiences on ground zero into their writings. I trust that this book will offer a clear road map of knowledge for those professionals who are seeking evidence-based interventions and the path of humanitarianism.

Syed Arshad Husain, MD, FRCPsych, FRCP(C)
24 March 2006
Columbia, Missouri

Preface

This book is the result of collaboration between professional colleagues (on both sides of the Atlantic) who have not only worked on or shared research interests in the area of trauma in children but have also been pioneer investigators in this fast-growing field. This whole project would not have been completed without their expertise and contributions. I have no claim to regard the project as a comprehensive account on responding to trauma but I have put together a stimulating, thought-provoking and evidence-based coverage in response to the publisher's original suggestions and the views of the anonymous reviewers who have read the submitted sample manuscript chapters at an early phase of this project.

However, the whole book has been structured (clustered) into two main sections. The first section is an overview which deals with ranges of trauma experienced by children, and possible evidence-based responses. It provides an in-depth introduction to the field and focuses on relevant responses or interventions that ought to be effective in addressing the needs of traumatized children. For example, Chapter 1 ('Responding to Traumatized Children: an Overview of Diagnosis and Treatment Options I', by Roy Lubit) and Chapter 2 ('Treatment Options for Young People and Refugees with Post-Traumatic Stress Disorder II', by Matthew Hodes and Angeles Diaz-Caneja) set the scene and discuss the diagnosis processes and a wide range of treatment approaches available to young and traumatized individuals. Chapter 3 (by Linda Chokroverty and her colleague Nalaini Sriskandarajah) is concerned with a model for acute care of children and adolescents exposed to trauma and life-threatening disasters. In Chapter 4, Natasa Ljubomirovic and Kedar Dwivedi look at outcomes of group work with traumatized children and their families in the southern Serbia and Kosovo regions. Further, Felicity de Zulueta focuses in Chapter 5 on the treatment of psychological trauma from the perspective of attachment research. Chapter 6 (Roy Lubit) provides guidelines on the cognitive behavioural therapy approach used in rehabilitation processes of traumatized children. Iyad Khreis and Rula Khreis (in Chapter 7) address the psychopharmacological treatment approach used with PTSD sufferers. Beyond treatment and interventions, Stephen Joseph and his colleagues Jacky Knibbs and Julie Hobbs (in Chapter 8) analyse the interplay between trauma, resilience and growth in children and adolescents. Roberto Danise (Chapter 9) has used the narrative approach while addressing the cultural perspective of healing trauma. In the concluding chapter of this section (Chapter 10), Kate Cairns presents an overview of her approach for caring for the carers and management of secondary traumatic stress.

The second section, meanwhile, expands the scope of the book to reflect on the applied context of trauma psychology and covers (in Chapter 11, by Liz Davies) responding to protection needs of traumatized and sexually abused children; legacies of conflict in Northern Ireland (Chapter 12, by Eve Binks and Neil Ferguson); and adjustment of both parents and children of exiled and traumatized refugees (Chapter 13, by Amer Hosin). The second section closes with a final chapter (Chapter 14, by Helen O'Nions) on national and international policies designed to deter vulnerable and traumatized asylum seekers and refugees. As can been seen, the focuses of the book are largely reflecting on efforts of effective interventions with references to risk factors. However, other aims of this book are to highlight current trends of morbidity and to bring out the underlying assumption which links both theories and applications.

This book is a suitable text for advanced undergraduates and postgraduate courses in psychology, social work, counselling, medicine (adult and child psychology), nursing, human development and family studies. Trauma psychology is growing rapidly and professional trauma experts have challenging roles, and are now vital members of multidisciplinary teams for child mental health clinics and other social or educational settings.

The choices of the assigned topics were determined by relevance, importance, application to real life situations and evidence-based research and practice. As an editor, I have tried to offer a range of topical coverage or options in an engaging, complementing fashion. The content of each chapter begins with an overview, coherent structure and depth that allow eventually the introduction of a specific option or intervention(s) to emerge. It is my understanding that this unique volume is the first to bring together optional interventions and treatment approaches for various traumatized children. That is to say after more than three decades of PTSD work, we are just beginning to realize the applied nature of the empirical research conducted in this area.

I wish to thank many people for their support and contribution to this scientific effort. First, the contributing authors of this volume for setting the agenda of this project and for their insightful contribution and cooperative spirit in joining me in this endeavour. Indeed, I was honoured and privileged to learn a great deal about their work and expertise while working with them and reviewing the current state of knowledge on trauma psychology. Second, I should also thank my publisher Palgrave for both the publication and the interest they have shown to promote and produce this volume. I must say, I owe the greatest thanks to my wife Sahar and our three children Reem, Ali and Feeras for their patience and support while I was working flat out on this project. Special thanks are also due to those colleagues and friends (namely Professor Ed Cairns and Professor Eileen O'Keefe) whose faith and spirit have proved to be inspirational. Indeed here I need to extend my appreciation and thanks to all of our friends at London Metropolitan University for their support and encouragement during the planning and writing of this project, particularly my colleagues Simon Moore, Nigel Marlow, Carina Browne, Jo Skinner and the late Jaye Daulphin. In fact, Jaye Daulphin was planning to contribute a chapter to this effort but her hospitalization, illness and recent premature death sadly made her unable to see the completion of this book. Dan Bunyard, Jo North and other editorial and production team members at Palgrave Macmillan deserve special praise for their skills, efficiency and experience. The editor would like to thank the *Journal of Family Therapy* (Blackwell Publishing) for permission to reproduce material appearing in Chapter 5 of this book by Felicity de Zulueta.

Finally, I hope that this book will attract and inspire the readers of various backgrounds to learn more about trauma and perhaps consider new approaches in intervention and/or explaining the consequences of traumatic events. The various perspectives that have been highlighted in this volume should also provoke thought, increase awareness and take professionals working in this area to a new level of understanding on life-threatening events.

Amer Hosin

Notes on the Contributors

Eve Binks is a lecturer in Psychology and the Beck Blanche Research Fellow at Liverpool Hope University. She also contributes to the programme delivered by the Desmond Tutu Centre for War and Peace Studies at Liverpool Hope University.

Kate Cairns is a social worker and teacher. With her partner Brian and their three birth children she shared in providing permanence to twelve other children. She also works as a Training Director for Akamas, a company producing and providing online accredited qualifications in child care and management.

Linda Chokroverty is an Assistant Professor of Psychiatry, Albert Einstein College of Medicine, Bronx, NY and chairperson, Child and Adolescent Committee, Disaster Psychiatry Outreach, New York, NY.

Liz Davies is a Senior Lecturer in Social Work, London Metropolitan University. With her main speciality in child protection and families, she teaches social work at both undergraduate and postgraduate levels. She also trains police and social workers in joint investigation and interview skills. She has extensive practice experience as a child protection manager and trainer who provides consultancy and writes widely on child protection issues.

Roberto Dansie is a Clinical Psychologist and director of the Center of Cultural Wisdom, Northern California, www.robertodansie.com. He is a member of the International Trauma Institute, University of Missouri and also a member of the National Center for Primary Care with the Morehouse School of Medicine. In 1997 he received the Golden Medallion from the National Indian Health Board for his contributions to health in Indian Country. In 2005 he was honoured by the University of Missouri with Humanitarian of the Year award for his work with traumatized children.

Dr Angeles Diaz-Caneja is a Consultant in Child and Adolescent Psychiatry, Spain, who formerly worked as a locum consultant, Northwick Park Hospital, Watford Road, Harrow, Middlesex HA1 3UJ, England.

Kedar Nath Dwivedi worked as a Clinical Lecturer (Honorary) in the University of Leicester and Consultant in Child, Adolescent and Family Psychiatry in Northampton until March 2005. He is also the Director of the International Institute of Child and Adolescent Mental Health, UK. He served as Assistant Professor in Social and Preventive Medicine in Simla before moving to psychiatry in the UK. He has been a member of more than a dozen professional associations, serves on the Court of Electors for the Royal College of Psychiatrists and convened the Child and Adolescent Overseas Working Party of the Royal College of Psychiatrists. He has contributed extensively to the literature (nearly forty publications) including editing of books on *Group Work with Children and Adolescents* (Jessica Kingsley), *The Therapeutic Use of Stories* (Routledge), *Enhancing Parenting Skills* (John Wiley), *PTSD in Children and Adolescents* (Whurr) and *Meeting the Needs of Ethnic Minority Children* (Jessica Kingsley), and co-editing, *Management of Childhood Anxiety Disorders* (Arena), *Depression in Children and Adolescents* (Whurr) and *Promoting Emotional Well Being of Children and Adolescents and Preventing their Mental Ill Health* (Jessica Kingsley). He is the Course Director for the Midland Course in Group Work with Children and Adolescents. He is also an examiner for both DCH and for MRCPsych. Dr Dwivedi has a particular interest in Eastern and Buddhist approaches to mental health.

Neil Ferguson is the Director of the Desmond Tutu Centre for War and Peace Studies and Associate Professor of Political Psychology at Liverpool Hope University. He has been a visiting lecturer to Lock Haven University of Pennsylvania, a Research Fellow at University of St Andrews and the Sr. Mary Linscott Fellow at Liverpool Hope University.

Dr Julie Hobbs is a Clinical Psychologist working at St Albans Child and Family Clinic with interests in childhood trauma, attachment, post-traumatic growth, vicarious traumatic growth and holistic psychology.

Matthew Hodes is Senior Lecturer in Child and Adolescent Psychiatry, Imperial College, London. His main research interest is in eating disorders and cultural psychiatry including refugee mental health. Dr Hodes has published many papers on these topics. He also served as a Guest Editor of *Clinical Child Psychology and Psychiatry* (2005), volume 10, number 2, special issue on Children and War. He also works as a Consultant in Child and Adolescent Psychiatry at St Mary's Department of Child & Adolescent Psychiatry, CNWL Mental Health Trust, Paddington Green, London.

Amer Hosin is trained in both psychology and child psychiatry and is currently a Senior Lecturer in Applied Psychology, London Metropolitan University. His previous publication is *Essay on Issues in Applied Developmental Psychology and Child Psychiatry* (Edwin Mellen Press) and numerous publications on traumatized children and childhood psychopathology. He is a consultative board member of the Arab Medical Union in Europe and is on the editorial board of the *Arab Medical Journal*. Dr Amer Hosin is also a member of the British Psychological Society and a fellow of both the American Academy of the Experts in Traumatic Stress and the Institute of Child and Adolescent Mental Health, UK.

Arshad Husain is Professor of Child Psychiatry and Child Health. He is also Chief of the Division of Child and Adolescent Psychiatry, Medical Director of Royal Oaks Hospital in Windsor, Missouri, and Director, International Center for Psychosocial Trauma (ICPT), University of Missouri, Columbia, School of Medicine Columbia, Missouri, USA.

Stephen Joseph is a Professor of Psychology, Health and Social Care in the Department of Sociology and Social Policy at the University of Nottingham. Professor Joseph is a senior practitioner member of the British Psychological Society Register of Psychologists Specialising in Psychotherapy. His research interests are in growth following adversity.

Iyad Khreis has obtained his medical qualification from the University of Damascus, Medical School 1984. His psychiatric training was then completed at the University of Missouri, Columbia, where he also completed his subspecialty on adolescent development, adjustment and problems. He is an American Board-certified psychiatrist and currently works as an Associate Medical Director of Royal Oaks Hospital in Windsor, Missouri. At the University of Missouri, Dr Khreis is the Associate Program Director of the Geriatric Psychiatric Program and is an active member of the International Center of Psychosocial Trauma, Missouri University, Colombia.

Rula Khreis is a biochemist who is pursuing her studies in the field of medicine and conducts research on the tumour-selectivity of S. Typhimurium at the Cancer Research Center of Columbia, Missouri.

Jacky Knibbs is a Consultant Clinical Psychologist working in Child & Adolescent Mental Health in South Warwickshire. She has a particular interest in the development pathways of children and in systemic interventions which maximize children's potential.

Natasa Ljubomirovic completed her medical training at the University of Sarajevo Medical School in 1990. She then specialized in child psychiatry at the Institute of Mental Health in Belgrade with special interest in the impact of war on adolescents. In 2001, Dr Ljubomirovic won a scholarship for further training in child and adolescent mental health and continued her training in the UK. She completed special training in group work with children and adolescents in Northampton, and the EMDR course in Edinburgh. She previously worked in conflict regions in southern Serbia and the Kosovo region and provided care for many Bosnian and Croatian refugees settled in collective centers in southern Serbia. Dr Ljubomirovic is a member of *Doctors without Borders – Belgium* and has worked in crisis areas in southern Serbia during 2003–5. Currently she is working as an NGO Amity's Project Coordinator and in partnership with UNICEF, and other NGO groups who deal with internally displaced refugees in southern Serbia.

Roy Lubit is a child and adolescent psychiatrist and a forensic psychiatrist practising in New York City. He specializes in the treatment of traumatized children, adolescents and adults. He is a member of the Disaster and Trauma Committee of the American Academy of Child and Adolescent Psychiatry. He is on the faculty of the Department of Psychiatry of New York University School of Medicine.

Helen O'Nions is a Senior Lecturer in Law at London Metropolitan University. She has published articles on deportation, asylum policy and the Roma. She is currently working on the publication of research examining minority rights protection and its application to Europe's Roma minority.

Nalaini Sriskandarajah is a psychiatrist in private practice in Poughkeepsie New York 75 miles north of Manhattan. She also consults and volunteers extensively with schools and child care agencies and is involved in the care and welfare of children and adolescents. She is a board member of Disaster Psychiatry Outreach (a volunteer organization based in Manhattan), and works with board liaison staff for the Child and Adolescent Committee. She provided volunteer work services to survivors after the 2001 attack on the World Trade Center, the South Asian tsunami in December 2004 and Hurricane Katrina in the autumn of 2005.

Felicity de Zulueta is a consultant psychiatrist in psychotherapy and head of the Traumatic Stress Service at the Maudsley Hospital, London. Dr de Zulueta is also an Honorary Senior Clinical Lecturer in Traumatic Studies at the Institute of Psychiatry, King's College, London. She studied biology at the University of East Anglia prior to doing medicine at Cambridge University and trained in psychiatry and psychotherapy at the Maudsley Hospital. As a consultant psychotherapist she founded and led the Department of Psychotherapy in Charing Cross Hospital where she also worked as a consultant psychotherapist. Dr de Zulueta is a group analyst, a systemic family therapist, psychoanalytic psychotherapist and EMDR therapist whose main interests lie in the study of attachment, psychological trauma as well as bilingualism. She is author of *From Pain to Violence: the Traumatic Roots of Destructiveness* (Whurr), 2nd revised edition (Wiley, 2006). Dr de Zulueta is also a founding member of the International Attachment Network, and a member of the European Society for Traumatic Stress Studies and the International Association for Forensic Psychotherapy and the British Neuro-Psychiatric Association.

Part I

An Overview of Trauma Psychology: Traumatic Experiences in Children and Responses

1

Responding to Traumatized Children: an Overview of Diagnosis and Treatment Options I

Roy Lubit

Introduction

Contrary to common belief, children are less resilient than adults to the impact of traumatic events. Children's coping skills are less effective than those of adults, making them more likely to become overwhelmed and traumatized. The potential impact of trauma on children goes well beyond the symptoms of Post-Traumatic Stress Disorder (PTSD). While adults' personalities are relatively formed and stable, those of children are still forming and their perceptions of the world and of themselves can be deeply impacted by undergoing a traumatic event. Traumatic experiences can interrupt normal developmental lines and cause problems with self-esteem, trust, interpersonal relations, the child's view of the world and affect regulation.

While an adult who suffers several months of impaired functioning after a trauma can generally return to the status quo, a child who is in such a position could fall behind peers and have a very hard time catching up. Hence, professionals need to understand the variety of impacts emotional trauma can have on an individual, each of which should be addressed in treatment. Depression, anxiety, withdrawal, difficulty concentrating, intrusive recollections and hyper-arousal are likely to interfere with a child's ability to participate in and maximally benefit from social and educational opportunities. A few months of traumatic or grief symptoms that interfere with a child's ability to benefit from these experiences can propel a child off the normal developmental curve. Once out of step with one's peers and schoolwork it may not be possible to catch up. As a result, the child may never attain the social and academic/work competence that would otherwise have been attained. These secondary problems may be more troublesome than the symptoms directly resulting from the trauma. To effectively help children who experience trauma, professionals need to understand the variety of impacts that trauma can have on an individual, each of which should be addressed in treatment.

There are many sources of emotional trauma. Two of the most common are child abuse and witnessing domestic violence. Sexual abuse, whether by a parent, relative, friend or stranger is generally traumatic. Natural and technological disasters affect millions of children each year. Transportation accidents, whether car accidents or ship sinkings, affect many people. Invasive medical procedures can cause PTSD. War and its resulting displacement affect huge numbers. Even simple bullying, a very common phenomenon, can be very traumatic.

Disasters, both manmade and natural, disrupt entire communities. Disasters create particularly serious problems for children. Children are severely impacted by the post-disaster crisis state and the tendency for adults to be preoccupied with rebuilding and being less able than usual to provide support. Parental anxiety and stress are common after disasters and compound the child's difficult task of rebuilding self-esteem and a sense of safety (Yule 1999). Furthermore, children tend to rely on routine and the structure of their world and find changes more difficult than do adults. In a disaster children often lose their schools, places of worship and social gathering places (Woodcock 2000).

Human suffering lasts long past the time of rebuilding and extends far beyond those directly affected. PTSD symptoms can persist and last for years, and some children will first develop symptoms years after the event (Dwivedi 2000; Sack et al. 1999). Two years after the bombing in Oklahoma City, 16 per cent of children who lived approximately 100 miles from Oklahoma City reported significant PTSD symptoms related to the event (Pfefferbaum et al. 2000). This is a remarkable finding because these youths were not directly exposed to the trauma or related to the deceased or injured victims. Two years after the Buffalo Creek Dam collapse, 37 per cent of children evaluated met 'probable' *DSM-III-R* PTSD criteria and 17 years after the collapse 7 per cent still met criteria (Green et al. 1994). Following Hurricane Andrew, 86 per cent of children met PTSD criteria at three months, 76 per cent met criteria at seven months, and 69 per cent met criteria at ten months (La Greca et al. 1996). Eighteen months after the 1988 Armenian earthquake 90 per cent of the children living adjacent to the epicentre and 30 per cent at the periphery met the diagnosis for PTSD (Pynoos et al. 1993). Six weeks after the 1999 Taiwan earthquake 22 per cent of adolescents aged 12–14 met criteria for PTSD (Hsu et al. 2002). The relatively low number may be a result of using psychiatric interviews rather than self-report forms to establish the diagnosis, the relatively high levels of support the country provided to those affected by the disaster, and cultural factors. Following the sinking of the *Jupiter*, 50 per cent of child survivors had PTSD shortly after the disaster and 15 per cent had PTSD 5–7 years later (Yule 1999). Fifteen years after being in Pol Pot's forced labour camps, 24 per cent of youths aged 17–24 met PTSD criteria (Hubbard et al. 1995). These data actually underestimate the number of children suffering significant emotional effects, since many children who do not have PTSD develop other anxiety disorders, depression, substance abuse, or show alterations in self-image and beliefs about the world that are detrimental to their emotional development and personality. Overall, individuals' function can be significantly impaired after a disaster (Giaconia et al. 1995).

The impact of trauma

Horowitz (1986, 1990) states that PTSD arises from an overwhelming, negative experience that is incongruent with existing schema. Traumatic events overwhelm the individual's ability to cope, leaving the individual feeling horrified, intensely afraid or helpless. Freud (1939/ 1962) noted that psychic trauma led to two types of symptoms: fixation to the trauma with subsequent repetition compulsion, and defensive reactions of avoidance, inhibition and phobia. Freud also noted the progressive weakening which follow traumatic events. Kardiner (1941) believed that trauma could lead to a 'physioneurosis' in which there is biological dysregulation and enduring hypervigilance to threat. Hosin (2001: 141) postulates that a traumatic experience may lead to extreme phobia reactions, that is, the anxious child feels continually on the verge of experiencing another trauma. Kardiner believed that the meaning the individual gave to the traumatic experience was a key mediating factor concerning its impact on the person. Combining these ideas, Van der Kolk (1994), and Van der Kolk et al. (1994b) proposed that PTSD involves a combination of a conditioned fear response to trauma-related stimuli, altered cognitive schemata and social apprehension, and altered neurobiological processes leading to increased arousal and unusual handling of memory. Each of these complex trauma, particularly early in the life traumatic events, can lead to problems with (a) regulation of affect and impulses, (b) memory and attention, (c) self-perception, (d) interpersonal relations, (e) somatization and (f) the creation of new systems of meaning (Van der Kolk et al. 2005).

Conditioned fear response

Following traumatic events, many people develop a conditioned fear response including marked anxiety and physiological arousal to things which remind them of the incident. Traumatic reminders may include returning to the location, smells or sounds that they encountered during the trauma, seeing people who were involved in the traumatic event or rescue operation, or simply thinking about what occurred.

Complicating the conditioned fear response is the unusual way the brain deals with traumatic memories, in comparison to normal memories. Traumatic memories appear to be stored largely in the amygdala rather than in the hippocampus. Recollection of the trauma feels like a re-experiencing of the event with all of the related emotional and physiological arousal, rather than simply thinking about what occurred. The conditioned fear response usually weakens over time, but for some it remains strong and expands to include increasing numbers of traumatic reminders, including any memory or discussion of the event. Such a reminder and condition can lead to a progressive restriction of the victim's activities. Frequent intrusive recollections can also exhaust the person. Many survivors become numb and withdraw from people and activities in general. Victims sometimes engage in increased risk-taking behaviour including substance abuse, either to deal with the feelings of withdrawal or to block out the painful intrusive memories.

Altered cognitions

Traumatic experiences can change children's perceptions of themselves and the world. Traumatic experiences often impair self-confidence and foster a more dangerous image of the world. Hence, trauma can catastrophically destroy a child's illusion of omnipotence and belief in his or her parents' protection. This combination can then significantly interfere with social and educational achievement. Trauma victims can also develop a sense of guilt or shame. Children's magical thinking leaves them particularly vulnerable to this. Changes in threat perception, a tendency to interpret other people's behaviour as aggressive and a predisposition to choose aggressive ways of dealing with conflict, impair social relationships and can lead to social isolation. Identification with the aggressor can occur in an attempt by some to gain control, and escape the horrifying world of the victim. A foreshortened image of the future can have a tremendous impact. Fearing that there may be little time left to experience life, teenagers may engage in risk-taking behaviour, for example by dropping out of school early or having family responsibilities and children prematurely.

Autonomic dysfunction and neurodevelopmental impact

A combination of neurobiological changes and a new cognitive schema depicting the world as a dangerous place, can lead to hyper-arousal (hyper-vigilance, increased startle reaction, irritability and difficulty sleeping). In children, the neurobiological changes may lead to long-term impact on the development of the brain. According to the cascade model, early trauma not only activates the stress response system, but leads to changes in brain development that affect later responses to stress. Stress hormones have a profound impact on the development of the brain of a child and affect patterns of myelination, neurogenesis, synaptogenesis and neural morphobiology. Enduring neurophysiologic impacts include reduction in the mid portion of the corpus callosum and decreased right/left hemispheric integration, electrical irritability of limbic circuits, decreased functional activity of the cerebellar vermis (and therefore decreased ability to inhibit limbic irritability) and attenuated left hemisphere development. Studies show mixed results of stress on the size of the hippocampus. These changes increase risks for PTSD, depression, dissociation, substance abuse and borderline personality disorder (Teicher 2002). Animal research has also shown that early stress interferes with the development of benzodiazepine and GABA receptors which inhibit the amygdala. As a result there is greater anxiety. In addition, prolonged stress or maternal inattention interferes with glucocorticoid receptors in the hippocampus that provide negative feedback to cortisol release, leading to augmented release of stress response hormones in the future. Early stress also results in decreased levels of oxytocin mRNA in the hypothalamus. Oxytocin is a critical factor in affiliative love, manintenace of monogamous relationships and normal non-sexual interactions (Liu et al. 1997; Carter 1998; Uvnas-Moberg 1998).

Who is at risk?

A number of factors affect who is most likely to be at risk and traumatized by an event. The intensity of trauma exposure – how serious the threat, how horrible the images witnessed, hearing cries for help, distance from the danger – are key issues. A history of previous trauma, abandonment, or insecure attachment also predisposes a child to developing PTSD. A prior history of anxiety and depressive symptoms, low resilience and high reactivity to stimuli also increase vulnerability. The parents' level of stress and their ability to respond to their children's needs and maintain normal routines and rules are also significant risk factors (Freud and Burlingham 1943). How quickly and fully children are brought to a safe and comfortable place, the unexpectedness and duration of a disaster, whether the disaster was an act of nature or of human cause, and whether the child feels guilty over acts of omission or commission associated with trauma are also influential factors affecting prognosis.

After a trauma most people have significant symptoms, but, after time, most recover without professional assistance. Therefore, chronic PTSD may be conceptualized as a disorder of recovery. Two factors that contribute to the ability of people to recover include the presence of supports and minimization of secondary stresses. For children, the presence of parents and their calm support is vital. Early signs that someone is at particularly high risk for later problems include: dissociation at the time of the trauma, having a prolonged startle reaction, and having negative thoughts about oneself (Pynoos 1993; Pynoos et al. 1995).

Developmental disturbance

Trauma can have a profound affect on a child's emotional and neurobiological development, including the development of affect and behaviour regulation, core identity and social skills (Gaensbauer 1994; Pynoos 1993; Pynoos et al. 1995; Perry et al. 1995, 1998). This impact however, is not captured by any of the DSM-IV-TR diagnoses. Traditional trauma treatment plans tend to overlook these sequelae and focus on symptoms such as intrusive recollections and sleep disturbance. As a result the child is less likely to fully recover and reach his or her pre-trauma potential.

Regulation of affect and behaviour

The intense negative emotions that arise in emotional trauma can interfere with a child's developing ability to regulate, identify and express emotions (Pynoos 1993; Pynoos et al. 1995). Flooded with painful feelings whenever traumatic reminders are encountered, children are unable to examine, reflect on, label and express their feelings in response to normal daily events. As a result, traumatized children often are unable to develop adequate control of their affective experiences and responses. Intensified startle reactions, hyper-vigilance, numbing and withdrawal also interrupt the acquisition of affect control. The frequent presence of intense negative emotions that are not appropriate reactions to current events can also lead to distrust and intolerance of one's emotions (Pollak et al. 1998). Another problem is that it is difficult to successfully engage in social and work activities when contending with hyper-vigilance, startle reflexes, numbness and withdrawal. Without normal developmental experiences, opportunities to habituate to stressful situations and to develop effective coping skill will be lost.

Hyper-vigilance can also lead to exaggerated perceptions of danger. Distortions of the intentions of others can markedly impair social relationships (Pynoos et al. 1995). Revenge and retaliation fantasies often occur, fostering identification with the aggressor and the self-righteous belief that one is entitled to behave violently. Even vicarious experiences of violence can lead to preoccupation with aggression, rumination on violent images, and a tendency to behave aggressively.

For some children the fear of aggression may promote inhibitions that can interfere with the appropriate use of assertiveness. Inability to be assertive can foster an image of oneself as a victim with periodic compensatory outbursts of aggression.

Some children and adolescents may turn to substance abuse in order to manage the painful emotions created by emotional trauma, impairing their self-control. Both Van der Kolk et al. (1991) and Pynoos et al. (1995) hypothesize that revenge fantasies, narcissistic rage, adolescent omnipotence, and access to drugs and weapons may result in an explosive combination that can lead the child to engage in violent behaviour, radical ideologies and hate groups.

Core identity

Emotional trauma can markedly affect a child's core identity through a variety of channels. Trauma can derail central organizing fantasies (unconscious meaning structures) around which the sense of self is established, leading to developmental arrest (Ulman and Brothers 1988: xiii, 2). The traumatic disruption of early narcissistic fantasies can cause a failure to resolve archaic grandiose fantasies and lead to a perpetual search to merge with powerful figures (Ulman and Brothers 1988: 17). Unable to resolve the tensions between the conflicting powerful images of him or herself the child may be unable to consolidate a coherent identity. In normal development, children slowly come to terms with the limited abilities of their parents. Trauma can cause the premature and sudden collapse of these images, weakening the child's attachment to parents and age appropriate identification. There are several alternative identifications. One is with rescuers leading to a long-term preoccupation with saving people (Pynoos et al. 1995). Another possibility is identification with the aggressor in order to avoid the painful sense of weakness. Anger and disillusionment with the parent and teachers who failed to protect him or her may support this negative identification. Revenge fantasies can also foster a combined identification with both aggressor and victim that can be disorganizing (Pynoos 1993; Pynoos et al. 1995).

Undergoing trauma can also damage self-esteem. There is a heightened realization of vulnerability and an enduring sense of weakness. The tendency of children to blame themselves for problems, along with magical thinking, can promote a deep sense of guilt or shame. Moreover, the belief that one did not perform well during the crisis, either due to a harsh superego, objective failure, or someone's unfortunate comment, can lead to further damage to self-esteem. This shameful or guilt-ridden self-image can become embedded into the core of the personality and have tremendous impact on personality development. Anger, disillusionment and narcissism can also interfere with the development of empathy and prosocial behaviour (Osofsky 1995). Anxiety, on the other hand, can block the child's engagement in the social relationships and experiences needed for development (Goenjian et al. 1999; Lubit et al. 2003; Garbarino and Kostelny 1992) and make it harder for a child to stand up to others and speak out for his or her beliefs.

Skills development

One of the most destructive aspects of PTSD is the delay and damage to the child's ability to engage in normal developmental experiences. For example, the child's anxiety, withdrawal, regression and difficulty concentrating interfere with participation in normal developmental activities such as socializing with other children and succeeding in school. The impact of this can be greater than the direct impact of the symptoms of PTSD. Once a child has fallen off his or her developmental path it is very difficult to get back, even after the symptoms of emotional trauma have resolved. A child that is behind his or her peers socially is likely to suffer rejection. A child that is no longer doing well in school may reformulate his or her self-image as no longer being a good student and cease trying. Catching up can also be very difficult.

Traumatic victimization fosters oppositional defiant behaviour. The oppositional defiant behaviour, in turn, can increase the risk of further victimization and lead to a cascade of problems including depression, engagement with a deviant peer group, wandering without adequate adult monitoring, substance abuse, truancy and problems with the law, and even aggressive delinquency (Patterson 1993; Magdol et al. 1998; Speltz et al. 1999; Ford et al. 2000; Ford 2002). Victimization predisposes children to see benign actions as hostile and to select aggressive responses, seeing them as either a good choice or the only choice possible (Dodge et al. 1995, 1997; Zelli et al. 1999; Cicchetti and Toth 1995; Ford 2002). Such children often have a resentful and resigned coping style (Chaffin et al. 1997).

Increased vulnerability to trauma

Sensitization and kindling make the traumatized person more vulnerable to further trauma in the future. 'Kindling' processes have been described as subclinical abnormal EEG activity. While 'temporal lobe kindling' has been associated with epilepsy, kindling in the amygdala has been associated with anxiety in animal models. Learned helplessness makes individuals less able to protect themselves in potentially dangerous situations. Research has shown (Post et al. 1995; Charney et al. 1993; Weiner 1992; Gill et al. 1990) that people who dissociate after a trauma have decreased blood flow to the frontal lobes when dissociating. Hence, a trauma victim's cognitive capabilities, and ability to get out of a dangerous situation, are impaired in future dangerous situations.

Indeed, traumatic experiences change our perception of the risk and dangers of the world. Some people face high levels of anxiety and become inhibited in a wide variety of situations. Others, in order to deal with the anxiety, use denial as a coping method. That is, in order to avoid facing the high levels of anxiety individuals face after a trauma, they deny the risks involved in these situations. Denial is less painful in the short run than experiencing anxiety, and it permits individuals to engage in some important developmental experiences. It can, however, lead some adolescents and children to become risk prone and place them in harm's way.

For example, children who have been abused or exposed to domestic violence are at increased risk for becoming involved in abusive relationships or abusing their own children. The early abuse provides them with a model of the world in which violence is used in intimate relationships. This leaves them at greater risk for becoming perpetrators or tolerating being abused. In addition, the fear and anger that result from the early trauma are likely to be played out in adult relationships.

Impact of different types of trauma

Although there is significant overlap of symptoms in response to different types of trauma, there are also differences. One of the most important differences concerns whether the trauma was a single event or multiple and frequently repeated events. The following paragraphs will cover the findings of symptoms in children traumatized in different ways.

Single event trauma symptoms

Following a disaster, accident or assault most children will develop significant psychiatric symptoms, and many will have a diagnosable disorder. The most common symptoms are fear, anhedonia, attention and learning problems (Anthony et al. 1999). New onset, reactivation or intensification of specific fears, along with dependent and regressed behaviour are also common (Goenjian 1993; Sullivan et al. 1991). As indicated in various chapters of this book, disasters can cause a wide range of anxiety symptoms, depressive symptoms, dissociative symptoms and behaviour problems including sleep problems, nightmares, trauma-related fears, repetitive trauma-related play, regression, clinginess, separation anxiety, intrusive recollections, numbing and withdrawal, hyper-arousal, problems with concentration, irritability, dysphoria, somatic complaints, substance abuse, and decreased ability to protect oneself from dangerous situations leading to revictimization (see also Yehuda et al. 2001; Cloitre et al. 1997; Widom 1999; Garrison et al. 1995; Perry 1999; Vogel and Vernberg 1993; Johnson et al. 2000). Belief that omens predicted the disaster, along with subsequent attention to possible warning signs and a sense of a foreshortened future, are also important (Terr 1979). While PTSD symptoms have a tendency to progressively lessen over time, anxiety and depressive symptoms and behaviour problems may well be greater after a few months than in the initial weeks (Vogel and Vernberg 1993; McFarlane 1987). Moreover, the onset of PTSD may be delayed (Sack et al. 1999).

  Children's symptoms vary as a function of age and developmental phase. Young children are not likely to report symptoms of numbing and withdrawal, but are likely to have the new onset of aggression or a fear not directly related to the trauma, such as separation anxiety or fear of the dark (Scheeringa et al. 1995). Numbing and withdrawal may appear as regression and loss of previously acquired skills. Intrusive memories in young children are likely to take the form of repetitive, joyless play with traumatic themes, or repetitively drawing pictures of the trauma or acting it out. Generalized anxiety, along with heightened arousal and exaggerated startle reactions, are common. Many children have sleep problems, nightmares without clear content, and somatic complaints. Regression, including loss of skills and increased attachment behaviour, is particularly common in young children. Young children develop renewed separation anxiety and new fears, avoid new activities, become aggressive and have temper tantrums, lose verbal skills and sphincter control, and wish to sleep in their parents' bed (Scheeringa et al. 1995; Bingham and Harmon 1996).

School age children may become obsessed with the details of the disaster in an attempt to cope, or enter a state of constant anxiety and arousal to prepare for future dangers. Some children withdraw into their own quiet world while others engage in increased aggressive behaviour. Concentration problems, distractibility, poor sleep and nightmares are common in this age group, along with preoccupation with danger and reminders. Somatic symptoms continue to be a common expression of distress at this age. School age children may become inconsistent in their behaviour, vacillating between being cooperative and argumentative, or from exuberant to inhibited. To avoid painful feelings associated with the disaster, children may avoid social activities and school. They may instead focus their energies on repetitive retelling of the event and traumatic play. School age children can also engage other children in playing out games recreating the trauma. Their play and comments may show misunderstandings about what occurred. School age children can have an inappropriate sense of responsibility for the disaster, reinforced by a tendency towards magical thinking. Time skew entails a child erroneously sequencing events when retelling what happened in a trauma.

As children move into adolescence, their reactions become similar to those of adults. They are likely to have several symptoms of numbing and withdrawal, as well as hyper-arousal and actual intrusive memories. To manage their painful feelings they may retreat from others or throw themselves into various activities. They may become unusually aggressive and oppositional. Adolescents develop a foreshortened view of the future and may precipitously enter into adult activities, leave school to find a job, or marry. They may engage in high-risk behaviour including life-threatening re-enactments of the trauma situation or using substance abuse to counter the pain of the trauma. They may harbour revenge wishes. Some become depressed and withdraw, and there may be sudden shifts in relationships. Eating disturbances, sleep problems and nightmares are common. The combination of concentration problems, hyper-arousal, dysphoria and irritability can simulate ADHD, oppositional defiant disorder, conduct disorder and even bipolar disorder.

Even single incident trauma can have a profound and long-lasting effect. Two years after the Buffalo Creek Dam collapse 37 per cent of children evaluated met 'probable' DSM-III-R PTSD criteria and seventeen years after the collapse 7 per cent still met criteria (Green et al. 1994). All of the children in the Chowchilla bus hijacking had post-traumatic symptoms four years later. Seven years after a bus–train accident, those having relatively high levels of exposure had relatively high levels of somatization, depression, phobic anxiety, psychoticism, and PTSD symptoms (Tyano et al. 1996). Half of victims recovered within three months, but many remained unwell for a year or more. Symptoms may re-emerge following a subsequent trauma, life stresses, or reminders of the original trauma.

Complex trauma

Complex trauma including repeated events, such as child abuse, can cause PTSD. In a group of severely maltreated children 40 per cent met criteria for PTSD upon removal from their parents' home and 33 per cent still met criteria two years later (Famularo et al. 1996). Widom (1999) found a 37.5 lifetime prevalence for PTSD in victims of substantiated childhood abuse and neglect. The primary symptoms in chronic trauma are impairment of affect regulation, chronic destructive behaviour (self-mutilation, eating disorders, drug abuse, oppositional behaviour, violence to others, risk taking, suicidality), problems with attention, somatization, problematic relationships, altered threat perception and shame (Van Der Kolk DSM-IV Field Trials 1994, 1996). These problems resulting from trauma have been referred to as 'disorders of extreme stress not otherwise specified' (DESNOS).

Complex trauma can lead to perceptual disturbances, possibly due to limbic system malfunction. Teicher et al. (1993) found that adult outpatients with childhood histories of physical and sexual abuse had significantly increased rates of limbic system symptoms commonly seen in temporal lobe seizures, including dissociative phenomena, perceptual distortions, and brief hallucinatory events.

Complex trauma can chronically adversely affect a child's affective state and ability to concentrate. Physically abused infants demonstrate high levels of negative affect and limited positive affect. Emotionally neglected infants tend to have blunted affect (Gaensbauer et al. 1980, 1984). Maltreated toddlers were found to be more angry, frustrated and non-compliant during an experimental task than were non-maltreated comparison children (Erickson et al. 1989). During the preschool years, these children were rated as more hyperactive, distractable, lacking in self-control, and evidencing a high level of negative affect. In kindergarten, the maltreated children were viewed as more inattentive, aggressive and overactive by their teachers (Erickson et al. 1989). As adults, maltreated children show increased rates of depression and domestic violence (Ciccetti and Toth 1995). Many children exposed to extreme violence under the Pol Pot regime in Cambodia which killed 10 per cent of the population of the country, did not reveal emotional problems until years later (Kinzie et al. 1986).

Maltreated infants and toddlers also show a preponderance of atypical attachment patterns. 'Internal representational models of these insecure and often atypical attachments, with their complementary models of self and other, may generalize to new relationships, leading to negative expectations of how others will behave and how successful the self will be in relation to others' (Cicchetti and Toth 1995: 541).

Physically abused children have heightened levels of physical and verbal aggression in peer interactions and some respond with anger and aggression to friendly overtures or signs of distress in other children. Maltreated toddlers have been shown to react to peer distress with anger, fear and aggression, rather than empathy and concern (Kelly and Regan 2000; Hartas and Parker-Jenkins 2000). Maltreated children are often avoidant of peer interactions (Mueller and Silverman 1989). In a new peer group, maltreated children show less social competence than controls, fewer positive emotions, direct less behaviour towards peers, initiate fewer interactions, and engage in less complex play (Howes and Espinosa 1985). Maltreated children are more attentive to and distracted by aggressive stimuli than controls (Rieder and Cicchetti 1989). Peers see maltreated children as evidencing more aggressiveness and disruptive behaviour and less leadership and sharing (Salzinger et al. 1993). A sixteen-year longitudinal study of maltreated preschool children showed that adolescent assaultive behaviour was related to severity of physical discipline, being sexually abused and a negative quality of the mother's interaction with the child (Herrenkohl et al. 1997). Maltreated preschoolers have a tendency towards aggression and lack of empathy to others, and are coercive and withdrawn in interactions with adults (Cicchetti and Toth 1995). Abused children tend to see their non-abusing mothers as unavailable, untrustworthy, unloving and unreliable and may develop an oppositional defiant stance as a defence against betrayal or vulnerability to any emotion (Lynch and Cicchetti 1998; Mulder et al. 1998).

Sexual abuse

Sexual abuse is traumatic in several ways and has profound effects on children (Briere and Runtz 1993). Traumatic sexualization occurs with subsequent aggressive sexual behaviour and inappropriate sexual activity. Sexual abuse also involves betrayal of a child's trust with subsequent depression, difficulty in trusting, feelings of shame, low self-esteem, weakness and vulnerability (De Young 1986).

It was noted (Yehuda et al. 2001; Veltkamp et al. 1994; Lindberg and Distad 1985; Rodriguez et al. 1997; Deblinger et al. 1989) that preschooler victims tend to suffer from anxiety, nightmares, PTSD, disruptive behaviour and inappropriate sexual behaviour. School age child victims tend to show fear, aggression, nightmares, school problems, hyperactivity and regressive behaviours. Adolescents (Schwarz et al. 1993; Schwarz and Perry 1994) show depression, withdrawal, suicidality, self-injury, somatic complaints, delinquency and substance abuse. Only 20–50 per cent showed no symptoms. Over time, 55–65 per cent of the abused did better but 10–24 per cent did worse. Survivors of sexual abuse often have poor social adjustment, fewer and less close friends, suffer binging and purging or self-mutilation, and see themselves as unworthy of healthy relationships (see also Chapter 11).

Some studies (Beitchman et al. 1992; Yehuda et al. 2001; Veltkamp et al. 1994) suggested that the full impact of abuse may not be experienced until the child reaches adulthood and engages in adult relationships and responsibilities and develops more sophisticated cognitive capabilities. However, research including adults who were sexually or physically abused as children shows significantly higher rates of PTSD (72–100 per cent) than studies of children who were abused (21–55 per cent) (Lindberg and Distad 1985; Rodriguez et al. 1997; Deblinger et al. 1989, Kiser et al. 1991). During adolescence or adulthood, a child who has been traumatized years before may suffer the onset of dissociation, disorganization, anxiety, depression, suicidal behaviour and aggression (Schwarz et al. 1993; Schwarz and Perry 1994). It was also claimed that sexual and physical abuse often lead to severe personality disturbances including borderline personality disorder (Polusny and Follette 1995; Weston et al. 1990). Joan McCord found that close to half of abused and neglected boys (45 per cent) were eventually either convicted of a serious crime, became alcoholic or mentally ill and died very young (McCord 1983)

Domestic violence

Witnessing domestic violence is a serious trauma for a child. Several studies (Fantuzzo and Lindquist 1989; Fantuzzo et al. 1991; Hughes 1988; Hughes et al. 1989; Adamson and Thomson 1998) have reported that children exposed to domestic violence exhibit more aggressive and anti-social behaviours (often called 'externalized' behaviours) as well as fearful and inhibited behaviours ('internalized' behaviours). When compared to non-exposed children exposed children also showed lower social competence than did other children (Fantuzzo et al. 1991), and were found to show higher average manifestation of anxiety, depression, aggression with peers, negative affect and less appropriate responses to situations than children who were not exposed to violence at home (Hughes 1988; Graham-Bermann and Levendosky 1998). The children tend to feel worthless, mistrust intimate relationships and be aggressive (Goodman and Rosenberg 1991). Very young children often identify with the aggressor and may lose respect for the victim (Crites and Coker 1988). Girls tend to become anxious, passive and withdrawn while boys demonstrate aggressive and disruptive behaviour (Pageloe 1990). Meanwhile, children who were exposed to and witnessed inter-parental violence were more likely to be convicted of crimes (e.g. car theft, burglary, assault, attempted rape, rape kidnapping, attempted murder or murder) than children who received corporal punishment. Spaccarelli et al. (1995: 173) found that among a sample of 213 adolescent boys incarcerated for violent crimes, those who had been exposed to family violence believed more than others that 'acting aggressively enhances one's reputation or self-image'; and holding this belief significantly predicted violent offending. Silvern's study of 550 undergraduate students found that exposure to violence as a child was associated with adult reports of depression, low self-esteem among women and trauma-related symptoms alone among men (Silvern et al. 1995).

Community violence

Community violence is an endemic problem in many of our cities. High levels of community violence exposure predicted peer-rated aggression alcohol and drug use, carrying knives and guns, defensive and offensive fighting, trouble in school, fear and anxiety, depression, helplessness and hopelessness, emotional withdrawal, somatic symptoms, impaired social relationships and increased general activity and restlessness (Cooley-Quille et al. 1995). The experience of chronic danger has a marked impact on a child's ability to explore the environment and develop skills, as well as impact on the child's views of the world. Seeing everyone as a potential threat, being hyper-vigilant has its toll (Marans and Cohen 1993).

Garbarino and Kostelny (1992) noted that preschool children exposed to community violence tend to have passive reactions and regressive symptoms in response. School age children tend to have aggression, inhibition, somatic complaints and learning difficulties. Adolescents tend to prematurely enter into adulthood, use substances, and display aggression, promiscuity and increased risk-taking behaviour.

We must also not forget that many of our children grew up in war-torn countries or experienced torture and loss of relatives before they migrated, became displaced and became refugees in Europe and the US.

Bullying

Bullying entails an abuse and harassment of vulnerable individuals. It differs from age-typical quarrelling or teasing by being prolonged, one-sided, and intending harm. It can be physical (hitting, kicking, robbing, pushing, unwanted sexual touching), verbal (insulting, threatening, taunting), or psychological torture (intimidation, spreading rumours, excluding). Bullying is also a serious problem for children and hurts both perpetrators and victims.

A recent study (Nasel et al. 2001) showed that around 17 per cent of school aged children had been bullied sometimes or weekly and around 19 per cent had bullied others sometimes or weekly. Six per cent of students were frequently both bullied and bulliers. Hence a considerable majority of children suffer bullying at some point.

Perpetrators fail to learn appropriate inhibitions against hurting others and instead receive gratification for being abusive. Victims often have problems learning in school, become depressed, may become isolated, suffer fear and anxiety, suffer humiliation and low self-esteem, fear going to school, and at times develop PTSD or turn to violence themselves. Students who are both bullied and bulliers (6 per cent) tend to have particularly problematic outcomes. Those who watch probably also suffer negative effects (Nansel et al. 2001; Olweus 1993; Fried and Fried 1996; Hawker and Boulton 2000 Kumpulainen et al. 1999; Batsche and Knoff 1994; Kochendorfer-Ladd and Wardrop 2001; Smith et al. 1999).

Death of a loved one

Bereavement and complex bereavement are very common problems. Bereavement affects 6 000 000 Americans a year. Around 20 per cent of these figures have complex bereavement. Complex bereavement (also known as traumatic bereavement) is a combination of a trauma reaction and bereavement. In classic bereavement one sees sadness or other dysphoria, social withdrawal, loss of interest in daily activities, and somatic symptoms. In complex bereavement, however, one sees a persistent intense grief reaction, unusual difficulty separating and a trauma reaction. Certain beliefs are common in complex grief including a sense of guilt and hopelessness, the feeling that one will not be able to cope, an abiding sense of the world as dangerous and unjust, and believing that the intensity and continuance of one's grief is a measure of love for the person and that ceasing to grieve would constitute betrayal of the lost loved one.

Adults often miss the fact that children are grieving because their reactions are different to those of adults. Children can fluctuate from playing to sadness. They may be preoccupied with who will take care of them. They lack a mature understanding of death and may note one minute that the loved one is lost and another minute ask if they will be back for the upcoming holiday. Complex grief is particularly likely under certain situations, i.e. if death is experienced as sudden. The individual feels that to cease grieving would be a betrayal or mean permanent loss. Complex grief is also common where the death was violent, witnessed by the bereaved, and there was either mutilation or no body; or it was a result of negligence by the bereaved.

The process of grieving for a loved one entails remembering the good and bad times, coming to a well-rounded picture of the relationship and changing the relationship from one in real life to a relationship in memory. When one has a trauma reaction, and one's thoughts of the person are preoccupied with violent images of how they died, it is not possible to go through the normal grieving process.

Invasive medical procedures

Invasive medical procedures and serious illness can also cause Post-Traumatic Stress Disorder. Children with cancer, children who suffer burns, children who undergo transplantation of bone marrow or livers are all at considerable risk for PTSD (Smith and Redd 1999; Sawyer et al. 1997; Slater 2002a, 2002b; Stoddard et al. 1989). Treatment of PTSD in these children can significantly improve medical compliance (Shemesh et al. 2000).

Inter-generational transmission of trauma

The inter-generational transmission of trauma is a particularly serious problem in our society. As a result, trauma has become an endemic problem in many parts of the world. Children who are abused are far more likely to abuse their own children than are non-abused children. Boys who witness domestic violence are more likely to abuse romantic partners than control groups, and girls who witness domestic violence have an increased rate of being abused themselves. In fact, the best predictor of whether an individual will be abusive is whether they had been abused as a child (Widom, 1999).

Several mechanisms are important. One mechanism is that experiencing trauma increases an individual's predisposition to behave aggressively by creating narcissistic injuries and predisposing the individual to feel threatened and violated by interactions with people. Trauma also interferes with the development of control of one's affective experience, as discussed above. Second, abuse interferes with the development of normal attachment. Insecure attachments are a prelude to later adult emotional problems. Third is the internalization of parental models of violence. Related to this, social learning theory provides a variety of pathways by which witnessing violence can lead someone to become a perpetrator in the future. Social learning theory (Bandura et al. 1961) argues that much of our behaviour is learned by observing others. People try out behaviours they have seen others model and then refine their own behaviour based on the feedback they receive. Internalization of observed behaviour is particularly likely if the model has high status and if the observer has low self-esteem. Behaviour is also influenced by the inner standards one develops about appropriate behaviour. These inner standards arise from the experience of having limits prescribed during childhood, and by seeing how peers and adults limit their own actions. In other words, according to social learning theory, people's behaviour is affected by direct reinforcement (being rewarded or punished), by vicarious reinforcement (seeing others rewarded or punished for a given behaviour), and by self-imposed standards.

Identification, children's assessment and treating trauma victims

The crucial issue in assessing the impact of trauma and deciding whether a child needs treatment is the degree of compromise in social and academic functioning and self-care (Lubit et al. 2003, 2002). Assessing and identifying the children who are having emotional problems as a result of emotional trauma can be very difficult. Children rarely maintain dysphoric affects in an uninterrupted fashion as adults do. Children tend to switch back and forth from dysphoria to play, leading parents incorrectly to assume that the child has recovered. Studies indicate that counsellors and teachers identify fewer than 50 per cent of adolescents with significant, treatable emotional problems. Paediatricians do even more poorly, probably due to their more limited time for interaction, and identify only 25 per cent of those with diagnosable mental disorders (Costello et al. 1988). Another problem in identifying those suffering from trauma is that PTSD is only one of several diagnosable disorders that can arise from trauma. Depression, anxiety disorders, dissociative disorders and disruptive behaviour mimicking ADHD, oppositional defiant disorder, conduct disorder, or even bipolar disorder are all common responses to trauma and can be very debilitating. Finally, the presentation of PTSD in children, especially in young children, differs from the presentation of PTSD in adults.

Scheeringa et al. (1995) recommend altering the criteria for PTSD when assessing very young children, in order to better fit both children's ability to report symptoms and the type of symptoms young children are likely to have. They would not require that the child be able to report fear, helplessness or horror in response to the trauma. They would require one of the following types of re-experiencing: post-traumatic play, play re-enactment, recurrent recollections, nightmares, episodes with objective features of a flashback or dissociation, or distress at exposure to reminders of the event. They would also require only one symptom of numbing/avoidance instead of three: constriction of play, relative social withdrawal, restricted range of affect, loss of acquired developmental skills. Moreover, only one symptom of hyperarousal would be required: night terrors, difficulty in going to sleep which is not related to being afraid of having nightmares or fear of the dark, night-waking not related to nightmares or night terrors, decreased concentration, hyper-vigilance and exaggerated startle response. Scheeringa et al. (1995) would add an additional class of symptoms to replace the modified C and D criteria, i.e. symptoms of fear and aggression marked by one of the following: new aggression, new separation anxiety, fear of toileting alone, fear of the dark, new fears of things or situations not obviously related to the trauma.

The hyperactivity, distractibility, impulsivity and interpersonal problems that often come from trauma can lead to a diagnosis of ADHD. Some trauma symptoms, such as loss of impulse control and aggression, can lead to diagnoses of oppositional defiant disorder (ODD) and conduct disorder. In teenagers, it can be difficult to distinguish between PTSD and borderline personality. Herman et al. (1989) report that 60–80 per cent of women with a diagnosis of borderline personality disorder report a history of childhood sexual abuse. Some researchers suggest that borderline personality disorder may be a severe, chronic manifestation of PTSD-related character pathology (Van Der Kolk et al. 1994b). Substance abuse is a common comorbidity that may represent a failed effort to relieve distress through self-medication. A study of 297 adolescents in a residential drug treatment programme reported that 30 per cent of the subjects met the diagnostic criteria for PTSD (Deykin and Buka 1997). Post-concussive syndrome (headaches, anxiety, emotional lability, concentration impairment, memory problems) and head injuries without loss of consciousness can be confused with PTSD (Lishman 1978; Trimble 1981). The aggression, difficulty concentrating, sleep problems, mood problems and risk-taking of PTSD can lead a clinician to diagnose bipolar disorder. The loss of interest in previously enjoyed activities, withdrawal from family and peers, and sleep problems may result in the diagnosis of major depression. Schwarz and Perry (1994) found that somatization is a prominent symptom in traumatized children and can lead to a focus on finding a medical problem.

Assessment

Children often avoid telling their parents and teachers about upsetting feelings because it is painful to talk about them, and because they do not want to worry their parents. Moreover, adults frequently assess changes in children's behaviour as simply being moodiness or a phase, rather than a reaction to a traumatic event. Teachers are often better at picking up the signs of a traumatized child than parents are, since they see the child interacting with others and attempting to concentrate over a period of several hours every day. Teachers, however, are mainly responsible for teaching their lessons and maintaining order in their classes. This leads them to pay more attention to the disruptive child and to overlook the child who is quietly in pain.

It is important to be alert to the possible signs of emotional trauma. Only by actively looking for them as a doctor would look for rashes or a teacher would be alert to a child who repeatedly failed to do their homework, can we begin to pick up on the numerous children who are suffering from trauma. Any time that a child has a negative change in behaviour you need to wonder if the child could have been subjected to a stressor or traumatic incident. The failure to do this is serious. We know, for example, that one-third of teenagers in serious car accidents develop PTSD. If we knew that one-third of a group developed TB we would screen them all actively. However, we don't do this with PTSD. Part of the solution involves an intensive education programme for paediatricians and schools. A great deal of medical time is wasted assessing and even treating non-existent medical problems whose symptoms are psychologically based. Children who are traumatized are disruptive and impaired in their ability to learn. They need to be recognized and treated.

After a disaster the community's resources are generally unable to recognize and treat all who need help. People are preoccupied with rebuilding basic services and taking care of the medically ill. Separating those with medical from psychiatric problems can be difficult. Intensive public awareness campaigns and training of teachers and medical personnel in the recognition of the symptoms of trauma are very important. In addition, paediatricians and paediatric dentists should be given checklists for signs of emotional trauma. Parents can then review the criteria themselves and be encouraged to discuss any potential signs with their paediatricians. Any negative change in the behaviour of a child should be considered as a possible sign of trauma and not simply that the child is entering into a phase he or she will grow out of. After a disaster large-scale screenings can occur in schools by having parents, teachers and children (when age appropriate) fill out checklists of symptoms several weeks after the disaster to see who is still having symptoms and would benefit from assistance. Child psychiatrists can be asked to address meetings to help educate parents. Radio, TV and print media can be encouraged to give brief reports on the wide variety of symptoms emotional trauma can present with and encourage people to consult with their paediatricians.

Debriefing

There has been considerable controversy concerning the issue of debriefing. Many feel that to pressure people to recount the worst things they saw and experienced, and to listen to the worst things others saw and experienced, can increase their trauma. Nevertheless, there is a great deal that mental health professionals can do immediately after a disaster, or immediately after someone has experienced a traumatic incident.

The likelihood of ongoing emotional trauma from an incident is greatly affected by the meaning the individual gives to the event and the speed with which the individual can reachieve a sense of safety and support. Therefore, helping the person to reach a safe place, reassuring them that their needs will be met, and surrounding them with supportive friends and family can do a great deal to help them. It is important to reassure them that the emotional turmoil they are experiencing is a normal reaction to an abnormal situation, and is not an indication that they are losing their mind or that they are weak. It is also important to find out the meaning they are giving to the event and to help them find a meaning that will facilitate the healing process. With children, people often encourage them to draw pictures of the disaster. To stop with their drawing a scene of the disaster or talking about what it was like can be counter-therapeutic. They need to be helped to move from the scene of the disaster to a more hopeful picture of the future and rebuilding. With a child one should ask them to draw a picture of the future. In exploring the meaning one should ask them why they think the event occurred and how it affects their view of the world and of their own safety.

Community interventions

Large-scale screening and focused intervention for traumatized children have been shown to be effective. Following a hurricane in Hawaii, elementary school children were screened and those with the most serious symptoms received treatment. Researchers found the intervention to be effective.

The researchers used manual-based treatment for four weekly sessions. The manual focused on helping children to restore a sense of safety, grieve for losses and renew attachments, adaptively express disaster-related anger, and achieve closure about the disaster and move forward. Children were given a safe place in which they could review their experiences and receive support. Treatment groups were conducted with four to eight children at a time. A combination of play, expressive art and talking was used to cover each of these issues. Both individual and group treatment were found effective (Chemtob et al. 2002).

Psychotherapeutic aspects of the interventions and treatment

It is destructive for children to suffer a significant period of poor psychosocial functioning. Poor social or academic functioning lasting a few months can cause a child to fall significantly behind peers. Once symptoms resolve it can still be difficult for them to catch up, particularly for those who sustain psychiatric sequelae from the trauma. Therefore, it is important for therapists to help their patients complete basic developmental tasks. Moreover, therapists should encourage parents to arrange for assistance in keeping their child from becoming developmentally derailed to prevent them falling behind their peers. Assistance may include social skills building and behavioural interventions that can disrupt the maladaptive coping patterns resulting from trauma. Creating a safety plan and helping children to deal with dangerous situations is also a fundamental part of treatment. Without this, it will be difficult for traumatized children to feel safe enough in their environment to learn, socialize and grow with full development. In addition, the child may need a safety plan for use in ongoing dangerous situations. Children from homes of domestic violence in particular, are in need of specific responses to risk situations. Coaching the child and appropriate family members in how to use the plan is part of the safety planning process. Role playing may be needed to induce behaviourally inhibited children to practise safety plans, so that they will actually use them when necessary.

It is important to work with the parents, and to treat the parents for their own trauma if necessary. Multiple studies have shown that parents' reactions are the most influential factors affecting a child's outcome. If the parents' stress, depression or anxiety is untreated, significant therapy for the child will be of limited help (Laor et al. 1997; Freud and Burlingham 1943; Janis 1951). However, it can be very helpful to have a joint session with the parent and child in which the therapist can 'teach' the parent about PTSD and relaxation techniques, cognitive processing (how our thoughts affect our feelings), and the impact the trauma has had. The child can share the narrative/story book of the trauma. All of this needs to be reviewed by the therapist and parents prior to the joint session. The joint session facilitates the ability of the child and parent to talk about what happened and to continue to work together to counter problematic cognitions and trauma symptoms.

All children with complex trauma should receive an assessment even if they do not manifest any symptoms. Adults often do not see children's internalizing symptoms because children deny that they are feeling bad. Hidden effects on the child's sense of self and views of the world may have a profound affect on development, but preventive work can help the child avoid serious problems in the future.

Complex bereavement also requires special techniques. Before helping the individual with grief, one treats the trauma reactions. In addition, the child needs help in working through ambivalent feelings about the lost person, guilt over unpleasant words or actions during the relationship, saying goodbye to the relationship, and reconnecting to life. Letters written to and imagined discussions with the deceased can be very helpful. Many trauma researchers note the value of using creative ways to help children tell the story of their traumatic event. Among the most innovative researchers is Bessel Van Der Kolk (1996, 2005). He suggests the use of dance, song and theatre to help children express themselves, rather than sitting and talking. He also argues for the critical role of helping children develop a sense of competence and achievement as they work in non-traditional creative ways on ameliorating the impact of their trauma (Van Der Kolk, personal communication).

Pharmacotherapy

Medications can be very helpful in the treatment of trauma. Many different medications have been researched, including SSRIs, mood stabilizers, beta blockers, and benzodiazepines. At this time it appears that SSRIs are the medication most consistently helpful. Long-term use of benzodiazepines may impede recovery, but brief use to help someone sleep is acceptable. Beta blockers may be helpful in decreasing future hyper-arousal (but not the rest of the syndrome of PTSD) when given in the first few hours to victims who are tachycardic. Further details on the use of pharmacotherapy can be found in Chapter 7 of this book

Prevention

Prevention of trauma is preferable to having to treat trauma sequelae. There is a strong tendency to rescue a particular individual with a name and face who has suffered a tragedy rather than taking actions to decrease trauma risk. Calabresi and Bobbitt (1990) notes this is neither cost-effective nor optimal for the well-being of children. Society can do far more to address child abuse. One approach is to encourage adolescent boys and girls to mentor young children. By learning about childhood development and becoming used to the normal behaviour of young children, those adolescents will develop invaluable patience and understanding before becoming parents themselves. We need to do far more to help parents and professionals learn how to help children in high conflict areas to develop without emotional scars (Osofsky and Fenichel 1994).

Anti-bullying programmes are effective and should be in place in every school. In such programmes, students and teachers are taught about the destructive effects of bullying. Children are also taught about respect, kindness, compassion, and to include rather than exclude others. Children also learn to negotiate conflict among peers, and to intervene safely in bullying situations. They are all taught that reporting on bullying is not tale-telling but protecting the rights of others. Effective programmes often involve surveys to assess the extent of the problem, role playing of difficult situations, individual work with bullies and the bullied, parental involvement, and increased supervision of areas and times in which bullying frequently occurs. Because bullying peaks between the fourth and seventh grade, efforts to prevent it should begin earlier and in the second or third grade (Hoover 1996; Garrity et al. 1994, 1996).

Programmes in social and emotional intelligence, such as those offered by the Center for Social and Emotional Education (Cohen 1999, 2001), may decrease the development of chronic PTSD and other emotional problems in traumatized children. Youths who can deal constructively with trauma, build relationships, access support, express feelings, and develop friendships with those who have experienced traumatic experiences, will be better able to minimize the harmful impact of the trauma.

Social and emotional intelligence programmes could address the most serious problem in helping traumatized children by giving them the skills to request help. The programmes in social and emotional intelligence shown to be effective are those which take a holistic approach. In addition to teaching, children can attend workshops and be given the opportunity to role play. Teachers and parents are taught to create a more supportive and caring environment, and issues around conflict resolution and understanding the feelings of others are brought into the social studies, language and arts curricula. Community support networks provide adults with the support they need, which can decrease their frustration, substance abuse, and related abuse of children.

Disasters' impact on families, schools and communities

Several studies (Freberg 1980; Nadler et al. 1985; Rose and Garske 1987; Sigal et al. 1988) have shown that the damage which disasters do to children, parents and community structures can not only last for years but also can be passed on to children and have a multi-generational effect. However, much of the impact of disasters on children is a secondary effect deriving from the disruptions of communities. Disasters have a tremendous emotional impact on children's caretakers. Disasters could undermine parents' ability to meet their children's emotional needs through traumatizing them and by diverting their attention to rebuilding their homes and addressing pressing financial concerns. Parents and teachers become anxious, depressed and irritable, increase their use of alcohol, and cannot maintain traditional styles of sup-port and discipline. They may be intolerant of their children's posttraumatic regression, may ignore them, or may flood them with their own anxiety. Traumatized parents and teachers find it very hard to reconstitute the setting necessary for children to heal.

Disasters often destroy the physical structures that children rely on for their daily activities: school, home, places of worship, and places of play. This imposes a serious burden on children, since they are generally unnerved by changes in the usual pattern of daily life. These structures form the basis for all life activities and constitute transitional objects. As such, children rely upon them for the integrity of their ego function. After a disaster, these normal structures of life are disrupted, destroyed or converted to traumatic reminders that induce stress reactions. For example, on 11 September 2001, the southern part of Manhattan was in disarray. Children were evacuated from their schools amidst images of burning buildings, smoke and panic. Furthermore, many children needed to relocate to temporary homes and temporary schools. Their personal belongings and places of play and worship were not available. When they did return home it was permanently changed. The air quality remained poor in southern Manhattan for months. Traditional places of play no longer existed. The landscape now contained military troops, rescue workers, large vehicles and poor air which served as unwelcome traumatic reminders.

Children, and the adults who care for them, can become further stressed and feel unsupported when disasters cause rifts in communities and families. Serious tension and splits can arise among people with different levels of symptoms. Those who are dealing with the disaster by denial and avoidance, along with those not greatly affected, often become impatient and insensitive to those who are more outwardly troubled and wish to converse about the disaster. Relations can degenerate from lack of understanding or insensitivity to irritation, teasing and anger. Following the World Trade Center disaster, major splits occurred among parents who disagreed about returning children to schools near Ground Zero. For example, in one elementary school there were angry confrontations between those who wanted their children to return to the former school several months after 11 September and those who felt that the air quality was not adequate and that returning would be too emotionally troubling for the children. The biggest splits were between the school board officials who insisted that the former schools reopen quickly and the parents who wanted to delay return until everything was back to normal.

There were also threats of divisions between those who had lost loved ones in the disaster and people who had lived in the area and had their community uprooted and severely damaged. Considerable political skill avoided a major battle over whether to place a memorial in Battery Park City. It would have drawn countless visitors to the small park used by residents of the area.

Splits in communities can also arise if victims are perceived as weak or defective. Those who suffered injury and property loss can be stigmatized and avoided lest their susceptibility to injury magically contaminate those who were less injured, or remind them of their own vulnerability. Stigmatization of victims sometimes occurs because nonvictims wish to maintain their vision that the world is predictable and fair, in order to maintain a sense of control. Splits can also arise when victims are seen as noble and acclaimed as heroes, leading some to engage in entitled behaviour that may alienate others.

Over time, some victims of disasters become disillusioned and angry with authority figures and aid workers. The emotional and concrete needs of people who survive disasters are so great that it is impossible to fully satisfy them since life can never be as it was before. In addition, the inevitable confusion that occurs in disasters leads to discontent. The anger of the victim towards rescue personnel who are attempting to help is generally very discomforting to those who are working hard to render aid.

Summary of essential steps to be taken for treatment of traumatized children

- Psychoeducation and parental guidance and counselling should be provided in parallel with individual treatment of the child.
- Coercing or forcing a child to talk about or recall trauma can make symptoms more intense and overwhelming.
- Creation of a narrative of the traumatic event is useful to help desensitize traumatized children.
- Safety planning with the traumatized child is particularly important in situations involving domestic and community violence.
- The treatment of traumatized children will often be unsuccessful if their traumatized parents are not treated also.

- Parents should be coached to avoid contaminating the child with their own feelings and verbalizing that their child may be damaged from the traumatic event.
- To prevent future symptoms and psychopathology, children with complex trauma should receive treatment even if they do not manifest any overt signs or symptoms.
- Care should be given to treating any secondary psychopathology and behavioural problems such as depression, phobias, aggression or school refusal or avoidance.
- Despite the paucity of research showing the efficacy of psychotropic agents for the treatment of trauma, treatment with psychotropic medications should be used as adjunctive treatment for clearly defined target symptoms.

References

Adamson, J. L. and Thomson, R. A. (1998) 'Coping with interparental verbal conflict by children exposed to spouse abuse and children from non-violent homes'. *Journal of Family Violence*, 13: 213–32.

Anthony, J. L., Lonigan, C. J. and Hecht, S. A. (1999) 'Dimensionality of post-traumatic stress disorder symptoms in children exposed to disaster: results from confirmatory factor analyses'. *Journal of Abnormal Psychology*, 108: 326–36.

Bandura, A., Ross, D. and Ross, S. (1961) 'Transmission of aggression through imitation of aggressive models'. *Journal of Abnormal and Social Psychology*, 63(3): 575–82.

Batsche, G. M. and Knoff, H. M. (1994) 'Bullies and their victims: understanding a pervasive problem in the schools'. *School Psychology Review*, 23(2): 165–74.

Beitchman, J. H., Zucker, K. J., Hood, J. E. et al. (1992) 'A review of the long-term effects of child abuse'. *Child Abuse and Neglect*, 16: 101–18.

Bingham, R. D. and Harmon, R. J. (1996) 'Traumatic stress in infancy and early childhood: expression of distress and developmental issues'. In C. Pfeffer (ed.), *Severe Stress and Mental Disturbance in Children*. Washington DC: American Psychiatric Association Press, pp. 499–532.

Briere, J. and Runtz, M. (1993) 'Child sexual abuse, long-term sequelae and implications for psychological assessment'. *Journal of Interpersonal Violence* 3: 312–30.

Calabresi, G. and Bobbitt, P. (1990) *Tragic Choices*. New York: W. W. Norton & Company, Inc.

Carter, C. (1998) 'Neuroendocrine perspectives on social attachment and love'. *Psychoneuroendocrinology*, 23: 779–818.

Chaffin, M., Wherry, J. and Dykman, R. (1997) 'School age children's coping with sexual abuse'. *Child Abuse and Neglect*, 21: 227–40.

Charney, D., Deutsch, A., Krystal, J., Southwick, S. and Davis, M. (1993) 'Psycho-biologic mechanisms of posttraumatic stress disorder'. *Archives of General Psychiatry*, 50: 294–30.

Chemtob, C., Joanne, P., Nakashima, M. and Roger, S. (2002) 'Intervention for postdisaster trauma symptoms in elementary school children: a controlled community field study'. *Archives of Paediatrics and Adolescent Medicine*, 156: 211–16.

Cicchetti, D. and Toth, S. L. (1995) 'A developmental psychopathology perspective on child abuse and neglect'. *Journal of the American Academy of Child and Adolescent Psychiatry*, 34: 541–65.

Cloitre, M., Scarvalone, P. and Difede, J. (1997) 'Posttraumatic stress disorder, self-and interpersonal dysfunction among sexually retraumatized women'. *Journal of Trauma Stress*, 10: 437–52.

Cohen, J. (1983) 'Practice parameters for the assessment and treatment of children and adolescents with posttraumatic stress disorder'. *Journal of the American Academy of Child and Adolescent Psychiatry*, 37(Suppl. 10): 4S–26S.

Cohen, J. (ed.) (1999) *Educating Minds and Hearts: Social Emotional Learning and the Passage into Adolescence*. New York: Teachers College Press.

Cohen, J. (ed.) (2001) *Caring Classrooms / Intelligent Schools: the Social Emotional Education of Young Children*. New York: Teachers College Press.

Colvin, G., Tobin, T., Beard, K., Hagan, S. and Sprague, J. (1998) 'The school bully: assessing the problem, developing interventions, and future research directions'. *Journal of Behavioral Education*, 8(3): 293–319.

Cooley-Quille, M. R., Turner, S. and Beidel, D. (1995) 'Emotional impact of children's exposure to community violence'. *Journal of the American Academy of Child and Adolescent Psychiatry*, 34: 1362–8.

Costello, E. J., Costello, A. J. and Edelbrock, C. et al. (1988) 'Psychiatric disorders in pediatric primary care: prevalence and risk factors'. *Archives of General Psychiatry*, 45: 1107–16.

Crites, C. and Coker, D. (1988) 'What therapists see that judges miss'. *The Judges Journal*, 27: 9–13, 40–1.

De Young, M. (1986) 'A conceptual model for judging the truthfulness of a young child's allegation of sexual abuse'. *Journal of Orthopsychiatry*, 56: 550–9.

Deblinger, E., McLeer, S. V, and Atkins, M. S. et al. (1989) 'Posttraumatic stress in sexually abused, physically abused and non-abused children'. *Child Abuse and Neglect*, 13: 403–8.

Deykin, E. Y. and Buka, S. L. (1997) 'Prevalence and risk factors for posttraumatic stress disorder among chemically dependent adolescents'. *American Journal of Psychiatry*, 154: 752–7.

Dodge, K., Lochman, J., Harnish, J., Bates, J. and Pettit, G. (1997) 'Reactive and proactive aggression in school children and psychiatrically impaired chronically assaultive youth'. *Journal of Abnormal Psychology*, 106: 37–51.

Dodge, K., Pettit, G., Bates, J. and Valente, E. (1995) 'Social information processing patterns partially mediate the effect of early physical abuse on later conduct problems'. *Journal of Abnormal Psychology*, 104: 632–43.

Dwivedi, K. (200) *Posttraumatic Stress Disorder in Children and Adolescents*. London: Whurr Publishers.

Erickson, M., Egeland, B. and Pianta, R. (1989) 'The effects of maltreatment on the development of young children'. In D. Cicchetti and V. Carlson (eds), *Child Maltreatment: Theory and Research on the Causes and Consequences of Child Abuse and Neglect*. New York: Cambridge University Press, pp. 647–84.

Famularo, R., Fenton, T., Augustyn, M. and Zuckerman, B. (1996) 'Persistence of pediatric post traumatic stress disorder after two years'. *Child Abuse and Neglect*, 20(12): 1245–8.

Fantuzzo, J. W. and Lindquist, C. U. (1989) 'The effects of observing conjugal violence on children: a review and analysis of research methodology'. *Journal of Family Violence*, 4: 77–94.

Fantuzzo, J. W., DePaola, L. M., Lambert, L., Martino, T., Anderson, G. and Sutton, S. (1991) 'Effects of interparental violence on the psychological adjustment and competencies of young children'. *Journal of Consulting and Clinical Psychology*, 59: 258–65.

Ford, J. (2002) 'Traumatic victimization in childhood and persistent problems with oppositional-defiance'. In R. Greenwald (ed.), *Trauma and Juvenile Delinquency: Theory, Research and Interventions*. New York: Haworth Press Incorporated.

Ford, J. D., Racusin, R., Daviss, W. B., Ellis, C., Thomas, J., Rogers, K., Reiser, J., Schiffman, J. and Sengupt, A. (1999) 'Trauma exposure among children with attention deficit hyperactivity disorder and oppositional defiant disorder'. *Journal of Consulting and Clinical Psychology*, 67: 86–789.

Ford, J. D., Racusin, R., Ellis, C., Daviss, W. B., Reiser, J., Fleischer, A. and Thomas, J. (2000) 'Child maltreatment, and other trauma exposure, and post-traumatic symptomatology among children with oppositional defiant and attention deficit hyperactivity disorders'. *Child Maltreatment*, 5: 205–17.

Freberg, J. T. (1980) 'Difficulties in separation – individuation as experienced by offspring of Nazi Holocaust survivors'. *American Journal of Orthopsychiatry*, 50: 87–95.

Freud, A. and Burlingham, D. (1943) *War and Children*. New York: Ernest Willard.

Freud, S. (1939/1962). *Moses and Monotheism*. In J. Strachey (ed. and trans.), *The Complete Psychological Work of Sigmund Freud*, Standard Edition, Vol 20. London: Hogarth Press.

Fried, S. and Fried, P. (1996) *Bullies and Victims: Helping your Child through the Schoolyard Battlefield*. New York: M. Evans & Co. Inc.

Gaensbauer, T. J. (1994) 'Therapeutic work with a traumatized toddler'. *Psychoanalytic Study of Childhood*, 49: 412–33.

Gaensbauer, T., Mrazek, D. and Harmon, R. (1980) 'Affective behaviour patterns in abused and/or neglected infants'. In N. Fred (ed.), *The Understanding and Prevention of Child Abuse: Psychological Approaches*. London: Concord Press.

Gaensbauer, T. J. and Hiatt, S. (1984) 'Facial communication of emotion in early infancy'. In N. A. Fox and R. J. Davidson (eds), *The Psychobiology of Affective Development*, Hillsdale, NJ: Erlbaum, pp. 207–30.

Garbarino, J. and Kostelny, K. (1992) 'Child maltreatment as a community problem'. *Child Abuse and Neglect*, 16(4): 455–64.

Garbarino, J., Dubrow, N., Kostelny, K. and Pardo, C. (1992) *Children in Danger: Coping with the Consequences of Community Violence*. San Francisco: Jossey-Bass.

Garrison, C. Z., Bryant, E. S., Addy, C. L. et al. (1995) 'Posttraumatic stress disorder in adolescents after Hurricane Andrew'. *Journal of the American Academy of Child and Adolescent Psychiatry*, 34(9): 1193–1201.

Garrity, C., Jens, K., Porter, W., Sager, N. and Short-Camilli, C. (1996) *Bully-Proofing your School*. Longmont, CO: Sopris West Press.

Giaconia, R. M., Reinherz, H. Z., Silverman, B., Pakiz, B., Frost, A. K. and Cohen, E. (1995) 'Traumas and posttraumatic stress disorder in a community of older adolescents'. *Journal of the American Academy of Child and Adolescent Psychiatry*, 34(1): 369–80.

Gill, T., Calev, A., Greenberg, D., Kugelmas, S. and Lerer, B. (1990) 'Cognitive functioning in posttraumatic disorder'. *Journal of Traumatic Stress*, 3: 29–45.

Goenjian, A. (1993) 'A mental health relief program in Armenia after the 1988 earthquake: implementation and clinical observations'. *British Journal of Psychiatry*, 163: 230–9.

Goenjian, A., Stilwell, B. M., Steinberg, A. M. et al. (1999) 'Moral development and psychopathological interference in conscience functioning among adolescents after trauma'. *Journal of the American Academy of Child and Adolescent Psychiatry*, 38(4): 376–84.

Goodman, G. and Rosenberg, M. (1991) 'The child witness to family violence: clinical and legal considerations'. In D. J. Sonkin (ed.), *Domestic Violence on Ttrial*. New York: Springer Publishing, pp. 97–125.

Graham-Bermann, S. and Levendosky, A. (1998) 'The social functioning of preschool-aged children whose mothers are emotionally and physically abused'. *Journal of Emotional Abuse*, 1: 59–84.

Green, B. L., Grace, M. C. and Vary, M. G. et al. (1994) 'Children of disaster in the second decade: a 17-year follow-up of Buffalo Creek survivors'. *Journal of the American Academy of Child and Adolescent Psychiatry*, 33: 71–9.

Hartas, D. and Parker-Jenkins, M. (2000) 'Child rearing practices and the development of social competence: a cross-cultural perspective'. In A. Hosin (ed.), *Essays on Issues in Applied Developmental Psychology and Child Psychiatry*. New York: Edwin Mellen Press.

Hawker, D. S. J. and Boulton, M. J. (2000) 'Twenty years of research on peer victimization and psychosocial maladjustment: a meta-analytic review of cross-sectional studies'. *Journal of Child Psychology and Psychiatry*, 41: 441–55.

Herman, J. L., Perry, J. C. and Van Der Kolk, B. (1989) 'Childhood trauma in borderline personality disorder'. *American Journal of Psychiatry*, 14: 490–5.

Herrenkohl, R., Egolf, B. and Herrenkohl, E. (1997) 'Preschool antecedents of adolescents' assaultive behaviour: a longitudinal study'. *American Journal of Orthopsychiatry*, 67: 422–32.

Hoover, J. H. (1996) *The Bullying Prevention Handbook: a Guide for Principals, Teachers, and Counselors*. Bloomington, Indiana: National Education Service.

Horowitz, M. J. (1986) *Stress Response Syndromes* (2nd edn). Northvale, NJ: Aronson.

Horowitz, M. J. (1990) 'Posttraumatic stress disorder: psyhcotherapy'. In A. S. Belleck and M. Herson (eds), *A Handbook of Comparative Treatments for Adult Disorders*. Chichester: Wiley.

Hosin, A. (2001) 'Children of traumatized and exiled refugee families: resilience and vulnerability'. *Medicine, Conflict and Survival*, 17: 137–45.

Howes, C. and Espinosa, M. P. (1985) 'The consequences of child abuse for the formation of relationships with peers'. *Journal of Child Abuse and Neglect* 9: 397–404.

Hubbard, J., Realmuto, G. M., Northwood, A. K. and Masten, A. S. (1995) 'Comorbidity of psychiatric diagnoses with posttraumatic stress disorder in survivors of childhood trauma'. *Journal of the American Academy of Child and Adolescent Psychiatry*, 34(9): 1167–73.

Hughes, H. M. (1988) 'Psychological and behavioural correlates of family violence in child witnesses and victims'. *American Journal of Orthopsychiatry*, 58: 77–90.

Hughes, H. M., Parkinson, D. and Vargo, M. (1989). 'Witnessing spouse abuse and experiencing physical abuse: a "double whammy"?' *Journal of Family Violence*, 4: 197–209.

Hsu,C. C., Chong, M. Y., Yang, P. and Yen, C. F. (2002) 'Posttraumatic stress disorder among adolescent earthquake victims in Taiwan'. *Journal of the American Academy of Child and Adolescent Psychiatry*, 41(7): 875–81, July.

Janis, I. (1951) *Air War and Emotional Stress*. New York: McGraw-Hill.

Johnson, J. G., Smailes, E. M., Phil, M. et al. (2000) 'Associations between four types of childhood neglect and personality disorder symptoms during adolescence and early adulthood: findings of a community-based longitudinal study'. *Journal of Personality Disorders*, 14: 171–87.

Kardiner, A. (1941) *The Traumatic Neuroses of War*. New York: Paul B. Hoeber.

Kelly, L. and Regan, L. (2000) 'Childhood marked by abuse and violence: legacies of harm'. In A. Hosin (ed.), *Essays on Issues in Applied Developmental Psychology and Child Psychiatry*. New York: Edwin Mellen Press.

Kinzie, J. et al. (1986) 'The psychiatric effects of massive trauma on Cambodian children'. *Journal of the American Academy of Child and Adolescent Psychiatry*, 25: 370–6.

Kiser, L. J., Heston, J., Millsap, P. A. et al. (1991) 'Physical and sexual abuse in childhood: relationship with posttraumatic stress disorder'. *Journal of the American Academy of Child and Adolescent Psychiatry*, 30: 776–83.

Kochendorfer-Ladd, B. and Wardrop, J. (2001) 'Chronicity and instability of children's peer victimization experiences as predictors of loneliness and social satisfaction trajectories'. *Child Development*, 72(1): 134–51.

Kumpulainen, K., Rasanen, E. and Henttonen, I. (1999) 'Children involved in bullying: psychological disturbance and the persistence of the involvement', *Journal of Child Abuse and Neglect*, 23: 1253–62.

La Greca, A., Silverman, W., Vernberg, E. and Prinstein, M. (1996) 'Posttraumatic stress symptoms in children after Hurricane Andrew: a prospective study'. *Journal of Consulting and Clinical Psychology*, 64: 712–23.

Laor, N., Wolmer, L., Mayes, L. C., Gershon, A., Weizman, R. and Cohen, D. J. (1997) 'Israeli preschool children under Scuds: a 30-month follow-up'. *Journal of the American Academy of Child and Adolescent Psychiatry*, 36(3): 349–56.

Lindberg, F. H. and Distad, L. J. (1985) 'Post-traumatic stress disorders in women who experienced childhood incest'. *Journal of Child Abuse and Neglect*, 9: 329–34.

Lishman, W. A. (1978) *Organic Psychiatry*. Oxford: Blackwell Scientific Publication.

Liu, D., Diorio, J., Tannenbaum, B. et al. (1997) 'Maternal care, hippocampal glucocorticoid receptors and hypothalamic-pituitary-adrenal responses to stress'. *Science*, 277: 1659–62.

Lubit, R., Hartwell, N., Van Gorp, W. G. and Eth, S. (2002) 'Forensic evaluation of trauma syndromes in children'. *Child and Adolescent Psychiatric Clinics of North America*, 11: 823–57.

Lubit, R., Rovine, D., Defrancisci, L. and Eth, S. (2003) 'Impact of trauma on children'. *Journal of Psychiatric Practice*, 19(2): 128–38.

Lynch, M. and Cicchetti, D. (1998) 'Trauma, mental representation, and the organization of memory for mother-referent material'. *Development and Psychopathology*, 10: 739–59.

Magdol, L., Moffitt Caspi, A. and Silva, P. (1998) 'Developmental antecedents of partner abuse'. *Journal of Abnormal Psychology*, 106: 375–89.

Marans, S. and Cohen, D. (1993) 'Children and inner-city violence'. In L. Leavitt and N. Fox (eds), *The Psychological Effects of War and Violence on Children*. Hillsdale, NJ: Lawrence Erlbaum, pp. 281–301.

McCord, J. (1983) 'A forty-year perspective on effects of child abuse and neglect'. *Journal of Child Abuse and Neglect*, 7: 265–70.

McFarlane, A. C. (1987) 'Posttraumatic phenomena in a longitudinal study of children following a natural disaster'. *Journal of the American Academy of Child and Adolescent Psychiatry*, 26: 764–9.

Mueller, E. and Silverman, N. (1989) 'Peer relations in maltreated children'. In D. Cicchetti and V. Carlson (eds), *Child Maltreatment: Theory and Research on the Causes and Consequences of Child Abuse and Neglect*. New York: Cambridge University Press, pp. 529–78.

Mulder, R., Beautrais, A., Joyce, P. and Fergusson, D. (1998) 'Relationship between dissociation, childhood sexual abuse, childhood physical abuse, and mental illness in a general population sample'. *American Journal of Psychiatry*, 155: 806–11.

Nadler, A., Kav-Venaki, S. and Gleitman, R. (1985) 'Transgenerational effects of the Holocaust: externalisation of aggression in second generation of Holocaust survivors'. *Journal of Counselling and Clinical Psychology*, 53: 365–9.

Nansel, T. R., Overpeck, M., Pilla, R. S., Ruan, W., Simmons-Morton, S. and Scheidt, S. (2001) 'Bullying behaviour among US youth: prevalence and association with psychosocial adjustment'. *Journal of the American Medical Association*, 25 April, 285(16): 2094–2100.

Olweus, D. (1993) *Bullying at School: What We Know and What We Can Do*. Cambridge MA: Blackwell.

Osofsky, J. D. (1995) 'The effects of exposure to violence on young children'. *The American Psychologist*, 50(9): 782–8.

Osofsky, J. D. and Fenichel, E. (eds) (1994) *Caring for Infants and Toddlers in Violent Environments: Hurt, Healing, and Hope*. Arlington VA: Zero to Three: National Center for Infants.

Pageloe, M. (1990) 'Effects of domestic violence on children and their consequences for custody and visitation agreements'. *Mediation Quarterly*, 7: 347–63.

Patterson, G. R. (1993) 'Orderly change in a stable world: the antisocial trait as chimera'. *Journal of Consulting and Clinical Psychology*, 61: 911–19.

Pelcovitz, D., Kaplan, S., Goldenberg, B. et al. (1993) 'Post-traumatic stress disorder in physically abused adolescents'. *Journal of the American Academy of Child and Adolescent Psychiatry*, 33: 305–12.

Perry, B. D. (1999) 'Memories of fear: how the brain stores and retrieves physiologic states, feelings, behaviours and thoughts from traumatic events'. In J. M. Goodwin and R. Attias (eds), *Splintered Reflections: Images of the Body in Trauma*. New York: Basic Books, pp. 26–47.

Perry, B. D., Polard, R. and Homeostasis, A. (1998) 'Stress, trauma and adaptation: a neurodevelopmental view of childhood trauma'. *Child and Adolescent Psychiatric Clinics of North America*, 7(1): 33–51.

Perry, B. D., Pollard, R., Blakely, T. et al. (1995) 'Childhood trauma, the neuro-biology of adaptation and "use-dependent" development of the brain: how "states" become "traits"'. *Infant Mental Health Journal*, 16(4): 271–291.

Pfefferbaum, B., Seale, T., McDonald, N. et al. (2000) 'Posttraumatic stress two years after the Oklahoma City bombing in youths geographically distant from the explosion'. *Psychiatry*, 63: 358–70.

Pollak, S., Cicchetti, D. and Klorman, R. (1998) 'Stress, memory and emotion: developmental considerations from the study of child maltreatment'. *Development and Psychopathology*, 10: 811–28.

Polusny, M. and Follette, V. (1995) 'Long-term correlates of child sexual abuse: theory and review of the empirical literature'. *Applied and Preventive Psychology*, 4: 143–66.

Post, R., Weiss, S. and Smith, M. (1995) 'Sensitization and kindling: implications for the evolving neural substrate of post-traumatic stress disorder'. In M. Friedman, D. Charney and A. Deutch (eds), *Neurobiological and Clinical Consequences of Stress: From Normal Adaptation to PTSD*. Philadelphia: Lippencott-Raven Publishers.

Prasad, K. (2000) 'Biologicial basis of posttraumatic stress disorder'. In K. N. Deivedi (ed.), *Post-traumtic Stress Disorder in Children and Adolescents*. London. Whurr Publishers.

Pynoos, R. S. (1993) 'Traumatic stress and developmental psychopathology'. In J. Oldham and M. Riba Tasman (eds), *American Psychiatric Press Review of Psychiatry*. Washington, DC: American Psychiatric Press, (12): 205–38.

Pynoos, R. S., Goenjian, A., Tashjian, M. et al. (1993) 'Post-traumatic stress reactions in children after the 1988 Armenian earthquake'. *British Journal of Psychiatry*, 163: 239–47.

Pynoos, R. S., Steinberg, A. M. and Wraith, R. (1995) 'A developmental model of childhood traumatic stress'. In D. Cicchetti and D. J. Cohen (eds), *Developmental Psychopathology: Risk, Disorder, and Adaptation*. New York: Wiley.

Rieder, C. and Cicchetti, D. (1989) 'An organizational perspective on cognitive control functioning and cognitive-affective balance in maltreated children'. *Development Psychology*, 25: 382–93.

Rodriguez, N. R., Ryan, S. W., Vande Kemp, H. and Foy, D. W. (1997) 'Post-traumatic stress disorder in adult female survivors of child sexual abuse: a comparison study'. *Journal of Consulting and Clinical Psychology*, 65: 53–9.

Rose, S. L. and Garske, J. (1987) 'Family environment, adjustment and coping among children of Holocaust survivors: a comparative investigation'. *American Journal of Orthopsychiatry*, 57: 332–4.

Sack, W. H., Him, C. and Dickason, D. (1999) 'Twelve-year follow-up study of Khmer youths who suffered massive war trauma as children'. *Journal of the American Academy of Child and Adolescent Psychiatry*, 38: 1173–9.

Salzinger, S., Feldman, R. S., Hammer, M. and Rosario, M. (1993) 'The effects of physical abuse on children's social relationships'. *Child Devevelopment*, 64: 169–87.

Sawyer, M., Antoniou, G., Toogood, I. et al. (1997) 'Childhood cancer: a two-year prospective study of the psychological adjustment of children and parents'. *Journal of the American Academy of Child and Adolescent Psychology*, 36: 1736–43.

Saylor, C. (ed.) (1993) *Children and Disasters*. New York: Plenum.

Sigal, J. J., DiNicola, V. F. and Buonvino, M. (1988) 'Grandchildren of survivors: can negative effects of prolonged exposure to excessive stress be observed two generations later?' *Canadian Journal of Psychiatry*, 33: 207–12.

Scheeringa, M. S., Zeanah, C. H., Drell, M. J. et al. (1995) 'Two approaches to the diagnosis of posttraumatic stress disorder in infancy and early childhood'. *Journal of the American Academy of Child and Adolescent Psychiatry*, 34: 191–200.

Schwarz, E., Kowalksi, J. and Hanus, S. (1993) 'Malignant memories: signatures of violence'. In S. Feinstein et al. (eds), *Adolescent Psychiatry*. Chicago: University Chicago Press, pp. 280–300.

Schwarz, E. D. and Perry, B. (1994) 'The post-traumatic response in children and adolescents'. *Psychiatric Clinics of North America*, 17(2): 311–26.

Shemesh, E., Lurie, S., Stuber, M. L., Emre, S., Patel, Y., Vohra, P., Aromando, M. and Shneider, B. L. (2000) 'A pilot study of posttraumatic stress and nonadherence in pediatric liver transplant recipients'. *Pediatrics*, 105(2): E29.

Silvern, L., Karyl, J., Waelde, L., Hodges, W. F., Starek, J., Heidt, E. and Kyung, M. (1995) 'Retrospective reports of parental partner abuse: relationships to depression, trauma symptoms and self-esteem among college students'. *Journal of Family Violence*, 10: 177–202.

Slater, J. (2002a) 'Psychiatric aspects of cancer in childhood and adolescence'. In M. Lewis (ed.), *Child and Adolescent Psychiatry: a Comprehensive Textbook*, 3rd edn. New York: Lippincott Williams and Wilkins.

Slater, J. (2002b) 'Psychiatric issues in pediatric bone marrow, stem cell, and solid organ transplantation'. In M. Lewis (ed.), *Child and Adolescent Psychiatry: a Comprehensive Textbook*, 3rd edn. New York: Lippincott Williams and Wilkins.

Smith, M., Redd, W., Peyser, C. and Vogl, D. (1999) '*Post-traumatic Stress Disorder in Cancer*: a review'. *Psycho-oncology*, 8(6): 521–37.

Smith, P. K., Morita, Y., Junger-Tas, A, Olweus, D., Catanano, R. and Slee, P. T. (eds) (1999) *The Nature of School Bullying: a Cross-National Perspective*. London: Routledge.

Spaccarelli, S., Coatsworth, J. D. and Bowden, B. S. (1995) 'Exposure to serious family violence among incarcerated boys: its association with violent offending and potential mediating variables'. *Violence and Victims*, 10: 163–82.

Speltz, M., McClellan, J., DeKlyen, M. and Jones, K. (1999) 'Preschool boys with oppositional defiant disorder'. *Journal of the American Academy of Child and Adolescent Psychiatry*, 38: 838–45.

Steiner, H., Garcia, I. G. and Matthews, Z. (1997) 'Posttraumatic stress disorder in incarcerated juvenile delinquents'. *Journal of the American Academy of Child and Adolescent Psychiatry*, 36(3): 357–65.

Stoddard, F. J., Norman, D. K., Murphy, J. M. and Beardslee, W. R. (1989) 'Psychiatric outcome of burned children and adolescents'. *Journal of the American Academy of Child and Adolescent Psychiatry*, 28(4): 589–95.

Sullivan, M. A., Saylor, C. F. and Foster, K. Y. (1991) 'Post-hurricane adjustment of preschoolers and their families'. *Advances in Behaviour Research and Therapy*, 13: 163–71.

Teicher, M. H. (2002) 'Scars that won't heal: the neurobiology of child abuse'. *Scientific American*, 286(3): 68–75.

Teicher, M. H., Glod, C. A., Surrey, J. et al. (1993) 'Early childhood abuse and limbic system ratings in adult psychiatric outpatients'. *Journal of Neruopsychiatry and Clinical Neurosciences*, 5: 301–6.

Terr, L. (1979) 'Children of Chowchilla: a study of psychic trauma'. *Psychoanalytic Study of the Child*, 34: 547–623.

Trimble, M. R. (1981) *Post-Traumatic Neurosis from Railway Spine to the Whiplash*. New York: Wiley.

Tyano, S., Iancu, I., Solomon, Z. et al. (1996) 'Seven-year follow-up of child survivors of a bus-train collision'. *Journal of the American Academy of Child and Adolescent Psychiatry*, 35: 365–73.

Ulman, R. B. and Brothers, D. (1988) *The Shattered Self: a Psychoanalytic Study of Trauma*. Hillsdale: The Analytic Press.

Uvnas-Moberg, K. (1998) 'Oxytocin may mediate the benefits of positive social interaction and emotions'. *Psychoneuroendocrinology*, 23: 819–35.

Van Der Kolk, B. A. (1994) 'The body keeps the score: memory and the emerging psychobiology of posttraumatic stress'. *Harvard Review of Psychiatry*, 1: 253–65.

Van Der Kolk, B. A., Herron, N. and Hostetler, A. (1994a) 'The history of trauma in psychiatry'. *Psychiatric Clinics of North America*, 17(3): 583–600.

Van Der Kolk, B. A., Hostetler, A., Herron, N. and Fisler, R. E. (1994b) 'Trauma and the development of borderline personality disorder'. *Psychiatric Clinics of North America*, 17(4): 715–30.

Van Der Kolk, B. A., McFarlane, A. C. and Weisaeth, L. (eds) (1996) *Traumatic Stress: the Effects of Overwhelming Experience on Mind, Body and Society*. New York. Guildford.

Van Der Kolk, B. A., Perry, C. and Herman, J. L. (1991) 'Childhood origins of self-destructive behaviour'. *American Journal of Psychiatry*, 148: 1665–71.

Van der Kolk, B. A., Roth, S., Pelcovitz, D., Sunday, S. and Spinazzola, J. (2005) 'Disorders of extreme stress: the empirical foundation of a complex adaptation to trauma'. *Journal of Traumatic Stress*,18(5): 389–99.

Veltkamp, L. J., Miller, T. W. and Silman, M. (1994) 'Adult non-survivors: the failure to cope of victims of child abuse'. *Child Psychiatry and Human Development*, 24(4): 231–43.

Vogel, J. M. and Vernberg, E. M. (1993) 'Children's psychological responses to disasters'. *Journal of Clinical Child Psychology*, 22: 464–84.

Weiner, H. (1992) *Perturbing the Organism: the Biology of the Stressful Experience*. Chicago: University of Chicago Press.

Weston, D., Ludolph, P., Misile, B., Ruffins, S. and Block, J. (1990) 'Physical and sexual abuse in adolescent girls with borderline personality disorder'. *American Journal of Orthopsychiatry*, 60: 55–66.

Widom, C. S. (1999) 'Posttraumatic stress disorder in abused and neglected children grown up'. *American Journal of Psychiatry*, 156: 1223–9.

Woodcock, J. (2000) 'Refugee children and their families: theoretical and clinical perspectives'. In K. N. Deivedi (ed.), *Post-traumtic Stress Disorder in Children and Adolescents*. London: Whurr Publishers.

Yehuda, R., Spertus, I. and Golier, J. (2001) 'Relationship between childhood traumatic experiences and PTSD in Adults'. In S. Eth (ed.), *PTSD in Children and Adolescents*. Washington DC: American Psychiatric Publishing, pp. 117–46.

Yule, W. (1999) *Posttraumatic Stress Disorders: Concepts and Therapy*. Chichester: Wiley.

Zelli, A., Dodge, K., Lochman, J. and Laird, R. (1999) 'Conduct problems prevention research group, the distinction between beliefs legitimizing aggression and deviant processing of social cues: testing measurement validity and the hypothesis that biased processing mediates the effects of beliefs on aggression'. *Journal of Personality and Social Psychology*, 77: 150–66.

Ziv, A. F. and Israel, R. (1973) 'Effects of bombardment on the manifest anxiety level of children living in kibbutzim'. *Journal of Consulting and Clinical Psychology*, 40: 287–91.

2
Treatment Options for Young People and Refugees with Post-Traumatic Stress Disorder II

Matthew Hodes and Angeles Diaz-Caneja

This chapter focuses on the effective treatments for Post-Traumatic Stress Disorder (PTSD) which are used with young people, particularly young refugees. Comprehensive accounts of treatments and treatment efficacy for PTSD in young people have been provided elsewhere (Dwivedi 2000; Perrin et al. 2000; Cohen and Mannarino 2004; National Collaborating Centre for Mental Health (NCCMH) 2005). The aims of this chapter are therefore twofold: first to describe the more established treatments for young people with PTSD, and second to look at all innovative treatment approaches that have been developed for young refugees. The chapter has an evidence-based perspective, and so provides data regarding the efficacy of the treatments described.

In order to achieve these aims, it was felt necessary to describe the background to evidence-based practice. This will be followed by a summary of children's and adolescents' reactions to traumatic events, and salient developmental factors. The description of treatments begins then with the therapies for which there is currently most evidence, e.g. cognitive behavioural and related treatments, including group CBT and exposure therapy.

Two other individual treatments – EMDR and psychopharmacology – will also be described in this chapter. There is then consideration of some innovative therapies that have been used for young refugees with PTSD, such as testimony therapy and narrative exposure therapy. Non-directive therapies such as art therapy are highlighted and discussed alongside the role of the family and its potential for involvement in treatment and any proposed management plan. Finally, attention is given to some contextual factors that will influence choice of treatments.

Evidence-based practice for PTSD

There is a burgeoning literature on the evidence base for treatment of post-traumatic stress, although only a small proportion of this has been directly concerned with children and adolescents. Nevertheless, in the last decade this topic has been the subject of much more intensive inquiry. This follows the relatively recent recognition that children may experience PTSD, and that it cannot be assumed that adult treatment research findings can be directly applied to the younger group.

Clinical guidelines for the treatment of PTSD in young people have existed for some years. The 'practice parameters' of the American Academy of Child and Adolescent Psychiatry (1998) were an important step. Other reviews consider treatment efficacy for PTSD (Cohen and Mannarino 2004; Perrin et al. 2000; Yule 2002). The NICE guidelines on PTSD published in March 2005 by the National Collaborating Centre for Mental Health addressed both adults and younger people with the disorder, and give details regarding methodological aspects of the studies (NCCMH 2005). High-quality studies have been carried out with young people exposed to single incident stressors, and a number of studies with children exposed to community violence include many ethnic minority children, including some who are refugees. Few high-quality studies (i.e. adequately large randomized controlled trials) have been carried out with young refugees suffering from PTSD. Thus the NICE guidelines suggested little about specific issues in the treatment of young refugees. In view of the need to 'follow the trail to the next best external evidence and work from there' (Sackett et al. 1996: 71), treatment studies with refugee children with weaker designs, such as open trials and multiple single case studies, are described.

PTSD in children and adolescents

The diagnostic criteria for PTSD are very similar in the two main classificatory systems used, which are the International Criteria for Diseases concerned with psychiatric disorders (World Health Organization 1993), and the system developed in the USA, the Diagnostic and Statistical Manual of Mental Disorders, DSM-IV (American Psychiatric Association 1994). The features are given in Table 2.1.

As can be seen, the cardinal features that are given in Table 2.1 include the experiencing of an unusually threatening or frightening event that would engender fear in practically everyone, followed by persistent remembering or reliving of the event, avoidance of reminders

Table 2.1: Diagnostic criteria for Post-Traumatic Stress Disorder: ICD-10 and DSM-IV

ICD–10 diagnostic guidelines	DSM–IV criteria
Stressor criterion	
A. The person must have been exposed to a stressful event or situation (either short – or long-lasting) of exceptionally threatening or catastrophic nature, which would be likely to cause pervasive distress in almost anyone	A.1. The person experienced, witnessed, or was confronted with an event or events that involved actual or threatened death or serious injury, or a threat to the physical integrity of self or others A.2. The person's response involved intense fear, helplessness or horror (or disorganized or agitated behaviour in children)
Symptom criterion	

Necessary symptoms
B. Persistent remembering or 'reliving' of the stressor in intrusive 'flashbacks', vivid memories, or recurring dreams, or in experiencing distress when exposed to circumstances resembling or associated with the stressor.
C. The patient must exhibit an actual or preferred avoidance of circumstances associated with the stressor, which was not present before exposure to the stressor.
D. Either of the following must be present:
  (i) Inability to recall, either partially or completely, some important aspects of the period of exposure to the stressor;
  (ii) Persistent symptoms of increased psychological sensitivity and arousal (not present before exposure to the stressor), shown by any two of the following:
	Necessary symptoms
	B. The traumatic event is persistently re-experienced in one (or more) of the following ways
	1. Recurrent and intrusive distressing recollections of the event, including images, thoughts or perceptions (or in children, repetitive play in which the themes or aspects of the trauma are expressed)
	2. Recurrent distressing dreams of the event (or in children frightening dreams without recognizable content)
	3. Acting or feeling as if the traumatic event were recurring (or trauma-specific re-enactment in children)
	4. Intense psychological distress at exposure to internal or external cues that symbolize or resemble an aspect of the traumatic event
	5. Physiological reactivity upon exposure to internal or external cues that symbolize or resemble an aspect of the traumatic event
	C. Persistent avoidance of stimuli associated with the trauma and numbing of general responsiveness (not present before trauma), as indicated by at least three of the following

Table 2.1: Diagnostic criteria for Post-Traumatic Stress Disorder: ICD-10 and DSM-IV – *continued*

ICD–10 diagnostic guidelines	DSM–IV criteria

Symptom criterion – *continued*

a. difficulty in falling asleep; b. irritability or outbursts of anger; c. difficulty in concentrating; d. hypervigilance; e. exaggerated startle response.	1. Efforts to avoid thoughts, feelings or conversations associated with the trauma 2. Efforts to avoid activities, places or people that arouse recollections of the trauma 3. Inability to recall an important aspect of the trauma 4. Markedly diminished interest or participation in significant activities 5. Feeling of detachment or estrangement from others 6. Restricted range of affect (e.g. unable to have loving feelings) 7. Sense of foreshortened future **D.** *Persistent symptoms of increased arousal (not present before the trauma) as indicated by two (or more) of the following* 1. Difficulty falling or staying asleep 2. Irritability or outbursts of anger 3. Difficulty concentrating 4. Hypervigilance 5. Exaggerated startle response

Time frame

Criteria B, C, D, must all be met within 6 months of the stressful event or the end of a period of stress. (For some purposes, onset delayed more than 6 months may be included, but this should be clearly specified.)	Duration of the disturbance (symptoms in Criteria B, C, and D is more than 1 month).

Disability criterion

Not specified	The disturbance causes clinically significant distress or impairment in social, occupational, or other important areas of functioning

of the event, and symptoms of high arousal. DSM-IV specifies that some of these symptoms may be manifest in specific ways in young children, so that the reliving may be apparent through repetitive play in which themes of the trauma are expressed. The DSM-IV criteria describe the ways in which the symptoms may be different for younger children. Young children may have less developed language skills than adults, and even those who have fluent speech may show their pre-occupation with the traumatic events only through their play and drawings. Furthermore, some symptoms require verbal expression of feelings that are contingent on an adequately mature cognitive development, such as a sense of a foreshortened future. Some recent studies of PTSD in younger children aged 2 to 6 years have sought to identify appropriate diagnostic criteria. It has been found that the optimum diagnostic algorithm was one cluster B symptom, one cluster C symptom, and two cluster D symptoms (Scheeringa et al. 2003, 2005). It was found that the loss of developmental skills, such as bladder and bowel control and speech, that may occur in young children following experience of traumatic events, were not required for the recognition of PTSD. It is also known that children after experiencing trauma may show the onset of, or significantly increased, anxiety regarding separation, aggression, and fears that are not obviously linked to the trauma, such as fear of the dark or of going to the bathroom alone (see Quota et al. 2005).

There has been criticism with regard to PTSD for two main reasons in the refugee mental health field (Hodes 2000, 2002a). Firstly, it has been argued that the disorder reduces human suffering to individual deviance and decontextualizes this from the broader political and social background. It is suggested that the dangers of this would be a focus on the individual and provision of services for individual distress when a collective response, such as community reconstruction and integration for asylum seekers in resettlement countries, might achieve a much greater impact on public mental health (Bracken et al. 1995; Summerfield 1999, 2000). Against this contention, is the view that the identification and awareness, e.g. through epidemiological investigation, of individual psychopathology is consistent with a public perspective and community intervention. Furthermore the diagnosis has value for the development of treatments and their provision in contexts when this is appropriate. A further criticism of PTSD has been that the disorder does not have cross-cultural validity (Summerfield 2000). However, PTSD has been identified in all language and culture groups (European and non-European) in which it has been investigated with similar symptoms in the diverse groups (Hodes 2002a; Mezzich et al. 1996). A number of the studies of the cross-cultural validity of PTSD have been carried out with young people (e.g. Sack et al. 1997).

Cognitive behavioural therapy (CBT)

Cognitive behavioural therapy is a structured, goal-orientated psychotherapy with a strong evidence base. It focuses on deficits or distortions in thinking (Beck 1991), which are postulated to maintain psychological problems. CBT contrasts with other types of treatment in that it views the young person as an active, equal partner, who collaborates with learning tools to prevent relapse after resolution of the presenting difficulties. Randomized controlled trials have shown its efficacy in depression and anxiety disorders in children and adolescents (Harrington et al. 1998; Kendall 1994). Many of the studies of PTSD are based on the outcome of treatment in sexually abused children and adolescents that included random assignments to well-defined manualized treatment. This type of intervention includes psychoeducation, training in coping skills to deal with disturbing memories of abuse and feelings of anxiety and guilt, correcting maladaptive cognitions, and gradual exposure/desensitization and relapse prevention (see Chapter 6 for more details). Parents or main caregivers may be involved in this approach.

Some other studies (Deblinger et al. 1996, 1999) have compared CBT (also known as trauma-focused CBT or TF-CBT) to other treatments, e.g. child-centred therapy, psychoanalytic psychotherapy and other control conditions. In fact, Deblinger et al. (1996, 1999) followed 100 sexually abused children who were randomly assigned to receive one of four provisions: standard community care, TF-CBT to the child, TF-CBT to the non-offending parent or TF-CBT to both child and parent. These researchers found that the child who receives TF-CBT (either with or without the inclusion of their parent in treatment) experienced significantly greater improvement in PTSD symptoms (approximately 59 per cent reduction in symptoms), whereas children whose parents received TF-CBT (with or without inclusion of the child in treatment) experienced significantly greater improvement in child-reported depression and parent-reported behavioural problems. These results were maintained at a two-year follow-up. In another study, 69 sexually abused preschool children were randomly assigned to TF-CBT or non-directive supportive therapy (NST). Children receiving TF-CBT experienced significantly greater improvement in PTSD symptoms including sexualized behaviours, and internalizing and total behaviour problems than children receiving NST. These differences were maintained over the course of a one-year follow-up (Cohen and Mannarino 1996, 1997; see also Chapter 6 of this book).

The same group of authors have published their findings on a large study involving 229 children aged 8–14 years who had experienced sexual abuse-related PTSD symptoms with 89 per cent met criteria for PTSD (Cohen et al. 2004). They were randomly assigned to trauma-focused CBT (providing 12 weekly sessions individual to child and parent) or child-centred therapy (12 sessions). The children receiving the trauma-focused CBT had significantly greater reduction in post-traumatic symptoms and depression, and improvement in interpersonal trust. These improvements were sustained at a 12-month follow-up (Cohen et al. 2005). However, two smaller studies evaluating TF-CBT did not show any differences (Berliner and Saunders 1996; Celano et al. 1996).

It is important to ascertain whether parental involvement improves the efficacy of the child therapy. In a study carried out by King et al. (2000), 36 sexually abused children (aged 5–17 years) were randomly assigned to a child-alone cognitive-behavioural treatment, a family cognitive behavioural treatment, or a waiting-list control. Compared with controls, children who received treatment exhibited significant improvements in PTSD symptoms and self-reports of fear and anxiety. Significant improvements also occurred in relation to parent-completed measures and clinician ratings of global functioning. In general, parental involvement did not improve the efficacy of cognitive behavioural therapy. Some research has been carried out with children exposed to natural disasters – which included young people who had PTSD as a result of exposure to the 1988 Armenian earthquake. This research concluded that children benefit from CBT intervention for both PTSD symptoms and related difficulties such as depression, social competence and behavioural problems (Goenjian et al. 1995, 1997).

Focusing on refugees or asylum seekers with PTSD, there are some case reports in adults using the CBT approach. Basoğlu et al. (2004) described how a 22-year-old Kurdish tortured asylum seeker living in Sweden received 16 sessions of CBT involving mainly self-exposure to trauma-related cues. Clinical measures completed at a six-month follow up showed significant improvement in PTSD symptoms including anxiety and depression. A study of adult refugees suffering from PTSD randomized to CBT or exposure therapy and treated for 16–20 sessions found that both treatments resulted in large improvements on all measures (Paunovic and Ost 2001).

A recent model to explain PTSD has been developed by Ehlers and Clark (2000). They suggested that PTSD becomes persistent when individuals fail to process the memory of the trauma, so that it comes to mind frequently and is experienced as a current threat. The sense of threat arises as a consequence of excessively negative appraisals of the trauma and/or its sequelae and a disturbance of autobiographical memory characterized by poor elaboration and contextualization, strong associative memory and strong perceptual priming. Changes in the negative appraisals and the trauma memory are prevented by a series of problematic and cognitive strategies. These three areas require modification during treatment. Using Ehlers and Clark's model with some modifications, Vickers (2005) described two refugee adolescents with PTSD. Both adolescents benefited from the therapy and showed a substantial reduction of the symptoms of PTSD. Cultural and language issues were considered using this model.

Group cognitive behavioural therapy

Group treatment becomes a practical way of helping large numbers of individuals at once. Therapeutic groups have the additional advantage of decreasing the sense of hopelessness and loneliness, as well as normalizing their reactions. CBT interventions have been adapted for delivery to groups of adolescents. They have been used in the treatment of depression (Lewisohn et al. 1990), poor anger control (Kellner and Bry 1999) and social phobia (Albano et al. 1995). This group treatment has been presented as a replicable, protocol-driven 'package' (March et al. 1998). The advantage of using group CBT is that it can also be implemented in schools, so that the barriers to accessing the health care system faced by children and adolescents, and particularly young refugees, may be overcome (Hodes 2000).

In children and adolescents with PTSD, this approach has been used when the PTSD symptoms have developed as a result of exposure to a single stressor (March et al. 1998), sexual abuse (Deblinger et al. 2001) or exposure to violence (Kataoka et al. 2003; Stein et al. 2003). All these studies showed that group CBT may be effective.

Seventeen children and adolescents with DSM-IV PTSD diagnosis following a single stressor from a school sample entered into an 18-week, group-administered CBT protocol (March et al. 1998). They used the Multi-Modality Trauma Treatment (MMTT) that adapts CBT protocols that have been shown to be effective in PTSD in adults (Foa et al. 1991) and for paediatric anxiety (Kendall 1994; March et al. 1994) protocol was developed. All but three of the seventeen enrolled patients completed the 18 weeks of treatment with significant improvement in all areas. No patient relapsed after discontinuation. However, there was no control group in this study.

Further, two school programmes using CBT group interventions for children and adolescents with PTSD have been evaluated in the USA. Stein et al. (2003) conducted a randomized controlled trial in children and adolescents with PTSD that resulted from personally witnessing or being exposed to violence. One hundred and twenty-six pupils (mean age 11 years) were randomly assigned to ten sessions of CBT group (Cognitive-Behavioural Intervention for Trauma in Schools or CBITS, Jaycox 2003) and 65 to a waiting list delayed intervention comparison group. After three months of intervention students who were randomly assigned to the early intervention group had significantly lower scores on symptoms of PTSD, depression and psychosocial dysfunction. At six months, after both groups had received the intervention, the differences between the two groups were not significantly different for symptoms of PTSD and depression; they showed similar ratings for psychosocial function and teachers did not report significant differences in classroom behaviours. Another study considered the school-based mental health programme for traumatized Latino immigrant children, many coming from countries with organized violence such as El Salvador and Guatemala, who had been exposed to community violence and had immigrated to the USA in the previous three years. Children were assigned to group CBT or waiting list comparison. Children (n = 152) offered the intervention showed a modest reduction in symptoms of PTSD and depression compared with a group allocated to a waiting list (n = 47) at a three-month follow-up (Kataoka et al. 2003). The intervention consisted of a manual-based eight-session group CBT delivered in Spanish by bilingual, bicultural school social workers. However, symptom changes remained in the clinical range at short-term follow-up.

Another study evaluated a newly designed psychosocial treatment programme for war traumatized child and adolescent refugees. The programme consists of individual, family and group sessions using a psychoeducational approach beside trauma and grief focusing activities, creative techniques and relaxation. Ten young Kosovan refugees (10–16 years) residing in Germany participated in this programme. All but four had PTSD diagnosis. Following the intervention, the overall psychosocial functioning increased substantially in nine of ten participants. The rate of PTSD diagnosis fell from 60 per cent to 30 per cent.

The number of patients with PTSD and a high rate of comorbid symptoms as well as a history of severe traumatization remained at 30 per cent (Möhlen et al. 2005).

In the UK, group CBT has proved to be effective in young refugees with PTSD (Entholt et al. 2005). Twenty-six children aged 11 to 15 years who were refugees or asylum seekers from war-affected countries participated. The manual-based intervention consisted of CBT techniques. The treatment group (n = 15) received six sessions of group CBT over a six-week period, while the control group (n = 11) were placed on a waiting list for six weeks and then invited to enter treatment. Children in the CBT group showed statistically significant but clinically modest improvements following the intervention, with decreases in overall severity of the post-traumatic stress symptoms compared with the waiting list group. However, this improvement was not maintained at a two-month follow up by a small subgroup (n = 8).

Eye movement desensitization and reprocessing

Eye movement desensitization and reprocessing (EMDR) is a newly developed treatment for PTSD. It involves bilateral stimulation when processing traumatic memories. It has been postulated that the trauma memories are not processed normally, and the bilateral stimulation makes a link between the two sides of the brain that enables the memories to be adequately processed (Shapiro 1995). Other researchers have considered EMDR to be a variety of CBT in the absence of eye movement (Cohen et al. 2000).

In adults, its use has been supported by a number of randomized controlled trials. No controlled studies have evaluated the benefits and risks of EMDR in children and adolescents. However, Chemtob et al. (2002) showed an improvement in PTSD symptoms after three sessions of EMDR in children presenting with PTSD symptoms a year after a disaster in an uncontrolled field study. Improvement was maintained after six months. A case series of young children with long-standing PTSD has also suggested improvement with two to four sessions of EMDR (Tufnell 2005).

One open study has reported the use of EMDR with thirteen refugee children aged 8–16 years (Oras et al. 2004). The EMDR was used in conjunction with conversational therapy for adolescents or play therapy for younger children (5–25 sessions) in a group of traumatized refugee children. The number of EMDR sessions was one to five. The young people showed significant improvement in social functioning, the GAF increased from 51.9 to 66.9 level, and all PTSS-C scale reduced by approximately 50 per cent. Other reports claim refugee children with PTSD have been helped with EMDR (Tinker 2002).

Psychopharmacological treatment

Psychopharmacological treatments are widely used to treat childhood PTSD, but no rigorous, empirical research has evaluated effectiveness. Medication may play a role in reducing debilitating symptoms of PTSD and providing a buffer for children while they confront difficult material in therapy and may help to improve their general functioning in day-to-day life. According to the American Academy of Child and Adolescent Psychiatry, medication (SSRIs) should be used adjuvant with psychological interventions, if depressive or panic symptoms are present (AACAP 1998). Anti-depressants may be used in treating conditions such as depression and anxiety disorders that commonly co-occur with PTSD. In a recent review of pharmacotherapy for PTSD in adults, SSRIs (sertraline and paroxetine) were the treatment of choice following successful controlled trials (Schoenfeld et al. 2004).

There are a few studies with children and adolescents with PTSD and use of medication. In a group of 25 paediatric burn patients, aged 2–19, with acute stress disorder received imipramine or chloral hydrate for seven days in a randomized double-blind design (Robert et al. 1999). Imipramine was more effective than chloral hydrate. An open study of children and adults with PTSD showed that citalopram decreased PTSD symptoms in children and adolescents to a comparable degree as it did in adults. However, cases of acute or chronic PTSD were not analysed separately (Seedat et al. 2002).

Carbamazepine (Loof et al. 1995), propanolol (Famularo et al. 1988), clonidine (Marmar et al. 1993; Harmon and Riggs 1996), guanfacine (Horrigan 1996) and risperidone (Horrigan and Barnhill 1999) have been reported to ameliorate PTSD symptoms in children in small open studies. No studies using medication in young refugees with PTSD have been published. Clinicians should be aware of the problems of sensitivity to medication and cultural aspects of taking psychotropic medication (see Chapter 7 for more details on psychopharmacological focused treatment).

Testimony therapy

Testimony therapy involves the telling of a series of events to the therapist who documents the narrative, and through a series of interactive discussions with the patient, expands it. During this process the testimonial may become more detailed and organized. This process involves the development of autobiographical memory. The written testimonial may be shared in the community, and contribute to the development of contemporary history, and towards inter-ethnic healing. The therapy may be suitable for people from cultures who are uninterested in discussing the affective components of PTSD, and have a strong tradition of storytelling, or who may want the testimonial to contribute to social integration or specific community tasks.

Most reports of testimony therapy are with adults. The first report involved treatment of 12 of 15 survivors of torture in Chile (Cienfuegos and Monelli 1983). This treatment was regarded as successful, in that there was reduction of symptoms. An open trial was carried out with 20 adult Bosnian refugees exposed to atrocities, all of whom had PTSD (Weine et al. 1998; Weine and Laub 1995). The intervention obtained almost 50 per cent reduction in symptoms as measured by standard rating scales of post-traumatic symptoms and depressive symptoms after six months. One study of testimony therapy with three Sudanese adolescents living in the USA who had been exposed to high levels of organized violence and losses suggests improvements (Lustig et al. 2004b). However, this small study did not have standardized outcome measures, and it was unclear how the testimony would be used in the wider socio-cultural community.

Narrative exposure therapy

In narrative exposure therapy the patient is requested to repeatedly talk about the worst traumatic events in detail, while re-experiencing all the emotions associated with it (Neuner et al. 2002, 2004). As most victims of organized violence have experienced many traumatic events, the patient is asked to talk about his/her whole life, focusing on the details of traumatic events. It is suggested that the therapy provides benefit because of the exposure, and also because of greater coherence in autobiographical memory. The therapy has some similarities to testimony therapy, and has also been developed specifically for refugees.

A study of six Somali adolescents aged 12–17 years suffering from PTSD resident in Uganda were treated with four to six individual sessions (Onyut et al. 2005). The therapy called KIDNET used illustrative material such as a life line, stones and flowers, as well as coloured drawings and role play. The adolescents showed a reduction in post-traumatic symptoms after treatment, which was sustained at the nine-month follow-up.

Non-directive therapies

Psychodynamic psychotherapy

There is a long history of the provision of psychodynamic psychotherapy for young people who have been abused and neglected. Despite this there are few systematic studies of the evidence for the therapy in the treatment of PTSD. The published studies have compared psychodynamic psychotherapy with other therapies. One study compared psychodynamic therapy to behavioural therapy for sexually abused children (Downing et al. 1988). Behavioural therapy was superior in improving sexualized behaviour but other aspects of PTSD were not measured. In another study carried out by Trowell et al. (2002), 71 sexually abused girls aged 6–14 years were randomly assigned to focused-individual psychoanalytical psychotherapy (up to 30 sessions) or group psychoeducation (up to 18 sessions). Both treatment groups showed a substantial reduction in psychopathological symptoms and an improvement in functioning, but with no evident difference between individual and group therapy. Although individual psychotherapy led to a great improvement in manifestations of PTSD, the small sample size and lack of a control group limit conclusions about changes attributable to treatment. No other studies with refugees or asylum seekers have been carried out to date.

There are accessible accounts of the use of psychodynamic psychotherapy with asylum seeking and refugee children (Melzak 1992; Shepperd 2001; Woodcock 2001). The specific features of these approaches are the focus on mental mechanisms such as denial and dissociation. In recent years there has also been consideration of the effect of societal abuse on relationship formation including attachment, and the experience of autonomy for the child and the various ways in which this may affect family life

Art therapy

Many young people who have experienced traumatic events find it difficult to verbalize their experiences. As has been described, this may be in part because memory of the event is associated with a high level of fear and avoidance behaviour may result to prevent that experience recurring. For some young people, play, and drawing and painting of traumatic events is easier (and indeed may reflect the preoccupation with events, see the section on diagnostic issues above). This provides a medium for exploring the events and creating a joint narrative within the containing therapeutic relationship with the art therapist (Wertheim-Cahen et al. 2004). Younger children will have immature speech, and others may have speech and language delay, so for these groups a non-verbal therapy appears advantageous. Another reason why art therapy may be considered is that recent migrants may not have fluency in the language of the host country including the involved mental health professionals.

Indeed, many refugee children will experience substantial mobility and changes in their cultural backgrounds. There may be differences within their families regarding these cultural and life changes, with challenges and threats to identity. Art therapy may help in the creation of new identities as well as have a beneficial effect on social and community ties (Rousseau et al. 2004). Art therapy has been provided in community settings and post-conflict situations to help with psychological adjustment and the creation of new meanings and ties in communities that have been damaged by organized violence (Kalmanowitz and Lloyd 1997; Wertheim-Cahen et al. 2004)

A recent evaluation has been carried out of school-based art therapy for refugee and immigrant children living in Quebec, Canada (Rousseau et al. 2005). A twelve-week programme was offered to 138 children aged 7–13 years, with a comparison group of children in the same schools. The children in the intervention group achieved lower mental health symptoms and higher popularity scores than those in the comparison group.

Working with families

Most young people will be brought to child and adolescent mental health services by their parents or carers. These adults will have observed the young person's psychological distress and will usually have more knowledge than the young person about how to access help. Obviously infants and young children will be brought for help, but even for adolescents parental support in getting help is important. Parents will be informants about the past problems, and may be able to help their offspring accept treatment.

With regards to young refugees, as described above, whole families, or survivors from families, may have been exposed to similar traumatic events. The level of children's psychological distress may be influenced by that of their parents (Quota et al. 2005; Smith et al. 2001). It has also been found that the quality of the relationship in families, as measured by the instrument expressed emotion predicts the treatment outcome in adults with PTSD (Tarrier et al. 1999). For these reasons consideration of the involvement of the parents in the therapy is important.

Few studies have specifically investigated the benefits of family intervention for PTSD. A recent study investigated child–parent psychotherapy for children aged 3–5 years who had been exposed to marital violence (Lieberman et al. 2005). The therapy had elements of cognitive behavioural and family therapy influences, including principles of attachment. The therapy was carried out with child and mother together in joint sessions and compared with individual therapy for mother and child, in a random allocation design. The child–parent psychotherapy was significantly more effective in reducing post-traumatic symptoms in the children, and mothers also had less psychological distress after one year of therapy.

Of special relevance here is a study of young children and their mothers in Bosnia who were exposed to many war events and were provided with a psychosocial programme (Dybdahl 2001). The active intervention involved improving the sensitivity of mothers to their children's needs and reinforcing good parenting. The intervention took place in groups, led by trained teachers. All mothers in the study were given basic medical care, but there was then random allocation to the psychosocial programme or no additional therapy. The mothers who received the active intervention had a greater reduction of post-traumatic symptoms, and the children also experienced greater reduction in anxiety symptoms and had greater weight gain. Family therapy with young refugees may be one element of a multimodal treatment programme. The study mentioned earlier on group CBT by Möhlen et al. (2005) included family sessions. Further work is required to investigate the place of family intervention for children with PTSD.

Treatments in clinical practice

Much of the accumulated evidence for PTSD is derived from studies carried out in research settings, with expert therapists following manualized treatments (Chorpita et al. 1998). Therapy will only involve volunteers who agree to be recruited to the trials. It will usually be necessary for patients to be able to speak the same language as the therapist. There are few evaluations of the applications of such research in ordinary clinical settings. For these reasons, the external validity of treatment research needs to be further assessed and care is needed in inferring the extent to which the evidence applies to treatment contexts in which young refugees will be seen.

In evidence-based medicine (EBM) external evidence from systematic research must be integrated with information regarding 'the patient's clinical state, predicament and preferences' (Sackett et al. 1996: 71). Patient (child and parent) preference is very important in influencing the treatment effectiveness, i.e. how it will be taken up and used.

However, there are a number of specific issues especially pertinent for refugees that will influence treatment choice. Firstly, consideration needs to be given to cultural and language factors. Many young refugees seeking help will not speak the same language as the therapist. Some treatments may be more accessible using interpreters or with limited ability to speak the host language. Thus art therapy, behaviour therapy (such as exposure) and drug treatment may be easier to carry out with interpreters than therapy in groups, and cognitive behaviour therapy involving cognitive restructuring. Cultural factors may influence attitudes to the various treatment modalities. In some cultures talking with 'strangers' in therapeutic groups may be regarded as threatening. For others, use of drug treatments may be more acceptable than psychological and 'talking' treatments (see Lustig et al. 2004a).

Individual and group CBT are based on the assumption that individuals want to talk about emotional responses to traumatic events, and are more easily carried out when there have been single incident stressors. However, refugees have often been exposed to multiple stressors and privations, which have taken place over a considerable length of time, and may not want to talk about emotional states in therapeutic settings. They may prefer to make disclosure of past abusive experiences as testimonies, which could be used for community integration, or inter-ethnic reconciliation, or in some circumstances the accumulation of evidence for prosecution. For such individuals testimony or narrative exposure therapy may be more suitable.

A second factor that is relatively specific to the asylum seeking and refugee population is their high mobility. Asylum seeking young people and families are placed in homeless accommodation and may then be rehoused, which can affect involvement in treatment. Those seeking asylum may not know how long they will be able to stay in the host country. This uncertainty may also affect their ability to focus on treatment. Anxiety symptoms and fear may be maintained and indeed increased if deportation is imminent.

These practical, but very real, issues of seeking asylum and obtaining adequately stable housing may result in young people and families in contact with mental health services seeking the support of clinicians. Clinicians may be asked to write psychiatric or medico-legal reports to support asylum applications (Tufnell 2003). Letters in support of rehousing applications are frequently requested. Even the initial settling-in period with the need to establish new social ties and links to various institutions including schools may result in a high level of distress. Treatment may progress more easily after appropriate support with these problems has been provided, as this will indicate to the families that the issues are being taken seriously, and a more holistic view of psychological distress is shared, rather than one that focuses largely on past traumatic events.

A third factor to take into account in selecting treatments for PTSD with young refugees is the extent to which they are able, or prepared, to look back and address past events, or whether they want to look at current and future difficulties and challenges. The evidence-based treatments described here that have the strongest evidence are trauma-focused therapies. Even those that have less robust evidence such as art therapy, and psychodynamic approaches, will involve reflecting on, or at least representing, past events. Individuals may not want to do this for many reasons. At a psychological level, doing this involves re-experiencing the traumatic events, which is distressing and aversive. The associated avoidance is a characteristic of the PSTD that the therapist is trying to treat. At a socio-cultural level, people from many cultures believe that dwelling on past events will not help them to function better, and that the adversities and hardship they experienced are not unusual. There may be feelings of inappropriate indulgence in focusing on individual suffering, There may be ambivalent feelings about discussing difficulties, arising in part because of guilt at survival, when many family or community members died, or could not escape terrible circumstances. It may be felt preferable to address present problems, which could relate directly to asylum or refugee status, or indirectly to this, e.g. bullying in school associated with cultural or language differences. For individuals who prefer to look forward, it may be preferable to provide a more symptoms-focused intervention, using appropriate social, family, psychological and psychopharmacological interventions.

The fourth factor in choosing treatment concerns psychiatric comorbidity. It is known that comorbidity is high with PTSD. Several studies of young refugees have shown that depressive disorder is frequently present with PTSD (Hubbard et al. 1995; Kinzie et al. 1986). Anxiety disorders, such as generalized anxiety disorder, separation anxiety disorder or agoraphobia may also occur (Brent et al. 1995; Goenjian et al. 1995; Yule and Unwin 1991). A study of children exposed to hurricane Andrew indicated that children's pre-disaster anxiety level predicted the presence of PTSD symptoms at three and seven months after the hurricane (La Greca et al. 1998). This suggested that anxiety disorders predispose to children to developing PTSD. The practical implications of the studies of comorbidity are that consideration needs to be given as to whether treatment for the PTSD will result in significant improvement of the comorbid disorder. This may be the case for mild depression and anxiety disorders. Severe comorbid disorders may require treatment in their own right. In planning treatment for the comorbid disorder it is important to consider whether that treatment may also ameliorate the PTSD. For example, in the case of severe depression, there is good evidence for benefit from psychopharmacological treatment with fluoxetine (TADS 2004). In the case of PSTD with comorbid psychosis, the anti-psychotic drugs may reduce arousal and other PTSD symptoms.

There are other factors that are not specific to refugees that need to be taken into account. These include the age and developmental stage of the child. Younger children may benefit from expressive methods such as drawing and play that represent their traumatic experiences, and are part of the exposure work. They may need a high level of support from parents and carers. By way of contrast, adolescents over 13 years will mostly be 'Gillick' competent and able to consent to treatment themselves, and express clear preferences for specific therapies. Unaccompanied asylum seeking children may be seen for treatment with relatively little support from adults, and approaches to therapy may be much more like those used with adults.

Service contexts and resources

Mental health interventions can only take place in societies that are adequately well functioning. Basic facilities need to be available, such as housing and essential commodities required for family life. Within the context of resettlement countries, a range of community supports are required for refugees (Hodes 2002b; Williams 1991).

The treatments described above require a relatively high level of resourcing, in terms of mental health professionals with appropriate skills. The treatments are best carried out within the context of a tiered system of care (Hodes 2002b). Even in the developed and affluent countries, it is beneficial to provide briefer, less intensive interventions in community settings such as schools (O'Shea et al. 2000). Brief family, individual or group cognitive behavioural therapy described here (Entholt et al. 2005; Stein et al. 2003) would be suitable for this context. Young refugees with more complex problems associated with greater functional impairment will require more intensive interventions. More intensive individual cognitive behavioural therapy (Vickers 2005) is associated with greater reduction in post-traumatic symptoms. Other treatments such as family intervention, or treatment for comorbid disorders such as depression, may need to be provided over a longer period. Such treatments may be best provided from mental health clinics that are staffed by multi-disciplinary groups of professionals.

Rather different considerations will apply to countries and communities that are in the grip of war. In such circumstances it may be unsafe for welfare organizations and mental health professionals to operate. When an adequate level of peace has been achieved, health care is needed that is appropriate for the countries' level of socio-economic development. The World Health Organization guidelines are important in this respect. They indicate the importance of mental health services that are culturally appropriate and sustainable, and take into account the range of health needs (Van Ommeren et al. 2005).

In many areas affected by conflict no child mental health professionals may be available. Nevertheless, there are reports of other professionals such as teachers who can be trained to deliver psychosocial interventions that may be based on group cognitive therapy principles or other approaches for children who have suffered psychological trauma (Dybdahl 2001).

Conclusions

The field of treatments for children and adolescents who have experienced psychological trauma is one that has received significant attention in recent years. The small number of adequate psychological treatment studies suggest that trauma focused cognitive therapy produces significant improvements, and children who have this therapy will have better outcomes than those who have no interventions or inactive therapies. Treatments for young refugees who have PTSD are similar to the treatments that may benefit non-refugee children who have had previously settled backgrounds. Nevertheless, young refugees may be living in very different circumstances, and this means that broader contextual issues, as well as their socio-cultural backgrounds, need to be taken into account. Of particular importance is that they may wish to focus on current and future adversities, rather than addressing past traumatic events. When considered in the international and global context, most psychological therapy will not be administered by mental health professionals, but there are approaches emerging that appear to be effective and that can be delivered by other professionals and will improve the adjustment of parents and children. Much more work is needed in developing treatments for children with PTSD in low-income countries, as well as the optimum mode of delivery. Further work is also required in the developed countries – particularly those regions which experienced natural or manmade disasters – to identify the most effective kinds of therapy and well as the need for sequencing therapies or multi-modal interventions. Finally, many of the above-mentioned issues highlighted so far will be revisited and discussed at length and with specific focus in the chapters of both parts of this book.

References

Albano, M. A., Marten, P. A., Holt, C. S. and Heimberg, R. G. (1995) 'Cognitive behavioural group treatment for social phobia in adolescents'. *Journal of Nervous and Mental Disease*, 183: 649–56.

American Academy of Child and Adolescent Psychiatry (1998) 'Practice parameters for the assessment and treatment of children and adolescents with posttraumatic stress disorder'. *Journal of the American Academy of Child and Adolescent Psychiatry*, 10 (supplement): S4–S26.

American Psychiatric Association (1994) *Diagnostic and Statistical Manual of Mental Disorders*. 4th edn. Washington DC: American Psychiatric Association.

Basoğlu, M., Ekblad, S., Bäärnhielm, S. and Livanou, M. (2004) 'Cognitive-behavioural treatment of tortured asylum seekers: a case study'. *Anxiety Disorders*, 18: 357–69.

Beck, A. T. (1991) *Cognitive Therapy and the Emotional Disorders*. London: Penguin.

Berliner, L. and Saunders, B. E. (1996) 'Treating fear and anxiety in sexually abused children'. *Journal of Interpersonal Violence*, 2(4): 415–34.

Bracken, P. J., Giller, J. E. and Summerfield, D. (1995) 'Psychological responses to war and atrocity: the limitations of current concepts'. *Social Science and Medicine*, 40: 1073–82.

Brent, D. A., Perper, J. A., Moritz, G., Liotus, L., Richardson, D., Canobbio, R., Schweers, J. and Roth, C. (1995) 'Posttraumatic stress disorder in peers of adolescent suicide victims'. *Journal of the American Academy of Child and Adolescent Psychiatry*, 34: 209–15.

Celano, M., Hazzard, A., Webb, C. and McCall, C. (1996) 'Treatment of trauma-genic beliefs among sexually abused girls and their mothers: an evaluation study'. *Journal of Abnormal Psychology*, 24: 1–16.

Chemtob, C., Nakashima, J. and Carlson, J. (2002) 'Brief treatment for elementary school children with disaster-related posttraumatic stress disorder: a field study'. *Journal of Clinical Psychology*, 58(1): 99–112.

Chorpita, B. F., Barlow, D. H., Albano, A. M. and Daleiden, E. L. (1998) 'Methodological strategies in child clinical trials: advancing the efficacy and effectiveness of psychosocial treatments'. *Journal of Abnormal Child Psychology*, 26: 7–16.

Cienfuegos, J. and Monelli, C. (1983) 'The testimony of political repression as a therapeutic instrument'. *American Journal of Orthopsychiatry*, 53: 43–51.

Cohen, J. A. and Mannarino, A. P. (1996) 'A treatment study of sexually abused preschool children: initial findings'. *Journal of the American Academy of Child and Adolescent Psychiatry*, 35: 42–50.

Cohen, J. A. and Mannarino, A. P. (1997) 'A treatment study of sexually abused preschool children: outcome during 1-year follow-up'. *Journal of the American Academy of Child and Adolescent Psychiatry*, 36: 1228–35.

Cohen, J. A. and Mannarino, A. P. (2004) 'Posttraumatic stress disorder'. In T. H. Ollendick and J. S. March (eds), *Phobic and Anxiety Disorders in Children and Adolescents: a Clinician's Guide to Effective Psychological Interventions*. Oxford: Oxford University Press, pp. 405–32.

Cohen, J. A., Berliner, L. and Mannarino, A. P. (2000) 'Treatment of traumatized children: a review and synthesis'. *Journal of Interpersonal Violence*, 8(1): 115–31.

Cohen, J. A., Deblinger, E., Mannarino, A. P. and Steer, R. A. (2004) 'A multisite, randomized controlled trial for children with sexual abuse-related PTSD symptoms'. *Journal of the American Academy of Child and Adolescent Psychiatry*, 43: 393–402.

Cohen, J. A., Mannarino, A. P. and Knudsen, K. (2005) 'Treating sexually abused children: 1 year follow-up of a randomized controlled trial'. *Child Abuse and Neglect*, 29: 103–5.

Deblinger, E., Lippman, J. and Steer, R. (1996) 'Sexually abused children suffering posttraumatic stress symptoms: initial treatment outcome findings'. *Child Maltreatment*, 6: 310–21.

Deblinger, E., Steer, R. and Lippman, J. (1999) 'Two-year follow-up study of cognitive behavioural therapy for sexually abused children suffering posttraumatic stress symptoms'. *Child Abuse and Neglect*, 23: 1371–8.

Deblinger, E., Stauffer, L. and Steer, R. (2001) 'Comparative efficacies of supportive and cognitive behavioural group therapies for young children who have been sexually abused and their nonoffending mothers'. *Child Maltreatment*, 6: 332–42.

Downing, J., Jenkins, S. J. and Fisher, G. L. (1988) 'A comparison of psychodynamic and reinforcement treatment with sexually abused children'. *Elementary School Guidance Counselling*, 22: 291–8.

Dwivedi, K. (2000) *Post-Traumatic Stress Disorder in Children and Adolescents*. London and Philadelphia: Whurr.

Dybdahl, R. (2001) 'Children and mothers in war: an outcome study of a psychosocial intervention program'. *Child Development*, 72: 1214–30.

Ehlers, A. and Clark, D. M. (2000) 'A cognitive model of posttraumatic stress disorder'. *Behaviour Research and Therapy*, 38: 319–45.

Entholt, K., Smith, P. and Yule, W. (2005) 'School-based cognitive-behavioural therapy group intervention for refugee children who have experienced war-related trauma'. *Clinical Child Psychology and Psychiatry*, 10: 235–50.

Famularo, R., Fenton, T., Augustyn, M. and Zuckerman, B. (1988) 'Propanolol treatment for childhood posttraumatic stress disorder, acute type: a pilot study'. *American Journal of Disease in Childhood*, 142: 1244–7.

Foa, E. B., Rothbaum, B. O., Riggs, D. S. and Murdock, T. B. (1991) 'Treatment of post-traumatic stress disorder in rape victims: a comparison between cognitive-behavioural procedures and counseling'. *Journal of Consulting Clinical Psychology*, 59: 715–23.

Goenjian, A. K., Pynos, R. S., Steinberg, A. M., Najarian, L. M., Asarnow, J. R., Karayan, I., Ghurabi, M. and Fairbanks, L. A. (1995) 'Psychiatric comorbidity in children after the 1988 earthquake in Armenia'. *Journal of the American Academy of Child and Adolescent Psychiatry*, 34: 1174–84.

Goenjian, A. K., Karayan, I. L., Pynoos, R. S., Minassian, D., Najarian, L. M., Steinber, A. M. and Fairbanks, L. A. (1997) 'Outcome of psychotherapy among early adolescents after trauma'. *American Journal of Psychiatry*, 154: 536–42.

Harmon, R. J. and Riggs, P. D. (1996) 'Clinical perspectives: clonidine for post-traumatic stress disorder in preschool children'. *Journal of the American Academy of Child and Adolescent Psychiatry*, 35: 1247–9.

Harrington, R., Whittaker, J., Shoebridge, P. and Campbell, F. (1998) 'Systematic review of efficacy of cognitive behaviour therapies in childhood and adolescent depressive disorder'. *British Medical Journal*, 316: 1559–63.

Hodes, M. (2000) 'Psychologically distressed children in the United Kingdom'. *Child Psychology and Psychiatry Review*, 5: 57–68.

Hodes, M. (2002a) 'Three key issues for young refugees' mental health'. *Transcultural Psychiatry*, 39: 196–213.

Hodes, M. (2002b) 'Implications for psychiatric services of chronic civilian strife or war: young refugees in the UK'. *Advances in Psychiatric Treatment*, 8: 366–74.

Horrigan, J. P. (1996) 'Guanfacine for posttraumatic stress disorder nightmares (letter to editor)'. *Journal of the American Academy of Child and Adolescent Psychiatry*, 35: 975–6.

Horrigan, J. P. and Barnhill, L. J. (1999) 'Risperidone and PTSD in boys'. *Journal of Neuropsychiatry and Clinical Neuroscience*, 11: 126–7.

Hubbard, J., Realmuto, G., Northwood, A. and Masten, A. (1995) 'Comorbidity of psychiatric diagnoses with posttraumatic stress disorder in survivors of childhood trauma'. *Journal of the American Academy of Child and Adolescent Psychiatry*, 34: 1167–73.

Jaycox, L. (2003) *Cognitive-Behavioral Intervention for Trauma in Schools*. Longmont, CO: Sopris West Educational Services.

Kalmanowitz, D. and Lloyd, B. (1997) *The Portable Studio. Art Therapy and Political Conflict: Initiatives in Former Yugoslavia and KwaZulu-Natal, South Africa*. London: Health Education Council.

Kataoka, S., Stein, B., Jaycox, L., Wong, M., Escudero, P., Tu, W., Zaragoza, C. and Fink, A. (2003) 'A school-based mental health program for traumatized Latino immigrant children'. *Journal of the American Academy of Child and Adolescent Psychiatry*, 42(3): 311–18.

Kellner, M. H. and Bry, B. H. (1999) 'The effects of anger management groups in a day school for emotionally disturbed adolescents'. *Adolescence*, 34: 645–51.

Kendall, P. C. (1994) 'Treating anxiety disorders in children: results of a randomized clinical trial'. *Journal of Consulting Clinical Psychology*, 62: 100–10.

King, N. J., Tonge, B. J., Mullen, P., Myerson, N., Heyne, D., Rollings, S., Martin, R. and Ollendick, T. (2000) 'Treating sexually abused children with posttraumatic stress symptoms: a randomized clinical trial'. *Journal of the American Academy of Child and Adolescent Psychiatry*, 39(11): 1347–55.

Kinzie, J. D., Sack, W. H., Angell, R. H., Manson, S. and Rath, B. (1986) 'The psychiatric effects of massive trauma on Cambodian children: I. The children'. *Journal of the American Academy of Child and Adolescent Psychiatry*, 25: 370–6.

La Greca, A. M., Silverman, W. K. and Wasserstein, S. B. (1998) 'Children's pre-disaster functioning as a predictor of posttraumatic stress following hurricane Andrew'. *Journal of Consulting and Clinical Psychology*, 66: 883–92.

Lewinsohn, P. M., Clarke, G. N., Hops, H. and Andrews, J. (1990) 'Cognitive behavioural group treatment of depression in adolescents'. *Behaviour Therapy*, 21: 385–401.

Lieberman, A. F., van Horn, P. and Ippen, C. G. (2005) 'Toward evidence-based treatment: child-parent psychotherapy with preschoolers exposed to marital violence'. *Journal of the American Academy of Child and Adolescent Psychiatry*, 44: 1241–8.

Looff, D., Grimley, P., Kuiler, F., Martin, A. and Shunfield, L. (1995) 'Carbamazepine for posttraumatic stress disorder (letter)'. *Journal of the American Academy of Child and Adolescent Psychiatry*, 34: 703–4.

Lustig, S. L., Kia-Keating, K., Knight, W.G., Geltman. P., Ellis, H., Kinzie, D., Keane, T. and Saxe, G. N. (2004a) 'Review of child and adolescent refugee mental health'. *Journal of the American Academy of Child and Adolescent Psychiatry*, 43: 24–36.

Lustig, S. L., Weine S. W., Saxe, G. N. and Beardslee, W. R. (2004b) 'Testimonial psychotherapy for adolescent refugees: a case series'. *Transcultural Psychiatry*, 41: 31–45.

March, J. S., Mulle, K. and Herbel, B. (1994) 'Behavioural psychotherapy for children and adolescents with obsessive-compulsive disorder: an open trial of a new protocol-driven treatment package'. *Journal of the American Academy of Child and Adolescent Psychiatry*, 33: 333–41.

March, J., Amaya-Jackson, L., Murray, M., Cathryn, M. A. and Schulte, A. (1998) 'Cognitive-behavioural psychotherapy for children and adolescents with post-traumatic stress disorder after a single-incident stressor'. *Journal of the American Academy of Child and Adolescent Psychiatry*, 37(6): 585–93.

Marmar, C. R., Foy, D., Kagan, B. and Pynoos, R. S. (1993) 'An integrated approach for treating posttraumatic stress'. In R. S. Pynoos (ed.), *Post-traumatic Stress Disorder: a Clinical Review*. Lutherville, MD: Sidran Press, pp. 239–72.

Melzak, S. (1992) 'Secrecy, privacy, survival, repressive regimes and growing up'. *Bulletin of the Anna Freud Centre*, 15: 205–24.

Mezzich, J., Kleinman, A., Fabrega, H. and Parron, D. (eds) (1996) *Culture and Psychiatric Diagnosis*. Washington DC: American Psychiatric Press.

Möhlen, H., Parzer, P., Resch, F. and Brunner, R. (2005) 'Psychosocial support for war-traumatized children and adolescent refugees: evaluation of a short-term programme'. *Australian and New Zealand Journal of Psychiatry*, 39: 81–7.

National Collaborating Centre for Mental Health (NCCMH) (2005) *Post-traumatic Stress Disorder: the Management of PTSD in Adults and Children in Primary and Secondary Care*. London: The Royal College of Psychiatrists and The British Psychological Society.

Neuner, F., Schaeur, M., Elbert, T. and Roth, W. T. (2002) 'A narrative exposure treatment as intervention in a Macedonian refugee camp: a case report'. *Journal of Behavioural Cognitive Psychotherapy*, 30: 205–9.

Neuner, F., Schauer, M., Klaschik, C., Karunakara, U. and Elbert, T. (2004) 'A comparison of narrative exposure therapy, supportive counselling and psychoeducation for treating posttraumatic stress disorder in an African refugee settlement'. *Journal of Consulting Clinical Psychology*, 72: 579–87.

Onyut, L. P., Neurer, F., Schauer, E., Ertl, V., Odenwald, M., Shauer, M. and Elbert, T. (2005) 'Narrative exposure therapy as a treatment for child war survivors with posttraumatic stress disorder: two case reports and a pilot study in an African refugee settlement'. *BMC Psychiatry*, 5: 7. www.biomedcentral.com/1471-244X/5/7

Oras, R., Cancela de Ezpeleta, S. and Ahmed, A. (2004) 'Treatment of traumatized refugee children with eye movement desensitization and reprocessing in a psychodynamic context'. *Nordic Journal of Psychiatry*, 58(3): 199–203.

O'Shea, B., Hodes, M., Down, G. and Bramley, J. (2000) 'A school-based mental health service for refugee children'. *Clinical Child Psychology and Psychiatry*, 5(2): 181–201.

Paunovic, N. and Ost, L. G. (2001) 'Cognitive-behaviour therapy vs exposure therapy in the treatment of PTSD in refugees'. *Behaviour Research and Therapy*, 39: 1183–97.

Perrin, S., Smith, P. and Yule, W. (2000) 'Practitioner review: the assessment and treatment of post-traumatic stress disorder in children and adolescents'. *Journal of Child Psychology and Psychiatry*, 41: 277–89.

Quota, S., Punamaki, R.-L. and El Sarraj, E. (2005) 'Mother-child expression of psychological distress in war trauma'. *Clinical Child Psychology and Psychiatry*, 10: 135–56.

Robert, R., Blackeney, P. E., Villareal, C., Rosenberg, L. and Meyer, W. J. (1999) 'Imipramine treatment in pediatric burn patients with symptoms of adult stress disorder'. *Journal of the American Academy of Child and Adolescent Psychiatry*, 38: 873–82.

Rousseau, C., Singh, A., Lacroix, L. and Measham, T., (2004) 'Creative expression workshops for immigrant and refugee children'. *Journal of the American Academy of Child and Adolescent Psychiatry*, 43: 235–8.

Rousseau, C., Drapeau, A., Lacroix, L., Bagilshya, D. and Heusch, N. (2005) 'Evaluation of a classroom program of creative expression workshops for refugee and immigrant children'. *Journal of Child Psychology and Psychiatry*, 46:180–5.

Sack, W. H., Seeley, J. R. and Clarke, G. N. (1997) 'Does PTSD transcend cultural barriers? A study from the Khmer adolescent refugee project'. *Journal of the American Academy of Child and Adolescent Psychiatry*, 36: 49–54.

Sackett, D. L., Rosenberg, W. M. C., Muir Gray, J. A., Haynes, R. B. and Richardson, W. S. (1996) 'Evidence based medicine: what it is and what is isn't'. *British Medical Journal*, 312: 71–2.

Scheeringa, M. S., Zeanah, C. H., Myers, L. and Putnam, F. W. (2003) 'New findings on alternative criteria for PTSD in preschool children'. *Journal of the American Academy of Child and Adolescent Psychiatry*, 42: 561–70.

Scheeringa, M. S., Zeanah, C. H., Myers, L. and Putnam, F. W. (2005) 'Predictive validity in a prospective follow up study of PTSD in preschool children'. *Journal of the American Academy of Child and Adolescent Psychiatry*, 44: 899–906.

Schoenfeld, F., Marmar, C. and Neylan, T. (2004) 'Current concepts in pharmacotherapy for posttraumatic stress disorder'. *Psychiatric Services*, 55(5): 519–31.

Seedat, S., Stein, D. J., Ziervogel, C., Middleton, T., Kaminer, D., Emsley, R. A. and Rossouw, W. (2002) 'Comparison of response to a selective serotonin reuptake inhibitor in children adolescents and adults with PTSD'. *Journal of Child and Adolescent Psychopharmacology*, 12: 37–46.

Shapiro, F. (1995) *Eye Movement Desensitisation and Reprocessing*. New York: Guildford Press.

Shepperd, R. (2001) 'Individual treatments for children and adolescents with post-traumatic stress disorder: unlocking children's trauma'. In K. Dwivedi (ed.), *Post-Traumatic Stress Disorder in Children and Adolescents*. London and Philadelphia: Whurr, pp. 131–46.

Smith, P., Perrin, S., Yule, W. and Rabe-Hesketh, S. (2001) 'War exposure and maternal reactions in the psychological adjustment of children from Bosnia-Herzegovina'. *Journal of Child Psychology and Psychiatry*, 42: 395–404.

Stein, B. D., Jaycox, L. H., Kataoka, S. S. H., Wong, M., Tu, W., Elliott, M. N. and Fink, A. (2003) 'A mental health intervention for schoolchildren exposed to violence: a randomized controlled trial'. *Journal of the American Medical Association*, 290: 603–11.

Summerfield, D. (1999) 'A critique of seven assumptions behind psychological trauma programmes in war-affected areas'. *Social Science and Medicine*, 48: 1449–62.

Summerfield, D. (2000) 'Childhood, war, refugeedom and "trauma": three core questions for mental health professionals'. *Transcultural Psychiatry*, 37: 417–33.

TADS (Treatment for Adolescents with Depression Study) (2004) 'Fluoxetine, cognitive-behavioural therapy, and their combination for adolescents with depression'. *Journal of the American Medical Association*, 292: 807–20.

Tarrier, N., Sommerfield, C. and Pilgrim, H. (1999) 'Relatives' expressed emotion (EE) and PTSD treatment outcome'. *Psychological Medicine*, 29: 801–11.

Tinker, R. H. (2002) 'EMDR for traumatized children around the world'. In J. Morris-Smith (ed.), *EMDR: Clinical Applications with Children*. ACPP Occasional Paper No 19. London: ACPP.

Trowell, J., Kolvin, I., Weeramanthri, T., Sadowski, H., Berelowitz, M., Glasser, D. and Leitch, I. (2002) 'Psychotherapy for sexually abused girls: psychopathological outcome findings and patterns of change'. *British Journal of Psychiatry*, 160: 234–47.

Tufnell, G. (2003) 'Refugee children, trauma and the law'. *Clinical Child Psychology and Psychiatry*, 8: 431–43.

Tufnell, G. (2005) 'Eye movement desensitization and reprocessing in the treatment of pre-adolescent children with posttraumatic stress disorder'. *Clinical Child Psychology and Psychiatry*, 10: 587–600.

Van Ommeren, M., Saxena, S. and Saraceno, B. (2005) 'Mental and social health during and after acute emergencies: emerging consensus?' *Bulletin of the World Health Organization*, 83: 71–7.

Vickers, B. (2005) 'A cognitive model of the maintenance and treatment of post-traumatic stress disorder applied to children and adolescents'. *Clinical Child Psychology and Psychiatry*, 10: 217–34.

Weine, S., Kulenovic, A. D., Pavkovic, I. and Gibbons, R. (1998) 'Testimony psychotherapy in Bosnian refugees: a pilot study'. *American Journal of Psychiatry*, 155: 1720–6.

Weine, S. and Laub, D. (1995) 'Narrative constructions of historical realities in testimony with Bosnian survivors of "ethnic cleansing"'. *Psychiatry*, 58: 246–60.

Wertheim-Cahen, T., van Dijk, M., Schouten, K., Rozen, I. and Drozek, B. (2004) 'About a weeping willow, a phoenix rising from its ashes, and building a house … art therapy with refugees: three different perspectives'. In J. P. Wilson and B. Drozek (eds), *Broken Spirits: the Treatment of Traumatized Asylum Seekers, Refugees, War and Torture Victims*. New York and Hove: Brunner-Routledge, pp. 419–41.

Williams, C. L. (1991) 'Toward the development of preventive interventions for youth traumatized by war and refugee flight'. In F. Ahearn and J. L. Athey (eds), *Refugee Children: Theory, Research and Services*. Baltimore and London: Johns Hopkins University Press, pp. 201–17.

Woodcock, J. (2001) 'Refugee children and their families: theoretical and clinical perspectives'. In K. Dwivedi (ed.), *Post-Traumatic Stress Disorder in Children and Adolescents*. London and Philadelphia: Whurr, pp. 213–39.

World Health Organization (1993) *The ICD-10 Classification of Mental and Behavioural Disorders. Diagnostic Criteria for Research*. Geneva: World Health Organization.

Yule, W. and Udwin, O. (1991) 'Screening child survivors for posttraumatic stress disorders: experiences from the "Jupiter" sinking'. *British Journal of Clinical Psychology*, 30: 131–8.

Yule, W. (2002) 'Post-traumatic stress disorder'. In M. Rutter and E. Taylor (eds), *Child and Adolescent Psychiatry*, 4th edn, Oxford: Blackwell, pp. 520–8.

3

A Model for Acute Care of Children and Adolescents Exposed to Disasters

Linda Chokroverty and Nalaini Sriskandarajah

Disasters have a devastating impact on the social and psychological well-being of children and their families. Many techniques (see Chapters 1 and 2 of this book) have been described as helpful in assisting affected individuals to cope with emotional well-being and other consequences following disasters. However, very little evidence-based research has been attempted particularly on the acute phase interventions with children. In planning for accessible psychosocial assistance in the acute phase that would help children cope with the stressful experiences, it has emerged that the use of play can be a valuable strategy. This became evident after the 11 September 2001 terrorist attacks in New York City, where a special environment for children and families was developed. The space was named the 'Kids' Corner' which utilized play as the primary mode of expression for children affected by the disaster. Its development was based on the premise that most children, given the opportunity to draw on their personal strengths and resources, will heal and recover from the effects of stressful experiences. This chapter will review the needs of children following a disaster, discuss the relevance of play in the healing process, describe the 'Kids' Corner' model, and discuss the benefits and drawbacks of such a model. In addition, suggestions for modifications that make it suitable for a variety of post-disaster situations will be offered.

According to the World Health Organization (WHO), a disaster is a disruption which can overwhelm the coping capacity of the affected community (WHO 1992). During and after a disaster, children remain vulnerable and at risk. Whether they will experience traumatic stress symptoms after a disaster, and for how long, depends on many variables (Pynoos and Nader 1988).

The effects of the disaster can interfere with children's social, psychological and physical development. Children who have survived a life-threatening traumatic event need to regain their normal developmental processes as early as possible. Governments of many countries now recognize this and have included mental health and psychosocial support into their emergency planning programmes (Civil Contingencies Secretariat 2004; Chatterjee 2005; Bisson et al. 2003). Provision of psychological support has also been integrated into disaster programmes of the WHO and other international organizations concerned with disaster relief efforts. The recent Asian tsunamis have heightened interest in post-disaster psychosocial services, especially for children. Many different theoretical models have been offered for conceptualizing the stages of disaster.

These may cover psychological stages as well as chronological stages and include both pre- and post-disaster events (Laor et al. 2003; Vernberg 2002). The duration of these stages can be defined, but where one ends and another begins is rather fluid. For this chapter, the acute stage of disaster is of interest. The acute stage is defined as the period from day one of the disaster until about three months after the event. This definition corresponds to the chronological stage, 'short-term adaptation phase', noted elsewhere in the literature (Vernberg and Vogel 1993).

Psychiatric sequelae and vulnerability

The literature on mental health responses following disaster is steadily growing, including research work involving children who have survived life-threatening events. It has been noted in several studies that elevated levels of post-traumatic symptomatology may occur in children for many months, even years, after the traumatic events. Some available studies (Cohen et al. 1998; Pynoos and Nader 1990; Lacey 1972; Morgan et al. 2003; Yule 1992a; Newman 1976; McFarlane 1987; Terr 1991) suggest that certain groups of children are vulnerable to future psychopathology. These studies include the well-known Aberfan coal mining tip accident in Wales, the *Jupiter* ship sinking disaster, the Buffalo Creek flood, Australian bush fires and the Chowchilla bus shootings (some of these studies were reviewed in Chapter 1).

Other research work indicates that psychological reactions in the aftermath of a disaster are commonly transient in nature. That is, most symptoms in the population subside over time, usually between sixteen months and three years (Solomon and Green 1992; Solomon 1999; Vogel and Vernberg 1993). Resilience research views this phenomenon as the trajectory of recovery, where normal functioning temporarily gives way to psychopathology, and gradually returns to pre-event levels (Bonnano 2004). However, some factors preclude recovery in children, including pre-existing psychopathology and multiple traumatic experiences that are highly distressing and severe in their nature (Lonigan et al. 1994; Earls et al. 1988; Vogel and Vernberg 1993; Yule 1992b: McFarlane 1987). Other factors which may increase the likelihood of prolonged distress among children are the degree of perceived life threat, serious injury to the child, or serious injury or death of a family member or close friends. The latter are more likely to increase the risk of symptoms of traumatic stress. In addition, environmental factors, such as substantial destruction, displacement and continued impact of the disaster on family functioning are also predictors of psychopathology.

A study of over 150 children who witnessed a shooting incident at a school playground revealed that the number of symptoms of Post-Traumatic Stress Disorder (PTSD) as well as their severity increased as the degree of exposure to the disaster increased (APA 1994; Pynoos et al. 1987; Pynoos and Nader 1990). Another study which assessed the needs of over 3000 children seven weeks after the 1995 Okalahoma City bombing in the United States indicated that female gender, level of personal exposure to the event, and incident-related television viewing correlated with higher rates of post-traumatic stress symptoms among the children (Pfefferbaum et al. 1999). McNally (1993), in a major review of the literature, noted that pre-existing psychopathology, level of intelligence, and availability of social support were associated with the likelihood of PTSD developing in children.

Despite distressing symptoms and the available resources, help is not always sought by disaster-affected individuals. However, children's psychological needs are hardly assessed by their care providers unless symptoms are overtly evident. In addition, abundance of mental health resources does not always guarantee that children in need will access them, suggesting stigma as a factor. Results of two major studies conducted in New York City following the 11 September 2001 attacks showed that many children who may have warranted mental health services did not receive them (Stuber et al. 2002; Hoven et al. 2002; Dodds Joyner and Cupit Swenson 1993). Lack of distinction between mental illness and mental health is also a factor in the avoidance of mental health assistance by disaster survivors as well as those planning and providing the services (Myers 1994). The mere mention of mental health to many people, regardless of culture, often sends these individuals into a defensive posture that 'they are not crazy' (Lindy et al. 1981). Sometimes the media perpetuates beliefs that mental health practitioners, particularly psychiatrists, should not do support work after a disaster. In a major newspaper in the United States following the Asian tsunamis, a psychiatrist wrote a lengthy editorial arguing against psychiatrists participating in disaster relief, further complicating the public debate about who should be engaging in the effort towards recovery (Satel 2005). The magnitude of the disaster itself (as in the aftermath of the Asian tsunamis where large areas were severely damaged and inaccessible), as well as geographical isolation, also deters individuals from accessing available services. In addition, low priority ascribed to mental health during the acute phase contributes to the low use of mental health services during this period. In some cultures 'feelings' do not have relevance unless there are behavioural problems, and therefore children's psychological needs may never be addressed or noticed. Also, in remote communities and of low socio-economic status, children may be expected to take part in the day-to-day chores of the family such as caring for younger children, cooking, working in farms and attending to animals. Under these conditions, unless the children verbalize their distress their needs will hardly be noticed. Cultural biases and beliefs also serve to perpetuate repression and denial as coping strategies which in some instances may be maladaptive.

Cultural considerations and sensitivity to local needs

After a disaster, as at any other time, the race, culture, religion, language and socio-economic status of the community all play important roles in the child's psychosocial development and recovery. For example, cultural assumptions of the care provider (the helper) as well as the recipient contribute to the use or under-use of available mental health services. Post-colonial developing societies may view mental health services as 'Western imported phenomena', which threaten indigenous healing efforts. Hence, mental health services provided by Western-based relief organizations and institutions that are seen to be lacking cultural understanding may be rejected. It should be noted here that local mental health professionals are most proficient in understanding the cultural environment of the child after a disaster. However, in many countries such professionals are not readily available because of inadequate pre-disaster mental health systems or due to economic reasons or cultural attitudes that hinder the development of mental health services. In these cases, outside experts in mental health often arrive to help in the relief effort. Given the possible biases and beliefs within affected communities, it is essential that visiting mental health professionals have a deep understanding and respect for the local culture, the individual child and his or her experiences, beliefs and values rather than assume common attributes of the community to which the child belongs. These professionals may work with available local people, who would serve as 'cultural consultants' in providing understanding about cultural values and settings, language and local resources. Cultures vary in their views about children, the role of the family, and the relevance of play in each specific culture; such variations are best understood by outside professionals when they employ a 'cultural consultant'.

Indeed, the subject of culture brings to awareness not just the social characteristics of communities affected by disasters, but also the different viewpoints that exist among those attending to the communities as they adjust and recover. Some view disaster survivors along perspectives of health, whereas others view them along illness. Critics of the medical (illness) model argue that symptoms perceived as PTSD may in fact be indicators of social suffering which are of social and political origin (Summerfield 1999). Researchers studying how individuals respond to traumatic events have observed that those with positive outcomes have preferred coping mechanisms that convert their traumatic experience into growth experiences (Horowitz 1986; Finkel and Jacobsen 1977). Tedeschi and his colleagues (Tedeschi et al. 1998) describe this process of recovery from trauma as post-traumatic growth (PTG), which fits into the health (wellness) model and is gaining increased support (Marsella and Christopher 2004; Tedeschi et al. 1998; North 2004). In fact, international relief organizations, by and large, have emphasized models of wellness and resilience (Brooks and Goldstein 2003) rather than the medical model of illness, in approaching post-disaster relief work. (See also Chapter 8 of this book.)

Resilience, which stems from individual, family and environmental attributes, should not be ignored while dealing with children in the acute phase or in the aftermath of a disaster. Bonanno (2004) describes resilience as the ability to maintain a stable equilibrium even in the face of adversity. Masten (2001: 227), on the other hand, defines resilience in children as a 'class of phenomena characterized by good outcomes in spite of serious threats to adaptation or development'. She further added that resilience derives not from 'rare and special qualities, but from the everyday magic of ordinary, normative resources in the minds, brains and bodies of children, from their families and relationships, and in their communities' (Masten 2001). The study of resilience in children has been growing fast during the last 30 years, and it is now felt by those interested in this field that resilience is common, thus lending further support to those communities and organizations that favour the wellness model in the post-disaster recovery effort. It is worth noting that the model for post-disaster care of children discussed later in this chapter is based on the concept of resilience.

Approaches and interventions during the acute phase

Working with families and children during the acute phase and beyond could be called the three-pronged approach. All three prongs are of equal importance. The first part of this approach is to assess for signs of maladjustment and the implication of these findings. The next part of the approach is the interventional aspect through psychosocial support. During this time, children are given an opportunity to express their feelings individually, in peer groups, with families, or in school, and if needed, undergo screening and treatment for mental health concerns. A less frequent, third prong of the work with children is treatment research where signs and symptoms among the affected population are noted, interventions are conducted and the effectiveness of the intervention is evaluated. So far, most literature on interventions with children are of the narrative and experiential type, rather than evidence-based. Methods used in such cases are based mostly on the clinical experience and training orientations of those initiating the interventions.

In the acute post-disaster phase, interventions should promote psychosocial well-being. These interventions could be very brief and informal, lasting only ten or fifteen minutes (Taxman 2004; Weaver 2002). Alternatively, work may be continued with interim appointments or sessions over a period of time lasting hours, days, weeks or longer. Interactions with children could be on an individual basis, as is often the case with older adolescents, or in the context of the family or other care providers. Group interactions soon after a disaster may also occur, and are best suited for displacement shelters and schools. In addition to the affected children, the target audience for these groups could include other children in school, parents and adult family members. In the case of schools, the target audiences would include school administrators, teachers and other school personnel as well. Psychosocial support methods used in such groups are variable, ranging from discussions, lectures and training, demonstrations on how to interact with children in play with toys and games, theatre, dance, music, storytelling and the employment of visual arts and crafts. Older children, teenagers, and adult family members as well as school personnel, are generally more able to engage in verbal groups, whereas younger children engage in play, art and drama. Individual interactions with children and parents may be in the form of discussion, consultation, and non-verbal techniques such as play. Such interactions could be with one child, one family, or the parent(s) of a particular child. In the case of a large-scale disaster such as the South Asian tsunamis with so many affected, and relatively few caregivers providing relief, the chance of providing individualized attention has been small. Rather, in these cases, semi-individual and small groups are more realistic approaches. Furthermore, group format activities may have more cultural validity and acceptance under these circumstances. Kao (2005), who used play therapy in her work with Asian children, found that group identity was favoured over individual identity. Hoffman and Rogers (1991) described a counselling programme after the Santa Cruz earthquake in California, where discussions, drawings and group play of games took place for several hours at a time with child survivors in a shelter.

Play intervention as a key element in post-disaster work with children

In planning to work with children in post-disaster situations, one must consider the special needs of children. Children have a few basic but important needs that distinguish them from adults. They need to feel safe and be with their parents and family, and they need to express their thoughts and ideas to their parents and others. Depending on their age, children use verbal and non-verbal communication skills. Regardless of whether the interactions with traumatized children are individualized or in groups, the most universal and culturally adaptable method involves the act of playing. Throughout the lifecycle, play (Carey 2004) is a universally important means for expression as well as recreation across cultures. For children, play is particularly meaningful, as it does not require the sophisticated use of language skill. Furthermore, play facilitates a child's physical, intellectual and social development, and it is an individual right and also an integral part of growth (Schaefer 1993; UN 1990).

Children not only communicate their needs but also their understanding of the world through play. Play provides them with the opportunity to reflect on their relationships and experiences with others, and also enables them to express pressing needs, release unacceptable impulses, and experiment with solutions when challenged with adversity. A child can move towards inner resolution of a frightening or traumatic experience through play by returning to the event again and again, and perhaps even changing the outcome in the activity (Hartley et al. 1952; Landreth 1993). In the healing process immediately after a crisis, the child, through play and replay, can transform and re-enact the passivity and impotence experienced into activity and power (Webb 1991). In a post-disaster setting, play serves both a normative and restorative function in the lives of children, whose existence has been otherwise thrown into disarray. In order to play, children need tools such as toys, creative materials and other props. In addition to physical materials, games and storytelling can serve as vehicles through which play can occur. Finally, it is the role of adult facilitators to set the stage on which children may express their intimate thoughts and feelings. The adults may observe and participate in the play, and when necessary, may reassure and perhaps put into words the unspoken and unthinkable feelings the child may be experiencing.

Indeed, play has real application in the healing process after disasters, especially when it occurs in a 'protected environment'. Winnicott (1953), in his description of transitional objects, concluded that physical objects represent primary attachment figures and the relationships a child has with those figures. A transitional object need not be something tangible to a child. Rather, it could be a place and its parts, or even an idea. Thus, for a child, a special area can represent the comfort and safety of being with those who love that child. After a disaster, this space can be an essential transitional object. To have real value as a transitional object, a child's space must also have adults incorporated into it, even if those adults are not their usual caretakers. After the World Trade Center attack in New York City on 11 September 2001, such a space was created for children by volunteer professionals. This area utilized play as the primary mode of expression for children affected by the disaster. The work done in this space was viewed as brief 'play therapy' when it was conducted by experienced mental health clinicians skilled in such techniques, or merely play that had therapeutic value, when it was conducted by less experienced relief workers and volunteers. In general, the use of play as a 'therapeutic approach' will vary depending on the characteristics of the particular disaster, the cultural context of where it occurs, the length and intensity of the interaction with the child or children, and the resources available to the community in the recovery effort.

Studies involving use of play as a therapeutic modality after disasters are rare, in comparison with studies of other techniques, such as cognitive behavioural treatments. Shen (2002) describes a short-term, school-based post-disaster group play therapy programme in Taiwan as being effective in reducing anxiety and suicide risk among children compared to controls. This study is especially meaningful, since it used Western play therapy techniques in an Eastern culture, suggesting the transcendent properties of play in post-disaster settings.

The 'Kids' Corner'

Play as a therapeutic approach for children in a time of crisis is hardly a novel concept. During World War Two, Freud and Burlingham (1943) made fundamental observations about young children and care providers in a nursery setting. Humanitarian aid groups have attended to the needs of children after disasters for many years, and some have understood the need for children to assemble and play. Raynor (2002) described play areas with child flood victims in Missouri, earthquake victims in Japan, and refugee centres in war-torn areas such as Bosnia and Zimbabwe. Lists and descriptions of therapeutic activities with children are also noted by Murthy and Mander (2002) and La Greca and Prinstein (2002). Despite the surge in the development of therapeutic approaches during the last three decades, therapeutic play milieu and guidelines for a disaster setting remain rare and are seldom found. After the 11 September 2001 attack, the notion of a therapeutic play area for children was conceptualized in the spirit of traditional play therapy using the experience of seasoned child specialists. The services of volunteer child psychiatrists and other professionals were coordinated by Disaster Psychiatry Outreach (DPO), a not-for-profit volunteer organization which worked in collaboration with the local office of mental health and other relief organizations (Chokroverty et al. 2002; Heath 2004; Disaster Psychiatry Outreach 2005). The therapeutic play area, named the 'Kids' Corner', was not just a place, but also a concept, from which lessons for the future have been learned. More recently, following the South Asian tsunamis of 26 December 2004, it has been replicated at a few sites in Sri Lanka. Throughout this chapter the 'Kids' Corner' in New York will be referred to as KC-NY, and those in Sri Lanka collectively as KC-SL. The general use of the phrase, 'Kids' Corner', will be referred to as KC.

At the KC-NY a wide range of therapeutic interactions occurred. Children engaged in the normative and therapeutic aspects of play while volunteers from mental health and other professions were present in the area. Although children were the primary recipients of attention from the volunteers, other beneficiaries of the space included adult family members of these children, and unrelated adults with concerns about their own children. The friendly atmosphere attracted many parents to seek their own counselling, participate in psychosocial interaction, obtain printed literature, and even receive mental health treatment referral when needed. Many parents were empowered by the guidance available at the KC-NY and in their ability to provide emotional support to their children. The volunteers (many of whom had been personally affected by the disaster), also benefited from working in the 'Kids' Corner'. Following the South Asian tsunamis, using the same blueprint, with a few modifications to make them suitable for very different conditions, KCs were created in affected areas in Sri Lanka during Disaster Psychiatry Outreach (DPO), and training of local volunteers was conducted in cooperation with local non-governmental organizations (NGOs). The KC-SL were assembled three to four months after the tsunami, and were set in a developing country, with scarce pre-existing resources, a rather large affected population, and overwhelming public health demands. This was in sharp contrast to the conditions of the KC-NY where a rich mental health infrastructure and other abundant resources were available. As a result, many modifications had to be made to accommodate the local cultural needs, and the level of expertise of the volunteers. Despite the main modifications that have been made, the basic concept of the KC remained unaltered as a place where play is a privilege and a right, and where adults serve to facilitate the act of playing. Furthermore, the fact that the KC could be replicated in the aftermath of disasters in various regions and for various conditions suggests that it is transcultural and universally applicable.

As previously noted, guidelines by various organizations (AACAP 2004; RCP 2004; Myers 1994), while emphasizing the special needs of children, and recommending special areas for children in the aftermath of disasters, have not described the essential components or methods to assemble such spaces. After a disaster, once a formal structure has been established and the needs of nutrition, clothing and refuge are in place, wherever families are gathered, be it at a shelter, camp, community centre or school, a KC could be assembled.

Focusing on resilience, it has been suggested (Masten 2001; Brooks and Goldstein 2003) that resilience depends not on the child's ability alone, but on a whole system that includes other people, especially adults, and factors such as opportunities, protection and past experiences. By drawing upon the innate tendency of children to play regardless of circumstances, the KC fosters resilience. In addition, by engaging adult family members and/or community members such as teachers and other child-friendly adults, it creates and strengthens relationships that are important to normal development in children who may be distressed. Finally, the KC utilizes materials and resources that are readily improvised, the familiarity of which serves to normalize an otherwise stressful situation.

The assembly of a 'Kids' Corner'

After a disaster, in order to develop a KC that is appropriate for the specific needs of the affected community, certain information will be necessary. This include the types of losses, the number of children and families affected, and the degree of social disruption due to the disaster. A suitable space for assembling the KC also has to be identified. By involving adults from the affected community in the selection of the space, ownership of the project will be brought to the local community, and will encourage sustainability of the space after the relief workers are long gone. Finally, coordinating with other local and visiting relief groups serving the children, as well as gathering information about available community resources for children, will facilitate cooperation and care of the children needing treatment. Since a KC can serve as a transitional object for a child after a disaster, an open and inviting space that conveys warmth should be selected. The KC-NY, by virtue of its openness and visibility, attracted child visitors easily. In addition to an open general space for play activities, having an adjacent, quiet space where adults or adult–child dyads can talk or play more privately is helpful for special circumstances. The quiet space should be near enough so that parents and children can have visual contact with one another. The power of such an arrangement was best demonstrated in the historic nursery of Margaret Mahler, where toddlers could see their mothers socializing separately but near their play area and feel independent yet reassured by the parents' proximity (Mahler et al. 1975). In keeping with expected reactions among children after a disaster (AACAP 2004), this arrangement can also provide security and reassurance to clingy and apprehensive children, while allowing them to participate in the activities of a KC.

The number of occupants of a KC should be carefully considered. At the KC-NY, occasions where adult volunteers heavily outnumbered the children only resulted in intimidating and scaring off the children (Heath 2004; Chokroverty et al. 2002). The reverse is also counterproductive. Too many children in proportion to the adults can be disruptive and distract from the focus of activity in the KC.

> **Case example 1:** In one of the KC-SL, so many children arrived at the same time that it became overwhelming to the adult organizers. Some of the extra children were removed and entertained elsewhere, so that sufficient space and attention were made available for a limited number of adults and children to engage in meaningful play. (S. Koyfman, personal communication, 15 April 2005)

The expectations of the local community, and the expertise available, will in part determine the size and objectives of a KC. If a community is replete with volunteers who are child specialists, as was the case in New York City, more intimate child–adult ratios are possible, and the interactions have more therapeutic potential. If, however, there are very few child specialists in a community, play may need to be encouraged in groups or as structured recreational activities to achieve therapeutic goals. This will allow higher child–volunteer ratios. The specific types of activities will also dictate the appropriate ratios. Games, talking or play groups allow for many children to fewer adults – between four and twelve children to one or two adults. However, if close facilitation of the process of play is desired, one adult for one to three children is needed. This ratio is based on practical experiences from KC-NY, KC-SL, and office-based play therapy.

Volunteers arriving at the scene of a disaster are not always experienced therapists. The creation of a therapeutic play area calls for additional training in various aspects of child development, and basic principles of play therapy for adults supervising this area, whether they are professionals or lay volunteers. A lack of understanding of a child's need to re-enact traumatic experiences could result in interference with that child's resolution of the stressful event.

> **Case example 2:** A psychiatrist at the KC-NY saw a lay volunteer interacting with a child. The little boy was playing aggressively with toy planes and crashed them repeatedly into one another. The adult told the child, 'that's not the right way to play', and suggested a 'nicer way' to play. The child was clearly not given permission to express freely his aggressive impulses during that time and attempt to process them. (H. Kandler, personal communication, February 2002)

Training should be provided to adult volunteers and teachers in basic child mental health and development. In cultures with generational hierarchy where children are expected to respect and obey adult directions, adults may have difficulty with cooperative play. At the KC-SL, local volunteers needed to be taught how to play with children rather than observe them for maladaptive pathology (J. Kearney, personal communication, 17 April 2005). Sometimes normal situational reactions can be interpreted as reaction due to the effects of the disaster, leaving the adults (who themselves are often dealing with the effects of the disaster) feeling helpless.

> **Case example 3:** A little girl playing in one of the KC-SL suddenly began crying and wailing while the adults stood around not knowing what to do. When asked by a child psychiatrist volunteer why she was crying, the adults informed her that the child's mother had died in the tsunami. Everyone assumed that she was crying because of the loss of her mother, and felt helpless and unable to console her. 'But she was playing earlier, what happened now to make her cry?', insisted the doctor. This inquiry eventually revealed that the girl's father had arrived to pick her up and finding her engrossed in play, had left after telling one of the adults that he would return later. The girl, however, suddenly finding her father gone, assumed that he wasn't coming back, and was crying because she thought she was not going home. Once the clarification was made that her father would return for her, the little girl stopped crying immediately, and returned to playing. This experience heightened the awareness among the adults that a grieving child's behaviour was still subject to the same variations as any other child's, but also that her sensitivity to abandonment may be easily missed. (J. Kearney, personal communication, 17 April 2005)

In spite of cultural variations and shortage of specialized training, the KC need not be devised only by outside relief workers, who may be temporary guests in a disaster region. It could be assembled by adult members of the community, who remain long after the flood of rescue teams has subsided. The desire of inexperienced volunteers to help could still be harnessed into positive roles as loving adults in the KC. A space of this nature can be valuable even in the absence of trained experts as long as the adults supervising the children are aware of the basic 'rules' of play, and the importance of relationships between children and adults.

Once the KC is conceptualized in a community, how will the children and their caregivers know of its existence? There needs to be appropriate advertising in the community through announcements in the media, posters, fliers, word of mouth, and public address systems. A lesson was learned about advertising the KC-SL in one particular village: a lack of clarification about how many children could attend at any one time resulted in about 65 children arriving at once; this volume far exceeded the capacity of the space and number of adult volunteers, requiring the group to be further broken down and reorganized (J. Kearney, personal communication, 17 April 2005). In addition to advertising, child-friendly signs depicting children or symbols of childhood are helpful means of identifying the location, and attracting children and families into a KC. In the case of the KC-NY and later KC-SL, a New York City artist volunteered her skills to create large, colourful posters depicting culturally appropriate children, which invited the children into the KC. Other creative modifications will depend on the planners and volunteers, as well as the children. Drawings by visiting children may be used to further adorn the space, as was the case at the KC-NY and at some of the 'child centred areas' in Sri Lanka after the tsunamis (Chokroverty et al. 2002; C. Katz, personal communication, 10 February 2005). Such artwork serves to personalize the KC and provides returning children with a sense of identification with the space.

The contents of a KC are crucial in determining its therapeutic potential. Comfort, safety and 'child-friendliness' are important factors in choosing appropriate material. Children often play on the floor of a play area and hence, adults should provide the resources, and also be able and willing to sit at the same level. This would require items such as carpets, pillows and blankets, or in the case of very basic conditions, mats or sheets. Perhaps the most important contents for a KC are the toys and other play materials. After disasters, well-intended donations of toys and other goods often flow heavily to affected communities. Not every toy or play material offered will facilitate meaningful therapeutic play for children, but may actually further perpetuate avoidance of and constriction of play. At the KC-NY, attempts were made by some adults to introduce a television into the area; it was quickly removed because of its potential contribution to passivity and inhibition of children's play (Chokroverty et al. 2002; Heath 2004). In some instances, toy gifts may represent physical restitution for children who have lost everything else. At the KC-NY, initial draws to the area were related to the availability of 'give-away toys'. When the 'give-aways' were removed the space evolved into the 'novelty of an enriched play experience' (Chokroverty et al. 2002). In Sri Lanka after the tsunamis, donated novelty items were found unused because local children and adults did not understand what they were (C. Katz, personal communication, 10 February 2005). Special care is necessary in selecting toys that are culturally appropriate, and whenever possible, locally derived.

Simple creative material such as crayons/markers and paper enhance the potential for therapeutic play at a KC. Representational toys such as hand and finger puppets of families and animals, routine and emergency vehicles (police cars, fire engines, ambulances, planes, trains, trucks, cars), doctor's kits, soft plush toys and various indigenous animals (especially wild ones), dolls-houses and doll families of culturally relevant ethnic backgrounds also provide for creative and therapeutic play. Other materials that are appropriate include toy weapons, large and small building blocks, and amorphous objects such as clay, sand and water (Landreth 1993; Raynor 2002; Webb 1991; Carey 2004). In an economically impoverished community, the presence of any toys can be a novelty.

> **Case example 4:** At the KC-SL, the children asked for permission to take home the toys that were meant for communal use. The volunteer doctor explained that the toys were her tools, like her stethoscope, and needed to stay behind in the KC for future use. This answer was acceptable to the children and staff. (J. Kearney, personal communication, 17 April 2005)

Even in impoverished communities, if the literacy rate is high, educational material and handouts for parents and older children could also be included in the supply list. Psychoeducational literature describing children's reactions following disasters provides the community with accurate information, and may help adults interpret children's behaviour more appropriately (Vernberg 2002). The KC-NY carried within it abundant psychoeducational literature for families (Chokroverty et al. 2002). At the KC-SL, educational handouts on child development were used in training volunteers about playing. Finally, name badges for children and adults can be an icebreaker, and also make the experience more personal. Children and adults could be creative in designing their own name badges using locally available material.

With regard to the interactions within a KC, the underlying philosophy with children should be: 'Be there, pay attention!' In short, the goals are to provide immediate support for the children and their parents or caregivers, as well as education of children and families about emotional reactions after a disaster. In addition, care should be taken not to ignore the maladaptive patterns that may emerge later in the acute phase, and appropriate referrals to available specialists should be made. The process of the interventions that can occur within the KC is beyond the scope of this chapter. Suffice it to say that play with children after a disaster must still reflect the appropriate developmental patterns of the children. Children between the ages of two and nine years like to engage in fantasy play, often with toys. As children grow older, the amount of verbal interactions accompanying play increases. By late childhood and into adolescence, play takes on a more organized form, usually as games, which involve a much higher degree of verbal and social interaction (Webb 1991). The appeal of toys may be far less in the older groups. This point is made because organizers of play activities need to be mindful that very young and more mature children will not derive the same benefit if placed together with the same props, toys or games.

> **Case example 5:** Five boys between the ages of 7 and 11 years were gathered in a corner at KC-NY. They were discussing the latest episode of *Dragonball Z* a Japanese cartoon series on television. The following discussion occurred:
>
> Boy 1: 'Goku died by exploding himself!'
>
> Boy 2: 'Why did he die?'
>
> Boy 3 (the oldest of the group): 'One minute he was there, and the next minute he was gone!'
>
> Author NS who had been observing the children's play in the KC that afternoon overheard this and asked if she could join them. The children politely made room on the sofa for her.
>
> Boy 3: 'It was too sudden ... they shouldn't have let him die.'
>
> NS: 'Do you mean you weren't expecting him to die in this episode?'
>
> Boy 4: 'He went into outer space and blew himself up so that the people on earth were not hurt.'
>
> Boy 1: 'Yeah, that was good. Goku saved the people on earth by dying like that.'

The children spent a few more minutes talking about death by discussing Goku's death, and then moved on to talk about something else on TV. Through their discussion of the Goku story with an adult, the boys poignantly alluded to the real life events of the suicide bombers and the victims of the World Trade Center explosions, and attempted to reassure and explain for themselves, the terrible and confusing act of 11 September 2001.

When grouping children together by age, and selecting age appropriate materials and methods for the groups some thought must be given to the fact that trauma may interfere with the developmental process. In some instances, children regress to exhibit behaviours of an earlier developmental stage. Terr (1991: 10) observed in her work with trauma victims that 'traumatized youngsters appear to indulge in play at a much older age than do non-traumatized youngsters'. Permission for even older children to participate in play activities reserved for younger ones may be considered in certain cases. Careful observation of play with the developmental stages in mind will identify these children.

As noted earlier, unstructured play, games, structured activities, art, storytelling and theatre, are among the specific types of play that fit well into a KC. Practitioners in the field of trauma and mental health have made further recommendations about interventions other than play with which to provide assistance. Some of these, such as recognizing and reaching out to traumatized parents (Koplewicz et al. 2004), also has application in a KC.

The KC offers something for every type of child including those with special needs, such as those who are disabled or ill. However, children with pre-existing emotional or cognitive disorders may need more attention and supervision than the average child. Similarly, chronically ill, injured or physically disabled children can also benefit from visiting the KC but may need more individualized attention and sensitivity to the physical limitations that these children may possess. Infants and toddlers need to have their parents near them or have constant adult supervision in order to ensure safety and comfort. A separate area within a KC and age appropriate toy selection is recommended for such young children. Furthermore, children who have been traumatized in the past or have had other previous losses may have special needs, and their play should be observed more carefully for maladaptive patterns (Doyle and Stoop 1991).

Media and its influences

In the aftermath of disasters, media can play an important role by providing rapidly available information to the affected community and elsewhere. Njenga and his colleagues described the positive influence of the media in using radio programming for public education after the attack on the American embassy in Nairobi (Njenga et al. 2003). As previously mentioned, advertisement of a programme or service such as a KC is another positive way in which media can be used. Also, photographs and video clips can have a powerful role in mobilizing communities to respond to the disaster. This was evident after the attack on New York City as well as the Asian tsunamis where the visual images on electronic and print media influenced response in the form of donations and volunteers. As noted elsewhere, psychological recovery among families can be mitigated by public educational documents, available from professional groups through the internet, and for use by individuals as well as the print and visual media (DPO 2005; AACAP 2004; RCP 2004). These documents can be printed and made available for affected individuals and families, or for professionals and paramedics to use in their work with affected groups. In many instances, such documents are already translated, or lend themselves to translation into local languages. Meanwhile, media can also have a distressing impact on viewers and listeners, as in the case of repeated emblazoned images of the Twin Towers after the New York City attack, or the devastation from tsunami waves sweeping away the Asian coastline. These images have far-reaching effects in traumatizing unaffected individuals, especially children. For this reason, after the 11 September 2001 attacks in the US, at the request of mental health professionals the media refrained from repeatedly showing these horrific images.

Limitations of the 'Kids' Corner'

While a KC is most suited for a displacement camp, shelter or recreation centre, it is not the only place to normalize and support children after a disaster. It is but one component of a larger ecologic system of interventions after a disaster (Laor et al. 2003). Since children spend a large part of their day in school, and because more children can be reached through school activities, the school has been suggested as an effective rehabilitation place for traumatized children (Koplewicz et al. 2004). Guidelines for intervention in schools, as another 'natural environment' following disaster, have been described in various places (Galante and Foa 1986; Klingman 1988; Chemtob et al. 2002; Saltzman et al. 2003; Goenjian et al. 1997; Pynoos and Nader 1990). Teachers and support staff at school can be trained in the facilitation of play. A school-based KC has the disadvantage of absent adult family members, while having the advantage that the teachers already know their students well, and could serve as adult references for the children. A KC can be dynamic only if the adults and facilitators have an understanding and appreciation of play. In the absence of proper guidance, the true potential of a KC cannot be harnessed.

> **Case example 6:** In one setting in Sri Lanka, parents and other adults (other than local volunteers) could not be engaged to join in interactions with the children. This resulted in a circle of adult observers surrounding the children. It was however remedied by creative minded trainers who invited everyone to engage in a game of 'falling' and 'catching' each other. The reluctant adults were coaxed into joining which then led to more energetic participation in other kinds of play. (J. Kearney, personal communication, 17 April 2005)

In order for a KC to operate successfully, training of volunteers and demonstrations in play techniques are essential. An additional challenge for non-local volunteers and relief workers is the language/culture gap that exists between visiting practitioners and relief workers and the disaster-afflicted communities. Experienced translators are much needed under these circumstances, and play a crucial role in accurately communicating the essence of the techniques needed. In communities with a scarcity of trained child therapists, the sustainability of a KC will be a challenge (although not impossible), when the 'outside experts' have left the disaster scene. Another major limitation of the KC is the need for continuous staffing and consistency in caretakers. With time, the flood of volunteers at a disaster runs dry, and those who remain could suffer stress and burnout (Creamer and Liddle 1990). Financial support can help address this problem by employing staff to offset the shortage left by transient volunteers.

From a clinical standpoint, the 'Kids' Corner' is an essential component in the stabilization and recovery of children after a disaster. However, like other post-disaster interventions, further evidence is required to reach the conclusion that this model is indeed a suitable post-disaster strategy in helping children. The notion of research is often received poorly in a disaster context, and more so when the research involves children. In the chaotic aftermath of a disaster, this problem is compounded by potential privacy violations and limited guarantees of confidentiality. Equally significant is the lack of quality assurance in relief efforts. No standards are known for the plethora of 'pychosocial trainings' that are now available for interested local volunteers following the Asian tsunamis. These trainings vary from one to two hour lectures to extensive training courses over several months including field supervision. Those providing such training are varied in their professional experiences. Furthermore, individuals receiving brief training in the aftermath of disasters cannot be considered experts in assisting affected individuals. Rather, their limited knowledge can lead to more harm than good, as is the case when an inexperienced therapist encourages excessive expression in a traumatized child and then is unable to cope with the emotional flooding that occurs as a result of such encouragement. They will need ongoing supervision by experts in child mental health. 'Child-centred areas' have now become clichés in disaster relief work (CCF 2005; Save the Children 2005). How these translate into the arena of post-disaster care for children is highly variable in nature, and usually dictated by the political climate of the relief effort as well as the interests of the affected communities. It was observed by the authors' colleagues in Sri Lanka, that some 'child-centred areas' for tsunami survivors had been created, but that these areas only hosted a few hours of structured purely recreational activities, lacking the dimensions of the KC concept (C. Katz, personal communication, 10 February 2005). Currently, no standards exist on what a 'child-centred area' should be or how it should be organized. The KC is an attempt to address this dilemma, at least in part.

Summary and concluding remarks

When disaster strikes at a community, the primary needs of the individuals and families are first and foremost a priority. If the adults are in obvious psychological distress they receive outside assistance. In the case of children, their parents and caregivers who themselves have been affected by the event are left to deal with their children's needs. Because most cultures are not comfortable discussing stressful events and grief with children, many distressed children often go unattended or unnoticed. The KC was first created by child mental health specialists who responded to the attacks on New York City, and later developed into a model for future applications. The authors of this chapter believe that its structure allows for easy replication with modifications to suit the post-disaster environment irrespective of cultural and economic variations. If conducted appropriately, it provides excellent support for children as well as adults in a caring, consistent and nurturing manner. By initiating the assembly of a KC in the acute phase of a disaster, future psychopathology may be avoided. In addition, it can act as a springboard for other preventive programmes for children. The

KC is a clinically sound idea, deriving from basic childhood needs and adults' response to these needs; it has been well received in the environments where disaster occurred. However, it is not yet a validated model, and further research using evidence-based and programme evaluation methods is needed to determine its effectiveness and wide application in disaster regions.

Note

The authors of this chapter are indebted to the DPO Child Mental Health Committee as well as DPO's other volunteers and collaborators, whose hard work allowed the concept of the Kids' Corner to evolve and be realized.

References

American Academy of Child and Adolescent Psychiatry (AACAP) Facts for Families Series. (2004) *Helping Children After a Disaster*, No.36 (Educational Handout). Online. Available at http://www.aacap.org/publications/factsfacm/disaster/htm (1 March 2005).

American Psychiatric Association (APA) (1994) *Diagnostic and Statistical Manual of Mental Disorders*, 4th edn. Washington DC: American Psychiatric Association.

Bisson, J. I., Roberts, N. and Macho, G. (2003) 'Service innovations: Cardiff traumatic stress initiative'. *Psychiatric Bulletin*, 27: 145–7.

Bonanno, G. (2004) 'Loss, trauma, and human resilience: have we underestimated the human capacity to thrive after extremely aversive events?' *American Psychologist*, 59(1): 20–8.

Brooks, R. and Goldstein, S. (2003) *The Power of Resilience: Achieving Balance, Confidence, and Personal Strength in Your Life*. New York: McGraw-Hill.

Carey, L. (2004) 'Sandplay art, and play therapy to promote anxiety reduction'. In N. Boyd Webb (ed.), *Mass Trauma and Violence: Helping Families and Children Cope*. New York: Guilford Press, pp. 216–33.

Chatterjee, P. (2005) 'Mental health care for India's tsunami survivors'. *The Lancet*, 365(9462): 833–4.

Chemtob, C. M., Nakashima, J. P. and Hamada, R. S. (2002) 'Psychosocial intervention for postdisaster trauma symptoms in elementary school children'. *Archives of Pediatric and Adolescent Medicine*, 156: 211–16.

Chokroverty, L., Heath, D. and Harwitz, D. (2002) 'The kids' corner: a safe haven for children and adults amidst disaster'. *Emergency Psychiatry*, 8(2): 49–54.

Christian Children's Fund (CCF) Australia website (2005) *India's Child Centered Spaces*. Online. Available at http://www.ccfa.org.au/ccrf/appeal/tsunami/ccf-in-action/india.cfm (23 April 2005).

Civil Contingencies Secretariat (2004) *UK Resilience: Dealing with Disaster*. Revised 3rd edn. Online. Available at http://www.ukresilience.info/contingencies/dwd/c4acare.htm (19 April, 2005).

Cohen, J. A., Bernet, W. B., Dunne, J. E., Adair, M., Arnold, V., Benson, R. S., Bukstein, O., Kinlan, J., Mcclellan, J. and Rue, D. (1998) 'Practice parameters for the assessment and treatment of children and adolescents with post-traumatic stress disorder'. *Journal of the American Academy of Child and Adolescent Psychiatry*, 38(Supplement): 1–51.

Convention on the Rights of the Child, Article 31 part 1. (1989) Online. Available at http://www.unhchr.ch/html/menu3/b/k2crc.htm (21 April 2005).

Creamer, T. L. and Liddle, B. J. (1990) 'Secondary traumatic stress among disaster mental health workers responding to the September 11th attacks'. *Journal of Traumatic Stress*, 18(1): 89–96.

Disaster Psychiatry Outreach (2005) Online. Available at www.disasterpsych.org (1 March 2005).

Dodds Joyner, C. and Cupit Swenson, C. (1993) 'Community-level intervention after a disaster'. In C. F. Saylor (ed.), *Children and Disasters*. New York: Plenum Press.

Doyle, J. S. and Stoop, D. (1991) 'Witness and victim of multiple abuses, collaborative treatment of 10-year old Randy in a residential treatment center'. In N. Boyd Webb (ed.), *Play Therapy with Children in Crisis: a Casebook for Practitioners*. New York: Guilford Press, pp. 111–40.

Earls, F., Smith, E., Reich, W. and Jung, K. G. (1988) 'Investigating psychopathological consequences of a disaster in children: a pilot study incorporating a structure diagnostic interview'. *Journal of the American Academy of Child and Adolescent Psychiatry*, 27: 90–5.

Finkel, N. J. and Jacobsen, C. A. (1977) 'Significant life experiences in an adult sample'. *American Journal of Community Psychology*, 5(2): 165–75.

Freud, A. and Burlingham, D. (1943) *War and Children*. New York: Medical War Books.

Galante, R. and Foa, D. (1986) 'An epidemiological study of psychic trauma and treatment effectiveness for children after a natural disaster'. *Journal of the American Academy of Child and Adolescent Psychiatry*, 25: 357–63.

Goenjian, A. K., Karayan, I., Pynoos, R. S., Minassian, D., Najarian, L. M., Steinberg, A. M. and Fairbanks, L. A. (1997) 'Outcome of psychotherapy among early adolescents after trauma'. *American Journal of Psychiatry*, 154(4): 536–42.

Hartley, H. E., Frank, L. K. and Goldenson, R. M. (1952) *Understanding Children's Play*. New York: Columbia University Press.

Heath, D. (2004) 'The World Trade Center Disaster and the Setting up of Kids' Corner'. In A. A. Pandya and C. L. Katz (eds), *Disaster Psychiatry: Intervening When Nightmares Come True*. Hillsdale, NJ: Analytic Press, pp. 203–10.

Hoffmann, J. and Rogers, P. (1991) 'Crisis play group in a shelter following the Santa Cruz earthquake. In N. Boyd Webb (ed.), *Play Therapy with Children in Crisis: a Casebook for Practitioners*. New York: Guilford Press, pp. 379–95.

Horowitz, M. J. (1986) 'Stress-response syndromes: a review of posttraumatic and adjustment disorders'. *Hospital and Community Psychiatry*, 37(3): 241–9.

Hoven, C. W., Duarte, C. S., Lucas, C. P., Mandell, D. J., Cohen, M.; Rosen, C., Wu, P., Musa, G. J. and Gregorian, N. (2002) *Effects of the World Trade Center Attack on NYC Public School Students – Initial Report to the New York City Board of Education*. New York: Columbia University Mailman School of Public Health – New York State Psychiatric Institute Applied Research and Consulting, LLC.

Kao, S. C. (2005) 'Play therapy with Asian children'. In E. Gil and A. A. Drewes (eds), *Cultural Issues in Play Therapy*. New York: Guilford Press, pp. 180–93.

Klingman, A. (1988) 'School community in disaster: planning for intervention'. *Journal of Community Psychology*, 16: 205–16.

Koplewicz, H. S., Cloitre, M., Reyes, K. and Kessler, L. S. (2004) 'The 9/11 experience: who's listening to the children?' *Psychiatric Clinics of North America*, 27(3): 491–504.

Lacey, G. (1972) 'Observations on Aberfan'. *Journal of Psychosomatic Research*, 16: 257–60.

La Greca, A. M. and Prinstein, M. J. (2002) 'Natural disasters: hurricanes and earthquakes'. In A. M. La Greca, W.K. Silverman, E. M. Vernberg and M. C. Roberts (eds), *Helping Children Cope with Disasters and Terrorism*. The American Psychological Association, pp. 107–38.

Landreth, G. L. (1993) 'Self-expressive communication'. In C. E. Schaefer (ed.), *The Therapeutic Powers of Play*. Northvale, New Jersey: Jason Aronson Inc., pp. 41–63.

Laor, N., Wolmer, L., Spirman, S. and Wiener, Z. (2003) 'Facing war, terrorism, and disaster: toward a child-oriented comprehensive emergency care system'. *Child and Adolescent Psychiatric Clinics of North America*, 12(2): 343–61.

Lindy, J. D., Grace, M. C. and Green, B. L. (1981) 'Survivors: outreach to a reluctant population'. *American Journal of Orthopsychiatry*, 51: 468–78.

Lonigan, C. J., Shannon, M. P., Taylor, C. M., Finch, jr., A. J. and Sallee, F. R. (1994) 'Children exposed to disaster II: risk factors for the development of post-traumatic symptomatology'. *Journal of the American Academy of Child and Adolescent Psychiatry*, 33: 94–105.

Mahler, M. S., Pine, F. and Bergman, A. (1975) *The Psychological Birth of the Human Infant: Symbiosis and Individuation*. Margaret S. Mahler, Basic Books 2000 Edition, Perseus Books Group.

Marsella, A. J. and Christopher, M. A. (2004) 'Ethno cultural considerations in disasters: an overview of research, issues, and directions'. *Psychiatric Clinics of North America*, 27: 521–39.

Masten, A. S. (2001) 'Ordinary magic resilience processes in development'. *American Psychologist*, 56(3): 227–38.

McFarlane, A. C. (1987) 'Posttraumatic phenomena in a longitudinal study of children following a natural disaster'. *Journal of the American Academy of Child and Adolescent Psychiatry*, 26: 764–9.

McNally, R. J. (1993) 'Stressors that produce post traumatic stress disorder in children'. In J. R. T. Davidson and E. B. Foa (eds), *Posttraumatric Stress Disorder: DSM-IV and Beyond*. Washington DC: American Psychiatric Association. pp. 57–74.

Morgan, L., Scourfield, J., Williams, D., Jasper, A. and Lewis, G. (2003) 'The Aberfan disaster: 33-year follow-up of survivors'. *British Journal of Psychiatry*, 182: 532–6.

Murthy, R. S. and Mander, H. (2002) *RIOTS: Psychosocial Care for Children*. Bangalore, India: Books for Change.

Myers, D. (1994) *Disaster Response and Recovery: a Handbook for Mental Health Professionals*. US Department of Health and Human Services, Public Health Service, Substance Abuse and Mental Health Services Administration, Center for Mental Health Services.

Newman, C. F. (1976) 'Children of disaster: clinical observations at Buffalo Creek'. *American Journal of Psychiatry*, 133: 312–16.

Njenga, F. G., Nyamai, C. and Kigamwa, P. (2003) 'Terrorist bombing at the US embassy in Nairobi: the media response'. *East African Medical Journal*, 80(3): 159–64.

North, C. S. (2004) 'Approaching disaster mental health research after the 9/11 World Trade Center terrorist attacks'. *Psychiatric Clinics of North America*, 27(3): 589–602.

Pfefferbaum, B., Nixon, S. J., Tucker, P. M., Tivis, R. D., Moore, V. L., Gurwitch, R. H., Pynoos, R. L. and Geis, H. K. (1999) 'Posttraumatic stress responses in bereaved children after the Oklahoma City bombing'. *Journal of the American Academy of Child and Adolescent Psychiatry*, 38(11): 1372–9.

Pynoos, R. S. and Nader, K. (1988) 'Psychological first aid and treatment approach to children exposed to community violence: research implications'. *Journal of Traumatic Stress*, 1(4): 445–73.

Pynoos, R. S. and Nader, K. (1990) 'Prevention of psychiatric morbidity in children after disaster'. In S. E. Goldstein, J. Yager, C. Heinicke and R. S. Pynoos (eds), *Preventing Mental Health Disturbances in Childhood*. Washington DC: American Psychiatric Association, pp. 226–71.

Pynoos, R. S., Frederick, C., Nader, K., Arroyo, W., Steinberg, A., Eth, S., Nunez, F. and Fairbanks, L. (1987) 'Life threat and posttraumatic stress disorder in school-age children'. *Archives of General Psychiatry*, 44(12): 1057–63.

Raynor, C. M. (2002) 'The role of play in the recovery process'. In W. Zubenko and J Capozzoli (eds), *Children and Disasters*. New York: Oxford University Press, pp. 124–34.

Royal College of Psychiatrists (RCP) (2004) *Traumatic Stress in Children – Mental Health and Growing Up*, 3rd edn, Factsheet 20, for parents and teachers. Online. Available at http://www.rcpsych.ac.uk/info/mhgu/newmhgu20.htm (10 April 2005).

Saltzman, W. R., Layne, C. M., Steinberg, A. M., Arslanagic, B. and Pynoos, R. S. (2003) 'Developing a culturally and ecologically sound intervention program for youth exposed to war and terrorism'. *Child and Adolescent Psychiatric Clinics of North America*, 12(2): 319–42.

Satel, S. (2005) 'Bread and shelter, yes. Psychiatrists, no'. *New York Times*, Section F, p. 5, 29 March.

Save the Children website (2005) *Indian Ocean Tsunami*. Online. Available at http://www.savethechildren.net/alliance/what_we_do/indian_ocean/emer_ne ws.html (23 April 2005).

Schaefer, C. E. (1993) 'What is play and why is it therapeutic?' In C. E. Schaefer (ed.), *The Therapeutic Powers of Play*. Northvale, New Jersey: Jason Aronson Inc.

Shen, Y. J. (2002) 'Short-term group play therapy with Chinese earthquake victims: effects on anxiety, depression, and adjustment'. *International Journal of Play Therapy*, 11(1): 43–63.

Solomon, S. D. (1999) 'Interventions for acute trauma response'. *Current Opinions in Psychiatry*, 12(2): 175–80.

Solomon, D. S. and Green, B. L. (1992) 'Mental health effects of natural and human-made disasters'. *PTSD Research Quarterly*, 3(1): 1–8.

Speier, A. H. (2000) *Psychosocial Issues for Children and Families in Disasters*, 2nd edn. DHHS Publication No. ADM 86-1070R. United States Department of

Health and Human Services, Public Health Service, Substance Abuse and Mental Health Services Administration, Center for Mental Health.

Stuber, J., Fairbrother, G., Galea, S., Pfefferbaum, B., Wilson-Genderson, M. and Vlahov, D. (2002) 'Determinants of counseling for children in Manhattan after the September 11 attack'. *Psychiatric Services*, 53(7): 815–22.

Summerfield, D. (1999) 'A critique of seven assumptions behind psychological trauma programmes in war-affected areas'. *Social Science and Medicine*, 48: 1449–62.

Taxman, J. (2004) 'An analyst's experience at ground zero'. In B. Sklarew, S. W. Twemlow and S. M. Wilkinson (eds), *Analysts in the Trenches: Streets, Schools, War Zones*. Hillsdale, NJ: Analytic Press, Inc.

Tedeschi, R., Park, C. and Calhoun, L. (1998) *Post-traumatic Growth: Positive Changes in the Aftermath of Crisis*. Mahway, NJ: Lawrence Erlbaum Associates.

Terr, L. (1991) 'Childhood traumas: an outline and overview'. *American Journal of Psychiatry*, 148: 10–20.

United Nations (UN) (1990) *Convention on the Rights of the Child and Youth: Universal Declaration of Human Rights, Part I; Article 31*. 1990. Online. Available at http://www.unicef.org/crc/crc.htm (1 August 2005).

United States (2004) Robert T. Stafford Disaster Relief and Emergency Assistance Act, as amended by Public Law 106–390, October 30, 2000, § 416, 'Crisis Counseling Assistance and Training', United States Code Title 42, § 5183. Washington, DC. (Laws). Online. Available at http://www.fema.gov/library/stafact.shtm#sec416 18 April 2005.

Vernberg, E. M. (2002) 'Intervention approaches following disasters'. In A. M. LaGreca, W. K. Silverman, E. M. Vernberg and M. C Roberts (eds), *Helping Children Cope with Disasters and Terrorism*. Washington DC: American Psychological Association, pp. 55–72.

Vernberg, E. M. and VogeL, J. M. (1993) 'Interventions with children after disasters'. *Journal of Clinical Child Psychology*, 22: 485–98.

Vogel, J. M. and Vernberg, E. M. (1993) 'Children's psychological responses to disaster'. *Journal of Clinical Child Psychology*, 22: 464–84.

Weaver, J. D. (2002) 'Disaster mental health – trauma relief, concepts and theory'. In W. Zubenko and J. Capozzoli (eds), *Children and Disasters*. New York: Oxford University Press, pp. 34–71.

Webb, Boyd N. (1991) 'Play therapy crisis intervention with children'. In N. Boyd Webb (ed.), *Play Therapy with Children in Crisis: a Casebook for Practitioners*. New York: Guilford Press, pp. 26–42.

Winnicott, D. W. (1953) 'Transitional objects and transitional phenomena: a study of the first not-me possession'. *International Journal of Psycho-Analysis*, 34: 89–97.

World Health Organization (WHO) (1992) *Psychosocial Consequences of Disasters: Prevention and Management*. Geneva, Switzerland: World Health Organization.

Yule, W. (1992a) 'Post-traumatic stress disorder in child survivors of shipping disasters: the sinking of the "Jupiter"'. *Psychotherapy and Psychosomatics*, 57: 200–5.

Yule, W. (1992b) 'Resilience and vulnerability in child survivors of disasters'. In B. Tizard and V. Varma (eds), *Vulnerability and Resilience: a Festschrift for Ann and Alan Clarke*. London: Jessica Kingsley, pp. 182–98.

4

The Outcomes of Group Work with Traumatized Children and their Families in the Southern Serbia and Kosovo Region

Natasa Ljubomirovic and Kedar Dwivedi

Introduction

The war in the Balkan region – which began in 1992 – inflicted a heavy suffering among the local population and displaced as many as 250 000 persons from their homes. Yet, over 600 000 have applied for refugee status and become exiled elsewhere in the neighbouring states. The conflict in that region and its aftermath have also exposed a large number of children and adolescents to immensely traumatic experiences and consequently to the vulnerability to mental disorders such as anxiety (Dwivedi and Varma 1997a), depression (Dwivedi and Varma 1997b) and other Post-Traumatic Stress Disorders (PTSD) (Dwivedi 2000).

Traumatic experiences in the context of war have been associated with a high risk of psychopathology (Bell et al. 2002; Cantor et al. 1993). These include experiences such as prolonged exposure to traumatic events, witnessing deaths, atrocity, torture, experience of severe injury, rape, captivity and losses. In addition to war trauma, conflicts also impose on individuals and civilians situational constraints including lack of medical supplies, inadequate immunization, food rationing, poor community support, overcrowding, inadequate hygiene and poor sanitation etc.

For many refugees post war may also associate with risk and vulnerability of being in a new and dissimilar host culture surroundings, isolation, unemployment, poverty, and institutionalized prejudice in the host culture. However, exposure to prolonged and multiple traumatic events – as emphasized above – leads to a high incidence of psychological and psychiatric disorders, including depression, anxiety and PTSD as well as low self-esteem and social dysfunction among refugees and similar exiled population (Hosin 2001). (See also Chapter 13.)

Exiled refugees are different from their counterpart group: internally displaced persons (IDP). Refugees often leave their native homeland for another country due to war, violence or disaster that either directly or indirectly threatens the safety of the individual, family or their community. IDP may leave their homes for the same reasons, but move to other locations within their own countries. However, displacement as accumulated losses presents a somewhat powerful risk factor for PTSD symptoms. For example, in a sample of Afghan and Cambodian refugees who live in the USA, PTSD symptoms were reported in 80 per cent of the individuals included in these studies (Blair 2000). Accumulated traumas and stressors during adaptation in the host culture could also contribute to increase vulnerability. Meanwhile, availability of resources and social support are very significant factors in coping with PTSD symptoms (Blair 2000; Cheung 1994). Reviewing other data relevant to the displacement of Bosnian refugees in Austria, Kucera and Lueger-Schuster (2000), for example, suggested that 63.6 per cent of their sample had mental health problems after the displacement, while another sizeable majority (76.4 per cent) declared having stressful lives in the host culture.

Oppedal et al. (2005: 646) went further to add that mental health is often affected by societal and individual factors. Such factors include the characteristics of the host culture (societies of settlement) compared to the societies of origin, the degree to which an individual travels (uprooted and forced to become a refugee), as well level of exposure to violence and/or threatening events. Ward (2001) found these factors important and to affect adjustment and well-being after resettlement in the host countries. It is also believed that the greater the culture distance between the host (receiving countries) and the original culture, the more challenging the adaptation process. Furthermore, in the host culture, attitudes and behaviour towards refugees, immigration policies and other political matters are among other risk factors that may influence psychological well-being and participation in the society of resettlement.

Focusing on long-term exposure to traumatic events, Djapic and Stuvland (2002), Jankovic (2002) and Ljubomirovic (1999) found that 78 per cent of the Bosnian children witnessed at least six traumatic experiences during the war. Most of these children and adolescents were confronted with bombings, shootings, cruelties to other people and experiences of losses, and some also had physical injuries and separation from family members. Other research (Karacic and Zvizdic 2002; Osmanovic and Zvizdic 2002) suggested that children who fled from Sarajevo seemed to have had fewer traumatic experiences than those who stayed. Further, Savic (2002) conducted work in the Republic of Srpska and found that all adolescents who were included in the survey had experienced war trauma, with adolescents in the collective centres having had the worst experience of all. Similarly, Ljubomirovic's (2002) study – which was conducted in the south of Serbia – seems to confirm these findings and indicates that children who were in collective centres had more traumatic events that those children who stayed in private accommodation. Milosavljevic and Turjacanin (2002) further support these findings and claim that two-thirds of adolescents in the Republic of Srpska reported witnessing seven or more war events.

On the overwhelming experience of many refugees, Jones (1998) describes the primary psychological experience as one of loss and uprooting, i.e. losses of family, home, school, town, friends or relatives together with other stressful war conditions including being in a refugee camp and being exposed to the shock of dissimilar culture. The individual experiences may also include the collective losses of the whole country, its community's culture and language etc. The term 'cultural bereavement' (Eisenbruch 1990) has been used to describe such losses, as these not only resonate with individual losses but also amplify them and limit the space in which individual grief may be expressed. If people do not readily express their grief, it is not because of denial and numbing but an appropriate restraint in the place of collective grief (Jones 1998). Children and adolescents seem to react quite differently to war events. Some of their reactions are associated with age, gender, emotional and cognitive development as well as level of proximity and whether they suffered physical injures or not (Gavranidou 2002). Moreover, it is also known that children and adolescents react to war stressors with different kinds of behavioural idiosyncrasies, disorders and psychological problems and do not respond to war trauma only with symptoms of PTSD (Jensen and Shaw 1993; Boardman 1994; Milgram 1982 Adjukovic and Adjukovic 1998).

Recent work by Lengua et al. (2005), who studied children's posttraumatic stress reactions following the 11 September 2001 terrorist attacks on the World Trade Center in New York City and the Pentagon in Washington and the main predictors of PTS among children, found a large majority of children included in their study – who were from Seattle, Washington – manifested worries and PTS symptoms in the week following the attacks. In fact, rates of worries, anxiety, upset, specific fears and PTS symptoms were similar to those found in studies that involved children directly exposed to and/or experiencing a disaster (e.g. Vogel and Vernberg 1993). Most children included in Lengua's study were found to have worries about the safety of friends, family and their own safety and future terrorist attacks occurring closer to home. Lengua et al. (2005) therefore suggested that communities should attend to children's mental health needs where there is a national or regional disaster, and that children who are geographically remote from the disaster nonetheless may be affected by it too. They also noted increases in symptomatology among children who were identified as high risk (previously manifested symptomatology) or special need persons who are more likely to develop problems following a trauma or disaster. The main findings of this particular study seem to confirm earlier results reported by several studies (e.g. Terr et al. 1999; Pfefferbaum et al. 2000; Pfefferbaum et al. 2001) that major traumatic or overwhelming events which affect entire communities do not need to be experienced directly to result in post-traumatic symptoms. Indeed, individual perception, fears, level of destruction, deaths and/or damage that can follow such events may be more important determinants of post-trauma reactions than direct exposure itself (La Greca et al. 1996). Some other studies (Schuster et al. 2001; Smith et al. 2001) added that exposure through television and media can lead to stress symptoms as some children may personalize the event. There is also evidence that distressed parents report greater symptomatology among their offspring following traumatic events. For further detail of risk factors and manifestation of post-traumatic stress symptoms among children following life-threatening events, including indirect exposure to a catastrophic event, see Lengua et al. (2005) and Resick (2001).

The development of resilience, support and rehabilitation

It becomes imperative for professionals working with traumatized children to consider the factors that strengthen individuals' inner resources and perhaps parenting functions (Dwivedi and Varma 1997a; see also Sephen Joseph and collegues, Chapter 8 of this book). This is to prevent deterioration and/or manifestation of further disorders from arising (Dwivedi and Harper 2004). Husain (2001: 9) who worked with traumatized children in Bosnia suggested that 'there is always hope and resiliency in the children and they do respond to both small and large efforts put to them by parents, teachers and humanitarian workers, and even in the most dire circumstances, there is so much that can be done to help.'

Dwivedi (2002), Kleinman (1988) and Lopez and Guarnaccia (2000) have noted and reminded professionals working in this area that cultural variations are often evident in the way people present their problems. That is to say, cross-cultural variations in the manifestation and meaning of mental disorders or psychiatric morbidity could be attributed to health beliefs, common practices and the possibilities of resilience among ethnic groups. Hence, somatization or somatic complaints have different meanings depending on a specific culture. In the developed world, a headache might be a manifestation of stress. But in Asia and other parts of the world parents still stigmatize mental illness and will usually avoid bringing a child to a psychiatrist due to the fear of stigma and blame of parenting practices (Hinshaw 2005). Awareness of the variation in meaning according to culture (see Chapter 5) is critical in understanding problems and developing effective interventions for survivors, refugees and other internally displaced people.

Many people in the Balkans were forced to start a new life. Indeed, the enormous upheaval in the former Yugoslavia – as indicated above – made people become either refugees or internally displaced persons elsewhere or in their own country. Being a refugee means a loss of friends, family members, property, neighbours, jobs and hope. Some feel that they are stigmatized with the new label as a 'refugee', with poor quality of life. It is also far more difficult when the individual is elderly and becomes a refugee. Some have no time to start a new life in humid, dirty, crowded conditions. Such places are so different from their homes in Kosovo or Croatia. Recollections of what happened in their homeland are told as stories to their children and grandchildren, who are fascinated by them (Dwivedi 1997b). Through these stories elderly people describe their memories in an extremely vivid manner and evoke images of their previous lives – the sea, coast lines, houses and so on.

However, the war in the Balkans broke out when different parts of the country wanted to show their strength and nationalism, or rather when national identity was an overriding factor and main seed of that particular conflict. Indeed, the real victims were innocent civilians, mainly children and women.

Besides displacement from their homes many children become 'unaccompanied' children, i.e. arriving to the host culture alone without their parents. The majority of this particular group have been exposed to death threats, violence, poverty, dead bodies, burnt houses and so on. They are no longer the members of the same family, neither pupils of the same school, nor inhabitants of the old, well-known neighbourhood. They find themselves wholly alone. They wear clothes which they didn't choose. They are exhausted by dramatic journeys and changes of living places. One child summarized this experience by

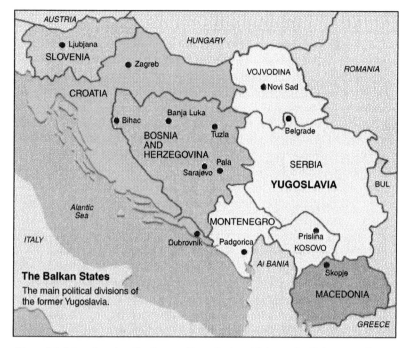

Figure 4.1: Map showing the former Yugoslavia with its main disintegrated parts including southern Serbia

noting: 'Belgrade is so ugly today that the sun doesn't shine as brightly as at my home.' Another 14-year-old refugee girl who was hosted in a boarding school in Belgrade wrote: 'I feel some strange restlessness. I know my worries; this one I cannot recognize. I suppose there is life worth living somewhere on this planet.'

A 15-year-old refugee boy, on the other hand, experienced at the beginning of war an immense fear while seeing corpses at the main town square which shocked him at a very deep level. He felt the murders as a part of his own self. The fear has not been worked through. It is kept alive by pictures of remembrance, but suppressed by the actual needs of living. These events and experiences contribute to the increased level of anxiety among children. The emotional reactions of their family members are also important as these have strong influence on children's behaviour. Some children's reactions – particularly those who were placed in collective centres – included clinging behaviour, fear of separation and sleeping problems as well as aggressive play.

Rehabilitation programmes and assistance offered to traumatized children of the conflict in southern Serbia

Several agencies were involved in helping traumatized communities in southern Serbia (see Figure 4.1). This chapter is mainly based on a project sponsored by Médecins Sans Frontières. Thus, an attempt was made to work through children's traumatic experience, and to help them build their inner resources to prevent disorders from arising. There were a large number of children with behaviour problems and mixed disorders of conduct and emotions. Some children had learning disabilities or other developmental disorders; hence most had not received any good quality care. They had had no ongoing professional treatment and there were no provisions to recognize their mental health needs or to develop a thera-peutic relationship with professionals. Eventually, children who were identified with mental health needs (during our visits) were offered treat-ment with the help of the mobile teams consisting of special therapists, psychologists and a psychiatrist or were referred to the state services. Psychosocial field visits were regularly conducted and children partici-pated in therapeutic groups managed by the teams with the main aims of highlighting children's difficulties and helping in the prevention of more severe psychiatric disorders. Various interventions were applied, includ-ing offering children appropriate schooling, psychological screening, individual therapy, group therapy, and therapeutic work with parents. However, the screening and assessment of children which lasted over three months revealed the following:

1. Families in the collective centres need to be offered psychosocial support and basic help during the visit.
2. Members of families need support through different group activities.

Depending on their needs, the IDP families which were hosted in the collective centres were divided into three categories:

- Red (severely vulnerable group)
- Orange (moderately vulnerable group)
- Yellow (mildly vulnerable group)

These categories were created using the parameters of (a) the traumatic experience of the families and (b) the inner resources and resilience each family has including their independent functions, network, cre-ativity, humour, initiatives, and positive approach to various aspects of life. The aim of each planned visit was to help many traumatized victims of war to deal with their present needs and to follow a planned therapeutic strategy related to such mental health needs detected during screening. Through active listening many families were encouraged to share their concerns and express their emotions. Thus, the process of psychological support and rehabilitation consisted of four main steps:

1. Assessment of mental health needs.
2. Debriefing.
3. Therapeutic strategy planning.
4. Intervention of both psychiatric and psychological programmes.

Group work activities and the underpinning theoretical perspective

Group work with children and adolescents can be of immense benefit, and should focus on the collective experiences of the survivors. It should be used to provide a space for the ventilation of feelings and exploration of identity, and to enhance problem solving and particularly the rebuilding of social ties (Dwivedi 1993; Jones 1998; Dwivedi and Harper 2004). However, the traditional approaches to group therapy may need to be adapted so that, for example, there is some flexibility about boundaries. It has also been pointed out that individuals may gain more from the repair of their social worlds than counselling for intrusive memories. That is to say, merely treating the symptoms of PTSD may be counterproductive as it can further alienate the person from a community in collective grief (Eisenbruch 1991; Summerfield 1996).

The surviving victims of war were from Kosovo villages; many owned large areas of land and big houses and had high social status. Post-war conditions left them alive but in unacceptable conditions; many were lacking self-confidence. Children meanwhile were neglected and their families had become passive, isolated, and kept in collective centres without any hope. However, some had good inner resources and great creative skills. It was therefore thought that implementation of group work as an activity would be very useful for children and their families. The idea was to help them to normalize their lives and show that they are similar to others. It was also important to understand their difficulties while being accommodated in these collective centres. The aims were therefore to help them to discover their inner resources, strengthen their well-being and to combat their emotional and psychological problems.

Preparations for group work were made with the help of a series of consultations. Before each group session a plan for the session was prepared. Plans were different for various groups because each group had different capabilities and affiliations (e.g. Serbian and Roma populations). The approach to group work was adapted to the context of the collective centres. Consultation helped the facilitators to share their impressions and feelings after group work, and also to learn from these experiences. This was then used to prepare reports and make plans for further activities. Different kinds of group work were organized: for example, mother and infants group, women's knitting group, 4–7-year-old children's groups (using play), 7–10-year-old children's groups (using board games), 10–15-year-old children/adolescents' groups (using games and sport). At the beginning of each group work session there were many difficulties. People felt that they didn't have time for this or that this was a waste of time. However, a few weeks later they began to appreciate the value and meaning of group work, and started to be open and accepting of the support. Many survivors began to feel that the group space and time truly belonged to them. They talked about different subjects during the groups. Sometimes the focus was on 'what happened to them during bombing', at other times on cultural similarities and differences. They began to feel respected by the group facilitators and fellow members and thereby became happy. Frequently they would not only share their own opinions but also they were curious about those of others.

As a result of the group work, both children and adults started to organize exhibitions, showing their creative work, feeling proud of their cultural traditions and also became more open to other people. This certainly made them feel better, less isolated and more similar to others. Children at this stage were interested and excited and would enjoy travelling in the jeeps from the collective centres to the activity room. Children began to sing and smile and look out through the car windows with great curiosity. They became again an active part of the real life in the environment. Through different kinds of games (sand play, drawing, painting, social games etc.) children also began to express their feelings and creativity and to develop various skills and take care of each other. Through this group work, team members then were able to identify children in both ethnic groups (Serbian and Roma) who needed specialist help. The group work was also useful as a preventive and curative measure.

For most children and adolescents, the small group became a natural and highly attractive group setting; they were taught in these groups, played and ate together. Group work is therefore an effective therapeutic tool for them because it recreates the important social aspects of their lives which include being at home with siblings and parents, at school with classmates and playmates, in the neighbourhood and so forth. Group work as a therapeutic approach is not only a cost effective measure (economical in terms of resources) but it is effective through the emphasis on different activities, peer support influence and reinforcement (Dinkmeyer and Muro 1971; Dwivedi and Mymin 1993; Glass and Thompson 2000). There are numerous possibilities for sharing problems, self-development, being accepted, improving coping mechanisms, detecting psychological problems, working on prevention of disorders, de-stigmatization and so on. However, group work may have a more limited value for the person with severe psychiatric illness and who has to be treated at the individual level.

It is important for the group facilitators to obtain prior experiential training in group work with children and adolescents (the Midland Course is useful and relevant in this regard: kedarnd@doctors.org.uk). Running groups without such training is like conducting surgery, driving or swimming without any experiential training, and may even be dangerous. Groups can unleash constructive, creative and therapeutic forces but could be destructive and damaging in unskilled hands.

Common problems in helping traumtized communities

Based on the experiences in Bosnia-Herzegovina, Kosovo/Albania and Rwanda, Baron et al. (2003) have identified some problems in the initial phases of interventions, which include the following:

- Inexperienced professionals with little knowledge about the information that already exists in the field of psychosocial assistance to refugees and IDP should be trained. Some offered 'help' based only on personal reasons or research.
- Lack of cooperation between national institutions and international organizations.
- Inhabitants of collective centres are very passive, waiting for a solution from others. They feel lonely and forgotten, and are depressed, anxious, sad, and fearful of their uncertain future.
- Professionals may face numerous neglected children without proper care and poor circumstances of living. Their parents have poor mental health and have difficulty bringing them up (Dwivedi 1997a).

Concluding remarks

In a society affected by war, displacement and deterioration of child mental health infrastructure, it is important to set up social, educational and psychological services that are comprehensive, community-oriented, potentially self-sustaining, empowering and adaptive rather than to focus purely on treatment of a single diagnosis due to traumatic stress.

References

Ajdukovic, M. and Ajdukovic, D. (1998) 'Impact of displacement on the psychological well-being of refugee children'. *International Review of Psychiatry*, 10: 186–95.

Baron, N., Buus Jensen, S. and de Jong, J. (2003) 'Refugee and internally displaced people'. In B. Green; M. J. Friedman, J. de Jong, D. Solomon, T. M. Keane, J. A. Fairbank and B. Donelan (eds), *Trauma Interventions in War and Peace, Prevention, Practice and Policy*. New York: Kluwer Academic/Plenum Publishers.

Bell, P., Bergeret, I. and Oruc, L. J. (2002) 'The effects of war trauma in Bosnian female civilians: a study description'. In E. Durakovic-Belko and S. Powell (eds), *The Psychological Consequences of War: Results of Empirical Research from theTterritory of Former Yugoslavia*. Sarajevo: UNICEF B&H, pp. 32–6.

Blair, G. R. (2000) 'Risk factors associated with PTSD and major depression among Cambodian refugees in Utah'. *Health and Social Work*, 25(1): 23–30.

Boardman, F. (1994) 'Child psychiatry in wartime Britain'. *Journal of Education Psychology*, 35: 293–301.

Cantor, J., Mares, M. L. and Oliver, M. B. (1993) 'Parents' and children's emotional reactions to TV coverage of the Gulf War'. In B. S. Greenberg and W. Gantz (eds), *Desert Storm and the Mass Media*. Cresskill, NJ: Hampton Press, pp. 325–40.

Cheung, P. (1994) 'Post traumatic stress among Cambodian refugees in New Zeland'. *International Journal of Social Psychiatry*, 40(1): 17–26.

De Jong, T. V. M. (ed.) (2002) *Trauma, War, and Violence: Public Mental Health in Socio-cultural Context*. New York: Kluwer/Plenum.

Dinkmeyer, D. L. and Muro, J. J. (1971) *Group Counselling: Theory and Practice*. Itasca, IL: F. E. Peacock.

Dixon, P., Rehling, G. and Sciwach, Raj (1993) 'Peripheral victims of the *Herald of Free Enterprise* disaster'. *British Journal of Medical Psychology*, 66: 193–202.

Djapic, R. and Stuvland, R. (2002) 'Longitudinal study of the war-related traumatic reactions of children in Sarajevo in 1993, 1995 and 1997'. In E. Durakovic-Belkom and S. Powell (eds), *The Psychological Consequences of War: Results of Empirical Research from the Territory of Former Yugoslavia*. Sarajevo: UNICEF B&H, pp. 156–60.

Dwivedi, K. N. (ed.) (1993) *Group Work with Children and Adolescents: a Handbook*. London. Jessica Kingsley.

Dwivedi, K. N. (ed.) (1997a) *Enhancing Parenting Skills*. Chichester: John Wiley.

Dwivedi, K. N. (ed.) (1997b) *Therapeutic Use of Stories*. London: Routledge.

Dwivedi, K. N. (ed.) (2000) *Post Traumatic Stress Disorder in Children and Adolescents*. London: Whurr.

Dwivedi, K. N. (ed.) (2002) *Meeting the Needs of Ethnic Minority Children*. 2nd edn. London: Jessica Kingsley.

Dwivedi, K. N. and Harper, P. B. (eds) (2004) *Promoting Emotional Well Being of Children and Adolescents and Preventing their Mental Ill Health: a Handbook*. London: Jessica Kingsley.

Dwivedi, K. N. and Mymin, D. (1993) 'Evaluation'. In K. N. Dwivedi (ed.), *Group Work with Children and Adolescents*. London: Jessica Kingsley.

Dwivedi, K. N. and Varma, V. P. (eds) (1997a) *A Handbook of Childhood Anxiety Mangagement*. Aldershot: Arena Publishers.

Dwivedi, K. N. and Varma, V. P. (eds) (1997b) *Depression in Children and Adolescents*. London: Whurr.

Eisenbruch, M. (1990) 'Cultural bereavement and home sickness'. In C. Fisher and C. L. Cooper (eds), *On the Move: the Psychology of Change and Ttransition*. London: Wiley.

Eisenbruch, M. (1991) 'From post traumatic stress disorder to cultural bereavement: diagnosis of Southeast Asian refugees'. *Social Science and Medicine*, 33: 673–80.

Gavranidou, M. (2002) 'Overview of results regarding children and young people'. In E. Durakovic-Belko and S. Powell (eds), *The Psychosocial Consequences of War: Results of Empirical Research From the Territory of Former Yugoslavia*. Sarajevo: UNICEF B&H, pp. 128–36.

Glass, D. and Thompson, S. (2000) 'Therapeutic group work'. In K. N. Dwivedi (ed.), *Post Traumatic Stress Disorder in Children and Adolescents*. London: Whurr.

Hinshaw, S. P. (2005) 'The stigmatization of mental illness in children and parents: developmental issues, family concerns and research needs'. *Journal of Child Psychology and Psychiatry*, 46(7): 714–34.

Hosin, A. (2001) 'Children of traumatized and exiled refugee families: resilience and vulnerability'. *Journal of Medicine, Conflict and Survival*, 17: 137–45.

Husain, S. A (2001) *Hope for the Children: Lessons from Bosnia*. Missouri: International Medical and Educational Trust.

Jankovic, J. (2002) 'Psychological consequences of the war and of displacement for child victims of war 1991–1995 in Croatia'. In E. Durakovic-Belko and S. Powell (eds), *The Psychosocial Consequences of War: Results of Empirical Research From the Territory of Former Yugoslavia*. Sarajevo: UNICEF B&H, pp. 203–5.

Jensen, P. S. and Shaw, J. (1993) 'Children as victims of war: current knowledge and future research needs'. *Journal of the Amercian Academy of Child and Adolescent Psychiatry*, 32(4): 697–708.

Jones, L. (1998) 'Adolescent groups for encamped Bosnian refugees: some problems and solutions'. *Clinical Child Psychology and Psychiatry*, 3(4): 541–51.

Karacic, S. and Zvizdic, S. (2002) 'The effect of war related trauma on the behaviour of adolescents'. In E. Durakovic-Belko and S. Powell (eds), *The Psychosocial Consequences of War: Results of Empirical Research From the Territory of Former Yugoslavia*. Sarajevo: UNICEF B&H, pp. 190–3.

Kucera, A. and Lueger-Schuster, B. (2000) 'The experiences of migrations and acculturation as reported by displaced people from B&H (Bosnia and

Herzegovina) living in Vienna (Austria)'. In E. Durakovic-Belko and S. Powell (eds), *The Psychosocial Consequences of War: Results of Empirical Research From the Territory of Former Yugoslavia*. Sarajevo: UNICEF B&H, pp. 84–8.

Kleinman, A. (1988) *Rethinking Psychiatry from Cultural Category to Personal Experience*. New York: Free Press.

La Greca, A. M., Silverman, W. K., Vernberg, E. M. and Prinstein, M. J. (1996) 'Symptoms of posttraumatic stress in children after Hurricane Andrew: a prospective study'. *Journal of Consulting and Clinical Psychology*, 64: 712–23.

Lengua, A., Long, A. C., Smith, K. I. and Meltzoff, A. N. (2005) 'Pre-attack symptomatology and temperament and predictors of children's responses to September 11 terrorist attacks'. *Journal of Child Psychology and Psychiatry*, 46(6): 631–45.

Lopez, S. R. and Guarnaccia, P. T. (2000) 'Cultural psychopathology: uncovering the social world of mental illness'. *Annual Review of Psychology*, 51: 571–98.

Ljubomirovic, N. (1999) *Stress and Youth*, Belgrade: Zaduzbina Andrejevic.

Ljubomirovic, N. (2002) 'Psychological reactions of adolescents to war-related stress'. In E. Durakovic-Belko and S. Powell (eds), *The Psychosocial Consequences of War: Results of Empirical Research From the Territory of Former Yugoslavia*. Sarajevo: UNICEF B&H, pp. 212–13.

Milgram, N. A. (1982) 'War-related stress in Israeli children and youth'. In L. Goldberg and S. Brenitz (eds), *Handbook of Stress: Theoretical and Clinical Aspects*. New York: Free Press, pp. 656–76.

Milosavljevic, B. and Turjacanin, V. (2002) 'Socio-demographic characteristics of children and their experience of war-related trauma'. In E. Durakovic-Belko and S. Powell (eds), *The Psychosocial Consequences of War: Results of Empirical Research From the Territory of Former Yugoslavia*. Sarajevo: UNICEF B&H, pp. 178–81.

Oppedal, B., Roysamb, E. and Heyerdahl, S. (2005) 'Ethnic group acculturation and psychiatric problems in young immigrants'. *Journal of Child Psychology and Psychiatry*, 46(6): 646–60.

Osmanovic, A. and Zvizdic, S. (2002) 'War-related traumatic experiences and psychosomatic reactions of younger adolescents'. In E. Durakovic-Belko and S. Powell (eds), *The Psychosocial Consequences of War: Results of Empirical Research From the Territory of Former Yugoslavia*. Sarajevo: UNICEF B&H, pp. 186–9.

Pfefferbaum, B., Nixon, S. J., Tivis, R. D., Daughty, D. E., Pynoos, R. S., Gurwitch, R. H. and Foy, D. W. (2001) 'Television exposure in children after a terrorist incident'. *Psychiatry*, 64: 202–11.

Pfefferbaum, B., Seale, T. W., McDonald, N. B., Brandt, E. N., Rainwater, S. M., Maynard, B. T., Meierhoefer, B. and Miller, P. D. (2000) 'Posttraumatic stress two years after Oklahoma City bombing in youths geographically distant from the explosion'. *Psychiatry*, 63: 358–70.

Resick, P. (2001) *Stress and Truma*. Hove: Psychological Press.

Savic, J. (2002) 'Psychological war trauma and achievement motive'. In E. Durakovic-Belko and S. Powell (eds), *The Psychosocial Consequences of War: Results of Empirical Research From the Territory of Former Yugoslavia*. Sarajevo: UNICEF B&H, pp. 174–7.

Schuster, M. A., Stein, B. D., Jaycox, L. H., Collins, R. L., Marshall, G. N., Elliot, M. N., Zhou, A. J., Kanouse, D. E., Morrison, J. L. and Berry, S. H. (2001) 'A national survey of stress reactions after the September 11, 2001, terrorist attacks'. *New England Journal of Medicine*, 345: 1507–12.

Smith; P., Perrin, S., Yule, W. and Rabe-Hesketh, S. (2001) 'War exposure and maternal reaction in the psychological adjustment of children from Bosnia-Herzegovina'. *Journal of Child Psychology and Psychiatry*, 42: 395–404.

Summerfield, D. (1996) 'The impact of war and atrocity on civilian populations: an overview of major themes'. In D. Black, J. Henry-Hendriks, G. Mezey and M. Newman (eds), *Psychological Trauma: a Developmental Approach*. London: Royal College of Psychiatrists, Gaskell.

Terr, L. C., Bloch, D. A., Michel, B. A., Shi, H., Reinhardt, J. A. and Metayer, S. (1999) 'Children's symptoms in the wake of the Challenger: a filed study of distance-traumatic effects and an outline of related conditions'. *American Journal of Psychiatry*, 156: 1536–44.

Vogel, J. M. and Vernberg, E. M. (1993) 'Part 1: Children's psychological responses to disasters'. *Journal of Clinical Child Psychology*, 22: 646–84.

Ward, C. (2001) 'The A,B,Cs of acculturation'. In D. Matsumoto (ed.), *The Handbook of Culture and Psychology*. New York: Oxford University Press, pp. 411–45.

5
The Treatment of Psychological Trauma from the Perspective of Attachment Research

Felicity de Zulueta

Most clinicians and professionals working in the field of trauma psychology are now familiar with the diagnosis of Post-Traumatic Stress Disorder (PTSD) as a constellation of symptoms. This chapter focuses on these symptoms and attempts to make the reader aware of the similarities between them and the psychobiological manifestations of a disrupted attachment system (Zulueta 1999, 2002, 2006). It is with such a conceptual formulation in mind that professionals can approach the treatment of PTSD in its more complex manifestations (Herman 1992). You may have noted these have not been addressed in the recent NICE guidelines for PTSD (NICE guidelines 2005).

Attachment behaviour and PTSD

Bowlby (1969, 1973, 1980) and his colleagues made us aware that, like all mammals, human infants are genetically predisposed to an attachment figure and seek proximity to the care-provider. And this behaviour is often triggered by fear.

Since the same emotion of fear and the accompanying sense of helplessness are inherent to the experience of psychological traumatization, it is perhaps not surprising to find that attachment theory and research provide a useful psychobiological framework to understand both the origin and the symptoms of PTSD and other forms of psychological trauma (Henry 1997; Wang 1997). It was in fact Lindemann, who as early as 1944, defined psychological trauma as 'the sudden uncontrollable disruption of our affiliative bonds'. Hence, and in order to both understand and treat patients suffering from PTSD and other forms of grief reactions, it appears there should be some level of understanding of attachment disorders (Zulueta 1999, 2006).

The psychobiological substrate of attachment behaviour

Since infants are totally dependent on their caregiver in early life, any threat to the child's sense of security will activate the attachment system resulting in a characteristic sequence of behaviours including protest and despair. It is on the basis of these reactions to separation that attachment behaviour has been studied in mammals and, in particular, primates (Harlow 1974). The separation studies carried out on primate infants removed from their mother reveal that:

(a) Attachment behaviour has a specific neuropsychological substrate in the brain. It involves, in particular, a great part of the right hemisphere and a part of the supra orbital area of the brain which, as Schore (2000: 30–2) noted, is:

> necessary to acquire specific forms of knowledge to regulate interpersonal behaviour through its position at the apex of the 'rostral limbic system' which processes facial expressions and adapts to changing environments. It is also deeply connected to the autonomic system and it is critical to the modulation of social and emotional behaviours, the affect regulating functions involved in attachment processes.

(b) Attachment behaviour is partly mediated by opiates, so much so that Panksepp once described social bonding as an opiate addiction (Panksepp et al. 1985: 25). Indeed distress symptoms produced by separation are similar to those seen in narcotic withdrawal states and plant opioids and endogenous opiates alleviate both physical pain and separation distress (Panksepp 2003).

Psychobiological attunement and the formation of 'internal working models'

Human infants are born without the capacity to regulate their arousal and emotional reactions. They cannot soothe or comfort themselves nor can they maintain their psycho-physiological homeostasis. However, through the development of attachment bonds a complex process of attunement takes place between infant and caregiver. This allows the infant's early physiological and hormonal systems to be regulated by his or her primary caregiver, functions s/he gradually acquires throughout early development. For example, the high reactivity of the hypothalamo-pituitary axis (HPA) at birth becomes better modulated so that initially high levels of cortisol become modulated to produce a normal response in relation to specific stressors in a securely attached child.

In this way, the attachment system not only provides protection for the infant but it enables the development of psychobiological attunement between infant and caregiver, a process that provides, from birth onwards, a matching of inner states between mother and infant described by Stern as 'affect attunement' (Stern 1985: 140–2).

As development takes place infants become alert to the physical and emotional availability of their caregivers: the latter may be either unpredictable or rejecting. These repeated experiences are synthesized in the infant's mind to become what Bowlby called 'internal working models' or internal representations of how the attachment figure is likely to respond to the child's attachment behaviour. These working models have become the focus of much research in the field of attachment using the Strange Situation (Ainsworth et al. 1978; Main and Hesse 1992). These researchers found that one-year-old infants responded in different ways to separation from their caregivers depending on how secure their attachment was to that caregiver.

Reflective functioning

Subsequent studies carried out by Fonagy and Target (1997) using the Adult Attachment Interview have shown that if the caregiver or another important individual to whom the child is attached demonstrates 'reflective functioning' by giving meaning to the infant's experiences and sharing and predicting his or her behaviour, the child can internalize this capacity. Such a developmental acquisition, described as 'reflective functioning' or 'mentalization', enables people to understand each other in terms of mental states and intentions. It is key to developing a sense of agency and continuity as well as enabling people to interact successfully with others. It does also protect children from some of the deleterious effects of abuse by reducing their risk of re-enacting past traumatic experiences.

Secure and insecure attachments and the representation of the self

Secure attachments

A securely attached child has a mental representation of the caregiver as responsive in times of trouble. Such children feel confident and are capable of empathy and of forming good attachments. The good enough mother of the securely attached infant is accessible to the child in need and shows a tendency to respond appropriately to her emotional expressions, be they positive or negative.

These regulated events allow for the expansion of the child's capacity to regulate his or her emotions and account for the principle that security of the attachment bond is the primary defence against trauma-induced psychopathology (Schore 2002: 15). The right hemisphere is heavily involved in determining the individual's characteristic approach to affect regulation. Meanwhile, in the securely attached individual, the attachment representation encodes an implicit expectation that homeostatic disruptions will be set right allowing the child to self-regulate functions that previously required the caregiver's external regulation. In addition, the activity of this hemisphere is crucial to the empathic perception of the emotional states of other human beings.

Insecure attachments

Insecure attachments develop when the infants do not have a mental representation of a responsive caregiver in times of need such as when they feel fearful or helpless. These infants develop different strategies to gain access to their caregiver in order to survive. Three types of insecure attachment behaviours have been recognized using the Strange Situation (Ainsworth et al. 1978):

1. The group C infants who show an anxious-ambivalent response;
2. The group A infants who show an avoidant type of response;
3. The disorganized infants (Main and Hesse 1992) who show an unpredictable response in relation to their caregiver and are seen to freeze in trance-like state, very much like adult sufferers of PTSD.

For those whose early experiences have meant fear, in particular fear without solution, such as is observed in infants with a 'disorganized' attachment pattern, the care-provider demonstrates not only less affect attunement, but he or she also induces traumatic states of enduring negative affect in the child, either by frightening or by being frightened. In the latter case, the caregiver suffers from PTSD and finds himself or herself reliving terrifying states of helplessness that may be induced by the infant. For example, the infant's eyes may remind his mother of the man who raped her. One mother who suffered from PTSD presented to us a small girl who showed a failure to thrive. She had been severely beaten by the child's father and, when the little girl became distressed, her eyes resembled those of her father, eliciting in the mother a fear response rather than the comforting behaviour the child required.

In both cases, the caregiver not only induces traumatic states in her child but she cannot interactively repair the infant's negative affective states. These experiences, central to the inter-generational transmission of psychophathology, are stamped into the insecurely attached infant's right orbito-frontal system and its cortical and sub-cortical connections (Schore 2002: 19). In addition, reflective functioning is severely impaired. As Van der Kolk (1996) reminds us, the loss of ability to regulate the intensity of emotions is the most far-reaching effect of early trauma and neglect.

Attachment and dissociation

The infant's psychobiological response to trauma is comprised of two separate response patterns: hyper-arousal and dissociation (Perry 1994; Perry et al. 1995; Prasad 2000).

1. Initial stage: the fight-flight response mediated by the sympathetic system. This blocks the reflective symbolic processing with the result that traumatic experiences are stored in sensory, somatic, behavioural and affective systems.
2. If the fight-flight response is not possible, a parasympathetic state takes over and the child 'freezes' which, in nature, may be linked to feigning death and thereby fostering survival. Vocalization is also inhibited: like young animals, human beings can lose the capacity to speak, a phenomenon that is related to the release of endogenous opiates and observed in the PET scans on patients with PTSD (Rauch et al. 1996).
3. In traumatic states of helplessness or 'fear without solution', both the above responses are activated leading to an 'inward flight' or dissociative response (information on the development of dissociation scale can be found in Bernstein and Putnam 1986).

Children in fear of their caregiver's hatred and violence will maintain their attachment to their desperately needed caregiver by resorting to what the psychoanalysts refer to as 'splitting' and neuropsychologists as 'dissociation', i.e. creating different representations of themselves in relation to their caregiver which results in a lack of self-continuity in relation to the 'other', such as is seen with patients suffering from a borderline personality disorder (Fonagy and Target 1997; Ryle 1997; Zulueta 1993, 1999). A 19-year-long follow-up study of infants with a disorganized attachment showed a tendency to develop dissociative disorders in adulthood ranging from borderline personality disorder to dissociative identity disorders (DID) (Ogawa et al. 1997). In other words, in order to maintain their attachment to their caregiver, the infant will develop an idealized attachment to the caregiver by dissociating off all their terrifying self–other interactions. At a cognitive level, these children will therefore blame themselves for their suffering and thereby retain the idealized version of their caregiver as well as retaining a sense of control. They are the cause of their misery and therefore one day, if they manage to behave better, they may finally get the love and care that they need. This powerful cognitive defence, called the 'moral defence' by Fairbairn (1952: 65–7), is ferociously maintained because not only does it ward off the unbearable sense of utter helplessness humans cannot bear, but it also gives the individual hope of something better. Unfortunately, it also reinforces the attachment and identification with the abusing parent. Addressing this 'traumatic attachment' and its cognitive distortions is central to the treatment of patients with a history of child abuse. A similar cognitive distortion takes place in adults suffering from late-onset trauma but it is more accessible to modification.

The psychobiology of neglect and abuse

Traumatization in early childhood results in damage to the right hemispheric cortical and sub-cortical limbic circuits limiting the child's capacity to play, empathize, form attachments and regulate emotions. This occurs through the over-stimulation or under-stimulation of the neuronal circuits at critical periods of brain growth by pruning or stimulation of the synapses (Schore 2001). PET scans carried out on patients with PTSD whilst they are reliving a traumatic experience highlight these changes by showing the shut down of Broca's speech area we referred to earlier and a marked shift of activity to the right limbic and paralimbic areas (Rauch et al. 1996).

As a result, these individuals have difficulties in modulating emotions such as sympathetic dominant affects like terror, rage and elation, or parasympathetic-dominant affects like shame, disgust and hopeless despair. This can leave victims of child abuse with a propensity to self-medicate with drugs or alcohol and a tendency to resort to violence. Similarly, the reliving of past traumatic experiences tends to produce an endogenous opiate release and resulting analgesia. Pitman et al. (1990) describe how a group of eight Vietnam veterans suffering from PTSD were exposed to a fifteen-minute film clip of the war in Vietnam; seven of them showed a 30 per cent reduction in the perception of pain and were found to have released the equivalent of 8 mg of morphine. This same phenomenon is also used by patients suffering from childhood-induced PTSD when they cut and self-harm as a form of relief.

One of the emotions that is particularly important in PTSD is that of shame. It is an unbearable emotional reaction in people who have been neglected or abused because it involves a sense of self that has been made to feel totally invalidated and humiliated. Failures in affect attunement lead to a belief that one's needs are shameful which in turn leads to self-loathing and feeling of being a social outcast. As Judith Herman says (personal communication) it is a very powerful emotion and a very powerful physiological experience as well. She points out that it is an emotion where 'the parasympathetic shutdown in profound. People go into freeze where they literally can't move'. As a result it can often lead to dissociative reactions and to violent acting out. As one patient with a history of murder said to his therapist: 'Better be bad than not be at all' (Gilligan 1996). Recognizing shame and attending to its manifestations is therefore very important in the treatment of PTSD (Block-Lewis 1981).

Enduring changes in the way the hypothalamo-pituitary-axis (HPA) functions do occur in infants in response to stress and separation. This leads to reduced levels of cortisol in relation to similar experiences later in life, as well as an increase in glucocorticoid receptors (Gunnar and Donzella 2002; Yehuda et al. 2005). Yehuda's study on road traffic accident victims showed that only those individuals whose response to the accident led to a lower than normal release of cortisol developed PTSD (Yehuda 1997). The author attributed this to an earlier sensitization of the HPA that can be ascribed to early attachment difficulties (Wang 1997: 164).

Treatment of PTSD

The input provided here and in the subsequent sub-sections is expected to complement the accounts covered in Chapters 1, 2, 6 and 7. PTSD is essentially a dissociative phenomenon since the patient is overwhelmed by vivid memories from the past. This appears to result from the failure to integrate trauma into the declarative memory system. As a result, trauma can become organized at a sensory and somatic level and the traumatic response can be unconsciously triggered off and physically re-experienced without the conscious memories to accompany it. This represents a somatic form of dissociation. As a result, the traumatized individual is likely to be repeatedly exposed to states of high arousal that cannot be handled because of an associated inability to modulate such experiences, both biologically and psychologically. This leads to attempts to self-medicate the pain and dysphoria by resorting to drugs or alcohol (Van der Kolk 1996).

Cognitive distortions are also used to ward off the unbearable sense of helplessness that results from the loss of what Ferenczi termed 'our secret psychoses', i.e. the beliefs that we are essentially invulnerable and in control of our lives. These are shattered by the experience of utter helplessness that is at the heart of PTSD. The first goal in treatment is to provide the traumatized patient with a secure base. Following the approach taken by Bloom (1997), treatment takes place in a series of stages, the first being that of ensuring safety, followed by affect modulation, grief and ending with evolution (SAGE).

Assessment

The assessment process is carried out with the following principles in mind. Firstly, a secure base has to be established before starting treatment. This requires an assessment of both the external system of social attachments and the internal system of 'working models' and resulting attachment behavioural patterns. The core of the therapeutic approach is to ensure that the patient is given a sense of control and responsibility thoughout the treatment programme. This is crucial to counteract the sense of helplessness induced by traumatic experience. This means that the patient and therapist are to become engaged in a 'journey of exploration' in which the therapist informs and guides the client. He or she does not take over the treatment or invite regression by adopting the conventional psychoanalytic stance of remaining silent – at least not in the early phase of treatment.

First and foremost, the victim of trauma wants to know that the therapist is affected and does care about what happened to him or her. This does not mean becoming emotional but simply and gently conveying compassion, respect and understanding of the victim's plight. The traumatic story is thereby validated.

Psychoeducation and empowerment

Many of our patients have avoided talking about their symptoms to medical staff because they fear they are going mad. This fear is particularly marked in people for whom the experience of flashbacks is tantamount to having hallucinations or going 'mad'. For this reason, one of the first tasks is to explain to patients and accompanied relatives or partners what are the symptoms of PTSD and why they occur. However, to counteract the overwhelming sense of helplessness experienced by sufferers of PTSD, they are given simple advice as to what they can do to feel more in control. They are taught relaxation techniques using tapes, guided imagery and the establishment of a safe place.

Risk assessment

Patients with complex PTSD often resort to destructive patterns of behaviour in order to cope with their symptoms. They may cut themselves, abuse drugs or alcohol or cling to destructive relationships. A thorough assessment needs to be done in relation to their capacity for self-harm or the dangers that they might bring upon themselves by engaging in treatment. When this isn't carried out, it can have tragic consequences.

For example, a black patient was taken on for the treatment of his childhood abuse whilst he was living in the home of one of his abusing parents. As he began to grow more independent and assertive during his treatment, his parent felt threatened and became very aggressive: our patient experienced this as the repetition of what happened to him when he had sought help as a child and ended up taking an overdose and being admitted to hospital. Battered women can face similar dangers if they embark on treatment without prior preparation. They can be given support and help in establishing a safety network before embarking on treatment. This may involve leaving, seeking a refuge, making contact with the police as well as seeking legal advice. It must be borne in mind that it is at the time when a woman seeks to leave an abusive relationship where domestic violence is taking place that she is in the greatest danger of being attacked or killed by her partner whose own dependency needs make him feel terribly threatened by her loss. In the case of substance abuse, patients will be advised to give up using alcohol or drugs and to seek specialized help if needed. If addicted, they will not be taken into therapy until their treatment is over.

Assessment of dissociative disorders

Dissociation refers to a wide variety of behaviours that represent lapses in the psychological and cognitive processing. Three main types of dissociative behaviour have been recognized: amnesia, absorption and depersonalization. Dissociative amnesia involves suddenly finding oneself in situations or faced with evidence that you have performed actions for which you have no memory. Absorption implies becoming so involved in what you are doing that you are unaware of what is going on around you. Depersonalization refers to experiencing events as if you are an observer, disconnected from your body or feelings. These various forms of dissociation are prevalent in people who suffer from childhood trauma or complex PTSD (Herman 1992) and can be assessed through the Dissociative Experience Scale (DES) with the patient. High scores (of 30 and above) mean measures need to be taken to deal with this phenomenon particularly when devising a treatment plan. For many patients, recognizing that they do suffer from a Dissociative Identity Disorder comes to them as a shock and, in our experience, we get very few individuals who present to us with a constellation of previously identified self–other states with named personalities.

In some cases, an awareness that therapy will involve exploring aspects of themselves they would rather not know about, leads patients to refuse therapy or to postpone it until such time as they can find no other solution to their problems. The strength of the early self is negatively related to the individual's capacity to dissociate; for Sroufe this underscores his view that dissociation is a self-related process (Ogawa et al. 1997: 877). The vulnerable self will tend to adopt dissociation as a defensive process because it does not have the belief in its worthiness gained from a loving and responsive early relationship.

Whilst the process of dissociation begins as a protective mechanism for the integrity of the self in the face of catastrophic trauma, it can become a direct threat to the optimal functioning of the self if it becomes a routine response to stress. There is therefore a need to help patients with a tendency to dissociate into different self-states to become aware of when this is happening, particularly if it is putting them at risk of being harmed or of harming others. In order to do this, there may be a need to establish a procedure whereby it is recognized that these patients will take responsibility for themselves and the management of their dissociated self-states. This can mean exploring triggers for dissociation in the therapeutic setting, particularly issues of shame. It may also mean involving friends, family or other carers in being available after therapeutic sessions and writing a diary between sessions to establish what are the triggers to these dissociative experiences.

Modulation of affect, attunement and the development of self-reflective functioning

Although affect modulation is inherent to the treatment process, it is important to remember that verbal interpretations processed by the patient's left hemisphere and the creation of insight are not going to access the right brain, the neurobiological repository of unconscious working models of insecure disorganized attachment schemas. As Schore (2002) states, it is the way negative moments between therapist and patient are addressed and repaired during the session that enables positively charged interactions to become central points of treatment. Humour has an enormous role to play in this process as does empathy and reflective functioning on the part of the therapist.

Standard trauma work usually requires a patient to confront their traumatic experience as well as the feelings and cognitive distortions that accompany it. In the Traumatic Stress Service, patients are offered a choice of psychoanalytic psychotherapy with a marked cognitive input, or Eye Movement Desensitization and Reprocessing (EMDR) (Shapiro 1995). This technique need not use eye movement but can use alternative forms of bilateral stimulation of the brain such as alternate hand tapping or sounds if the patient prefers. In many cases this approach produces rapid results. It is particularly useful for patients who tend to experience a lot of physical symptoms or who tend to intellectualize and also in cases where patients find it hard to talk about their traumatic experience because of language difficulties or because of the humiliation and shame involved, such as victims of rape or torture.

We also use EMDR when patients involved in other therapies appear to be stuck or as an adjunct to the treatment of patients with complex PTSD. In these cases, the patient's therapist may accompany the patient during this stage of treatment so that the information that is brought up in the EMDR session can be integrated into the ongoing therapy.

One foot in the past and one foot in the present

The slow and painful reconstruction of the patient's narrative requires the patient to focus on the past whilst recognizing the presence of the therapist in the here and now of the present. Many patients suffering from complex PTSD will tend to dissociate and get lost in the horrors of their past – thereby recreating their past trauma within the therapeutic setting. In order to prevent this, the therapist may keep in verbal contact with the patient by commenting on what he sees or hears and reminding the patient that the event was in the past. Patients can be helped to stay in the room through various grounding techniques such as keeping eye contact, holding onto something and, most important, by both becoming aware of and working through with the therapist his or her feelings of shame.

Some patients simply forget what took place in the sessions. In such cases, the use of tape-recordings of the session has proved to be very helpful with some people. The patients take the tape home and listen to it before the next session. Some will comment about what was said, check out misperceptions and probably use the tape as a transitional object. However, this process could facilitate the capacity for self-reflective functioning. Fonagy and Target (1997) have emphasized how important it is for an individual to put himself in the mind of another in reducing the tendency for self-destructive repetition of earlier experiences. They ascribe the internalization of this capacity as taking place when an infant has the experience of being in the mind of another – be it caregiver or anyone involved with them. In listening to the recording of a therapeutic interaction, the patient can observe two minds interacting with the other, and one of them attempting to have the other in mind, something they have rarely known. Knowing how important it is for these individuals to feel that they are not over-dependent nor abused or helpless, it is important to look out for therapeutic situations that may precipitate destructive behaviour and, at the same time, help with the reintegration of earlier self–other experiences. In some cases, the damage perpetrated on the wife and children by the sufferer's irritability and even violence may make it essential to involve the family using a systemic approach.

Knowing how PTSD can negatively affect people's capacity to express themselves emotionally, a phenomenon described as alexythimia (Henry 1997), it is no surprise to find that art therapy can also be extremely helpful in enabling some patients who appear stuck in one therapeutic modality, to move on.

Team work

Whatever the form of therapy being offered to a patient, the team approach remains central to our service to reduce dependency on the part of the patient and to support the therapists. Psychiatrists will offer patients the possibility of taking medication, such as an SSRI, to help with their symptoms: it is offered as a 'life jacket' to cope with the difficulties of the therapeutic journey. In this way more than one member of the team becomes involved with most patients.

Problems around avoidance

Most patients are ambivalent about coming for treatment. They may attempt to avoid any reminders of their traumatic experience either by bringing up different issues and problems in their treatment sessions, or by failing to attend sessions or by not carrying out the tasks they agreed to do. If this avoidance pattern persists, the therapist needs to clarify what may lie behind this behaviour. In some cases, the client clearly believes that the therapeutic journey is too dangerous or too painful and they cannot make a commitment. These individuals may be told that they are not yet ready for the journey but that they can return when and if they change their minds. Many patients make a stronger commitment at this point. In other cases, their diagnosis of PTSD has clearly given them a role in the system that they do not want to lose, either for legal reasons or for family reasons. In the first case, they are advised to return when their compensation has been resolved, and in the second, offered a systemic family assessment followed in many cases by a combined approach of family therapy and/or individual work.

Problems associated with ending

The ending of treatment is always a major step in the therapy of patients suffering from complex PTSD. For many, the gains experienced in the treatment may seem to disappear and very child-like wishes to be cared for emerge. The prospect of ending brings back childhood experiences of rejection, loss and abuse that need to be worked through. These problems can be significantly minimized by offering time-limited therapy and by addressing the need for reintegration into the family and community right from the beginning of treatment. At an individual level, if feelings of pain and rage can be directly expressed in the therapy this bodes well for these patients who have spent their lives either suppressing their anger or expressing it inappropriately.

Problems relating to the false memory syndrome

The subjective reality of the patient's experience is central to the therapeutic process but it is important to make it clear that memories may not always reflect what actually took place in the past. The therapist will withhold any ideas he or she may have about what took place in their patients' lives so as not to influence their patients in any particular direction; this also helps their patients stay with the experience of not knowing. In the later phases of treatment, the therapists may support patients who wish to seek external confirmation and validation of their abusive experiences. However, the therapists won't endorse such behaviour before they know that their patients are prepared to face the possibility that these abusive experiences may be denied and that they may face rejection and attack. If patients later want to confront their abusers by taking legal action, the therapist will strongly recommend that no such action is taken before corroborative evidence has been obtained by the patient and that he or she has good legal support.

Taking care of the therapist

There is no doubt that secondary or vicarious traumatization is a very dangerous aspect of working with this particular group of patients, In order to work in this field, it is important for therapists to develop other activities and interests both within and outside their professional life (see also Chapter 10 of this book on managing secondary and traumatic stress).

Supervision should be provided on a weekly basis and the team members need to feel that they can express themselves freely. They may feel anger or disgust, frustration and helplessness and, in many cases, doubt as to whether they are doing the 'right thing'. Whilst supervision tends to take place in a group setting, a therapist should feel free to talk to her supervisor about more personal issues that may arise when a patient touches a personal wound in the therapist. The latter must know that she can seek guidance and support, as well as therapy outside the work context. Ensuring the safety of the therapist is of primary concern with patients who are at risk of being violent.

Concluding remarks

The treatment of patients suffering from childhood trauma or complex PTSD is one of the most interesting and challenging areas of work in the field of mental health. Professionals are not only dealing with a disorder that is only just beginning to be recognized but they are also constantly learning new forms of treatment – each one of which opens up new perspectives as to how the mind responds in relation to a traumatic experience. An attachment perspective helps to make sense of what takes place among the sufferer of PTSD, both from a psychobiological perspective and in terms of the meaning he or she gives to such an experience. It also bridges the gap between the experience of the individual and his or her social community. For example, a supportive community can act as external protective buffer and prevent the emergence of PTSD in traumatized individuals just as an internalized secure attachment can act as an internal protective buffer for the individual who would otherwise develop PTSD (Zulueta 1993).

To those for whom life has become a nightmare from the past, the provision of safe and consistent professional attachments can provide these desperate individuals with a sense of hope and the possibility of healing their emotional wounds.

References

Ainsworth, M. D. S., Blehar, M. C., Waters, E. and Wall, S. (1978) *Patterns of Attachment: a Psychological Study of the Strange Situation.* Hillsdale, NJ: Lawrence Erlbaum Associates.

Bernstein, E. M. and Putnam, F. W. (1986) 'Development, reliability and valididty of a dissociation scale'. *Journal of Nervous and Mental Disease*, 174: 727–35.

Block-Lewis, H. (1981) 'Shame and guilt in human nature'. In S. Tuttman, C. Kaye and M. Zimmerman (eds), *Object and Self: a Developmental Approach.* New York: International Universities Press.

Bloom, S. (1997) *Creating Sanctuary: Toward the Evolution of Sane Societies.* London: Routledge.

Bowlby, J. (1969) *Attachment*, Vol. 1, *Attachment and Loss*, 2nd edn. London: Hogarth Press.

Bowlby, J. (1973) *Separation: Anxiety and Anger*, Vol. 2 *Attachment and Loss*. London: Hogarth Press.

Bowlby, J. (1980) *Loss, Sadness and Depression*, Vol. 3, *Attachment and Loss*. London: Hogarth Press.

Fairbairn, R. (1952) *Psychoanalytic Studies of the Personality.* London: Routledge & Kegan Paul.

Fonagy, P. and Target, M. (1997) 'Attachment and reflective function: their role in self organization'. *Development and Psychopathology*, 9: 679–700.

Gilligan, J. (1996) *Violence: Our Deadly Epidemic and its Causes.* New York: G. P. Putnam's Sons.

Gunnar, M. R and Donzella, B. (2002) 'Social regulation of the cortisol levels in early human development'. *Psychoneurendocrinology*, 27: 199–220.

Harlow, H. F. (1974) *Learning to Love*, 2nd edn. New York and London: Jason Aronson.

Henry, J. (1997) 'Psychological and physiological responses to stress: the right hemisphere and the hypothalamic-pituitary-adrenal-axis, an inquiry into problems of human bonding'. *Acta Physiologica Scandinavica*, 161: 164–9.

Herman, J. (1992) *Trauma and Recovery: the Aftermath of Violence from Domestic Abuse to Political Terror.* New York: Basic Books.

Lindemann, E. (1944) 'Symptomatology and management of acute grief'. *American Journal of Psychiatry*, 101: 141–9.

Main, M. and Hesse, E. (1992) 'Disorganized/disorientated infant behaviour in the strange situation, lapses in monitoring of reasoning and discourse during the parent's adult attachement interview, and dissociative states'. In M. Ammanati and D. Stern (eds), *Attachment and Psychoanalysis.* Rome: Gius Laterza and Figli, pp. 86–140.

NICE (2005) Guidelines on post-traumatic stress disorder. *The Management of PTSD in Adults and Children in Primary and Secondary Care.* Clinical Guidelines 26, March 2005 (http://www.nice.org.uk) accessed May 2005.

Ogawa, J. R., Sroufe, L. A., Weinfeld, N. S., Carlson, E. A. and Byron, E. (1997) 'Development and the fragmented self: longitudinal study of dissociative symptomatology in a non-clinical sample'. *Developmental Psychopathology*, 9: 855–79.

Panksepp, J. (2003) 'Feeling the pain of social loss'. *Science*, 302: 237–8.

Panksepp, J., Siviy, S. M. and Normansell, L. A. (1985) 'Brain opioids and social emotions'. In M Reite and T. Field (eds), *The Psychobiology of Attachment and Separation*. London: Academic Press, pp. 3–49.

Perry, B. D. (1994) 'Neurobiological sequelae of childhood trauma: post-traumatic stress disorders in children'. In M. Murberg (ed.), *Catecholamines in Post-traumatic Stress Disorder: Emerging Concepts*. Washington, DC: American Psychiatric Press, pp. 253–76.

Perry, B. D., Pollard, R., Blakely, T., Baker, W. and Vigilante, D. (1995) 'Childhood trauma, the neurobiology of adaptation and "use-dependent" development of the brain: how "states" become "traits"'. *Infant Mental Health Journal*, 16(4): 271–91.

Pitman, R. K., Van der Kolk, B. A., Scott, P. O. and Greenberg, M. S. (1990) 'Naloxone-reversible analgesic response to combat-related stimuli in post traumatic stress disorder'. *Archives of General Psychiatry*, 47: 541–4.

Prasad, K. (2000) 'Biological basis of post-traumatic stress disorder'. In K. N. Dwivedi (ed.), *Post-traumatic Stress Disorder in Children and Adolescents*. London: Whurr Publishers.

Rauch, S. L., Van der Kolk, B. A., Fisler, R. E., Alpert, N. M., Orr, S. P., Savage, C. R., Fischman, A. J., Jenike, M. A. and Pitman, R. K. (1996) 'A symptom provocation study of post traumatic stress disorder using positron emission tomography and script driven imagery'. *Archives of General Psychiatry*, 53: 380–7.

Ryle, A. (1997) 'The structure and development of borderline personality disorder: a proposed model'. *British Journal of Psychiatry*, 170: 82–7.

Schore, A. N. (1996) 'Experience dependent maturation of a regulatory system in the orbito-frontal cortex and the origin of developmental psychopathology'. *Development and Psychopathology*, 8: 59–87.

Schore, A. N. (2000) 'Attachment and the regulation of the right brain'. *Attachment and Human Development*, 2: 23–47.

Schore, A. N. (2001) 'The effects of early relational trauma on right brain development, affect regulation, and infant mental health'. *Infant Mental Health Journal*, 22: 201–69.

Schore, A. N. (2002) 'Dysregulation of the right brain: a fundamental mechanism of traumatic attachment and the psychogenesis of post-traumatic stress disorder'. *Australian and New Zealand Journal of Psychiatry*, 36: 9–30.

Shapiro, F. (1995) *Eye Movement Desensitization Reprocessing: Basic Principles, Protocols, and Procedures*. New York: Guilford Press.

Stern, D. (1985) *The Interpersonal World of the Infant: a View From Psychoanalysis and Developmental Psychology*. New York: Basic Books.

Van der Kolk, B. A. (1996) 'The body keeps the score: approaches to the psychobiology of post traumatic stress disorder'. In B. A. Van der Kolk, A. C. McFarlane and L. Weisaeth (eds), *Traumatic Stress: the Effects of Overwhelming Experience on Mind, Body, and Society*. New York: Guilford Press, pp. 214–41.

Wang, S. (1997) 'Traumatic stress and attachment'. *Acta Physiologica Scandinavica*, 161: 164–9.

Yehuda, R. (1997) 'Sensitization of the hypothalamic-pituitary axis in post-traumatic stress disorder'. In R. Yehuda and A. C. McFarlane (eds), *Psychobiology of Post Traumatic Stress Disorder* vol. 821. New York: Annals of the New York Academy of Sciences, pp. 157–82.

Yehuda, R., Engel, S. M., Brand, S., Seckl, J., Marcus, S. M. and Berkowitz, G. S. (2005) 'Transgenerational effects of posttraumatic stress disorder in babies of mothers exposed to the World Trade Center attacks during pregnancy'. *Journal of Clinical Endocrinology and Metabolism*, 90(7): 4115–18.

Zulueta, de F. (1993) *From Pain to Violence: the Roots of Human Destructiveness*. London: Whurr.

Zulueta, de F. (1999) 'Borderline personality disorder as seen from an attachment perspective: a review'. *Criminal Behaviour and Mental Health*, 9: 237–53.

Zulueta, de F. (2002) 'From post traumatic stress disorder to dissociative identity disorder: the traumatic stress service in the Maudsley Hospital'. In Valerie Sinason (ed.), *Attachment Trauma and Multiplicity: Working with Dissociative Identitiy Disorder*. London: Brunner-Routledge.

Zulueta, de F. (2006) *From Pain to Violence: the Roots of Human Destructiveness*. Chichester: John Wiley and Sons.

6
Cognitive Behavioural Therapy Approach (CBT) Used in Rehabilitation Processes of Traumatized Children

Roy Lubit

Research has shown that structured treatment focusing on PTSD and trauma symptoms can ameliorate the effects of trauma (Taylor and Chemtob 2004). Even complex PTSD is ameliorated by CBT (Resick and Schnicke 1992; Resick et al. 2003). It is important to remember in treating PTSD in children that the impact goes far beyond the *DSM-IV* diagnostic criteria of intrusive recollections, numbing/withdrawal and hyperarousal, particularly if the symptoms have persisted for a period or if there were multiple traumatic incidents such as one finds in child abuse.

Trauma experiences impact what children focus their attention on and how they interpret and think about the world. Their general emotional state, behaviour and even their biology are affected. The task of therapy is to help them regain a sense of mastery and of efficacy, and to enable them to interact effectively with the world rather than recreate their trauma (Van der Kolk 2003). This chapter will outline the use of CBT in the treatment of children suffering from emotional trauma. The use of CBT in children requires some modifications from its use in adults (Friedberg et al. 2002; Grant et al. 2004). Cognitive behavioural therapy (CBT) techniques integrate the following five components.

The first is a combination of psychoeducation, stress inoculation, and relaxation training. In addition, some children will need help in feeling identification – learning to put feelings into words. The second component is the creation of a narrative of what occurred and gradual exposure. This helps to desensitize the child to painful memories and traumatic reminders, and decrease the child's withdrawal and avoidance. Depending upon the child's age, professionals may talk directly about what occurred, or create a book, or create a make-believe radio show about the events.

The third component of the CBT treatment of emotional trauma is exploring the way in which the child has been affected by the trauma and replacing unhelpful thoughts with more helpful ones. The fourth component is working on social skills so that the child's relationships improve and he or she can catch up with peers who have continued to develop and learn. The fifth and final component is safety planning: what active steps can the child take to deal with dangerous situations in the future.

Whenever possible, parents should receive guidance in parallel with the child's therapy (see Cohen 2002; Deblinger and Heflin 1996; Van der Kolk et al. 1996; Cloitre et al. 2002; Resick et al. 2002, 2003). Regardless of the specific treatment protocol one uses, it is crucial to remember that *the most important factor in healing is the development of a trusting relationship in which patients feel that their therapist truly understands and is concerned about them.*

Phase I: Orientation to CBT and stress inoculation

Therapy begins by providing an orientation to CBT and stress inoculation. The indications for therapy are discussed. If the child has a limited understanding, the clinician or the therapist can acknowledge that the child has been through a traumatic experience, and that when terrible things happen people have strong feelings and often do not want to talk about them. When a child is able to talk about the event it helps them to feel better. People often suggest that it is better to forget or that it is very hard to talk about what occurred and makes them more upset. One might think that the point of therapy is to put the trauma behind them, not think about it a lot and move on. The problem is that avoiding talking about it has not worked. The memories come back outside of the child's control and make him or her very upset when thought about. The point of therapy is to detoxify them so that the child can think about her experiences when and if she wishes, not have the memories force themselves on her, and not be overwhelmed with painful feelings when she thinks about them. Building a solid therapeutic alliance is key to keeping traumatized individuals in therapy and to helping them deal with the stress involved in it (Cloitre et al. 2004).

Stress inoculation involves a variety of means of dealing with stress. Breathing control is a particularly common method. You can have a child lie on his or back, place a book on his or her stomach and watch it go up or down. You can ask the child to notice how she feels calmer when breathing slowly and deeply than when breathing rapidly.

Having the child teach her parents the exercise is often a useful way of helping the child master the technique.

Progressive muscle relaxation takes longer, but can be very helpful at times. In progressive muscle relaxation the child goes through each part of her body first tensing and then relaxing: feet, lower legs, upper legs, bottom, stomach, chest and shoulders, arms, hands, neck, face.

Thought stopping is an important technique when the child is dealing with disruptive intrusive thoughts. The child could say no to herself or could imagine a stop sign rapidly coming towards her whenever faced with intrusive thoughts. With time the child will become better at it. It is important to keep practising. For children having nightmares, dream control techniques in which the child tells him or herself before going to bed that a repeating painful dream will now end in a better way can be very helpful. Having the child say positive things to herself/himself about the ability to cope and about the eventual outcome of the situation can also be useful, as are role playing situations. Practising going to the doctor or answering questions people may ask about the traumatic event can be helpful in inoculating people to stress. Young children can play out scenes with a doll's house or stuffed toys and animals.

Another crucial part of the introduction to CBT is explaining the cognitive triangle. The cognitive triangle is a diagram in which the words thoughts, feelings and behaviour are written at each of the three corners. Two-way arrows connect each of the words. How we think about things, how we interpret events, determines how we feel. For example, if someone walks by us without saying hello and we believe they are doing it because they don't like us we are likely to feel sad. If we think they are doing it because they are preoccupied with something it is not likely to bother us. If we think that we are unlikable we will blame ourselves. If we think they do it to everyone it will bother us much less. To give another example, if a child asks a teacher for help and the teacher asks the child to do it him- or herself the child's emotional reaction will be very different if the child feels the teacher thinks he is able to do it himself and wants to encourage autonomy rather than not liking the child. How we feel also affects how we think. Once we slide into depression we tend to interpret things in negative ways rather than in neutral or positive ways. People often receive unclear signals from the environment and can interpret them in various ways. Both how we think and how we feel affects how we behave. The reverse occurs as well, as we see from the work of Ben on self-perception theory. If we avoid something which makes us anxious, we will often become increasingly fearful over time and tend to see it as more than we can cope with. If we engage in activities that make us anxious, in doses that we can handle, our discomfort will generally decrease.

Feeling identification is important for many children. By putting words to feelings a child is generally able to gain greater self-control. Rather than feeling overwhelmed by feelings they do not understand and can't cope with or communicate they can tell you about them. You can also ask the child to provide examples of situations that would lead to various feelings. Another exercise is to draw a feeling thermometer and to ask the child how intense the feeling is. The Story Telling Card Game and the Talking, Feeling and Doing Game can be very useful in these circumstances.

Phase II: Telling the narrative and gradual exposure

After the child and his or her parents understand the reason for therapy, have formed an alliance and engaged with the therapist, and have worked on feeling identification and relaxation techniques it is time to work on creating the narrative and gradual exposure. This step generally begins with explaining the reason for this process. The child, and possibly his or her parents, are likely to be very wary of gradual exposure. Many people would like to simply push the event under the rug and cease thinking about it. Trying to talk about it can seem to be going in the wrong direction. It is sometimes helpful to draw an analogy to an infection. It hurts to clean out a scrape. But, if you do not, an infection can set in and that can cause far more problems. The treatment of PTSD involves detoxification of the memories of the event. The individual needs to become able to think about it without experiencing a flood of disruptive feelings. Being able to tell the story, seeing that they can survive in doing so and finding out that it does not lead the individual to disintegrate, is a very crucial experience. The child here may use the relaxation techniques learned to modulate his or her emotions.

Children can retell stories in a variety of ways. Some children write a book or create a picture book about the experience. Others may pretend to put on a radio show. The form doesn't matter. What matters is being able to tell the story. The child needs to talk about the feelings involved, and not simply the events. Unhelpful beliefs and perceptions need to be worked on. Some children feel that they behaved badly during the crisis or that somehow they caused it or caused someone to be hurt. They may feel that the world is an uncontrolled dangerous place or that they will never be happy again. If a loved one died they may believe that their last moments were agony or that they cannot go to heaven because their body was damaged in the disaster.

To work through and undo some of the damage of a traumatic incident, it is not enough to have the child simply tell the story or draw pictures. Children also need a corrective experience. They need to be left with a peaceful and hopeful picture in their minds, rather than one of pain and despair. Therefore, it is very important to have the child write a corrective story or draw a corrective picture of what they want things to be like in the future, of how to build a better community and a better life.

Once the child has done this, he or she has a joint session with his or her parents. The therapist should prepare a quiz for them to see what they know, and teach them about relaxation techniques, the cognitive triangle, the symptoms of PTSD, aspects of the trauma the child is unsure of, and discuss the parents' thoughts about what happened. Parents should be well prepared for the joint session. They should read the child's book in advance and be prepared to answer the child's questions. The parents need to listen to the retelling and provide copious positive feedback for the child's bravery in doing so. There should be no criticism of the child or correction of details at this point, unless the child asks for clarification. If the child has misinformation leading to disruptive fantasies, it can be corrected later. It is often necessary to work with parents to desensitize them to what occurred so that they can listen to their child's retelling of the events without being flooded by emotions. Professionals should offer the parents another joint session, and actively encourage them to attend if communication did not go smoothly.

Phase III: Evaluating the impact on the child

Big, visual events can have an impact on us that goes well beyond their likelihood of recurring or the concrete impact on our lives. They can affect our images of ourselves, our ability to trust others, our sense of safety, and images of and plans for the future. To undo the damage that can result from a traumatic incident one needs to assess how these areas have been impacted and work with the child to rebuild their cognitive map and new images.

Many children develop negative self-images or negative images about the world after a trauma. They may feel that they are partly to blame or that they cannot trust the world. The child's ability to socialize, succeed in school and enjoy life can all be significantly compromised. The child will fall increasingly far off his or her previous developmental path. Unless specifically addressed, these beliefs can profoundly affect their future development and adjustment long after the symptoms of withdrawal, intrusive recollections and hyper-arousal have cleared, or even if they never occurred. With a young child these self-images and beliefs about the world can come out in play. With older children they may emerge through talking. You can also surmise that they have occurred by observing the child's behaviour. Information needs to be obtained directly from the child as well as from parents, teachers and others who know the child well.

Once you understand how the child now sees the world and herself you can work together to question those views. In fantasy play, for example, you can encourage the child to find happier endings and situations in which she is in control. In talking therapy you can help the child to re-evaluate their current perceptions of themselves and others and form more balanced views. Also one can promote the idea that there are people you can't trust and things that are dangerous, but there is also a lot we can do to protect ourselves short of isolation from the world.

Marylene Cloitre (2002) has developed the STAIR method for treating trauma. It is particularly valuable for those whose relationships and ability to cope with feelings and the world have been adversely affected. Adolescents who sustained multiple traumas are often unable to adequately regulate their emotional state and can benefit greatly from this approach.

A professional staff here works together to assess the child's current method of coping and regulating his or her mood – what leads the child to become upset and how the child responds to crisis and tries to self-soothe. You suggest alternative, better ways. The child is helped to accept his or her feelings and to increase tolerance in dealing with painful feelings. You discuss the relationship between emotions and interpersonal problems, using role play to develop assertiveness and flexibility.

Phase IV: Social and academic skills

While other children are continuing to develop social and academic skills, the traumatized child is stagnating or falling backwards. After a few months, or years, of compromised social and academic learning it becomes almost impossible to catch up without considerable help. The therapist of a traumatized child needs to help the child's parents understand this and arrange for remedial assistance.

Phase V: Safety planning

Safety planning may occur in Phase III as part of helping the child to feel more secure about the world. Sometimes, children respond to trauma by closing their eyes to dangers in the world and becoming reckless. Wholesale denial of danger may be less painful than the anxiety they would otherwise face. These children need help in learning to be more careful. Studies have shown decreased blood flow to the frontal lobes in people who have been traumatized and are facing traumatic reminders (Van der Kolk 2003; see also Chapter 5 in this book). Such individuals need help in tolerating the anxiety inherent in thinking about the dangers in the world as well as help in recognizing the situations in which they close their eyes to dangers and to learn how to better deal with them.

Working with parents

It is important to work with the parents, and to treat the parents for their own trauma if necessary. Multiple studies (Ziv and Israel 1973; Freud and Burlingham 1943; Janis 1951) have shown that parents' reactions are the most influential factors affecting a child's outcome. If the parents' stress, depression or anxiety is untreated, significant therapy for the child will be of limited help

Once the parents are able to handle their own trauma it can be very helpful to have a joint session with the parent and child in which the child can share with the parent the PTSD experience, relaxation techniques, cognitive processing (how our thoughts affect our feelings), and the impact the trauma has had. The child can also share the narrative/storybook of the trauma. All of this needs to be reviewed by the therapist and parents prior to the joint session. The joint session facilitates the ability of the child and parent to talk about what happened and to continue to work together to counter problematic cognitions and trauma symptoms.

Treating traumatic grief

Traumatic grief, also known as complex bereavement, involves the loss of a major loved one in a traumatic way. As a result, the child is unable to mourn the loss of the loved one and move on with life. The treatment of complex bereavement requires special techniques. Specifically, before helping the individual with their grief reaction one needs to treat the trauma reaction. In addition, the child needs help in working through ambivalent feelings about the lost person, perceived guilt over unpleasant words or actions during the relationship, saying goodbye to the relationship, and reconnecting to life.

The process of mourning the loss of a loved one entails remembering positive times together, remembering what you learned together, making peace with the loss, stepping away and forging ties with others. When a loved one has died in a violent way, particularly if their body has been mutilated, the images of the trauma and horror of their death can so overwhelm the child that he or she can't think about their positive times together and mourn the loss. Once the emotional trauma and painful images of how they died are worked through you can move on to do the grief work.

Sometimes ambivalent feelings about the person who died or guilt over angry things the child said to them prevents mourning. Mourning requires a sense of peace in the relationship. In these situations it can be very helpful to write letters to the person who died or imagine discussions with the deceased in which the child makes peace with the person. The mourning process involves remembering the good times you had with someone, the things you learned, disengaging and saying goodbye, and connecting to those aspects of the real world that are still available to you. When a child is filled with an image of how a parent or sibling died in a violent way this is often impossible. Rather than happy images the child can hold onto in memory while he or she says goodbye to their concrete relationship, the child is filled with violent images that are too painful to think about. The emotional trauma needs to be worked through before the mourning process can occur. Ambivalent, angry or guilty feelings can also complicate the grieving process and therefore need to be resolved. The process for doing this entails exploring the negative feelings, discussing the intervention with the parent to see if there are objections, and using imaginary conversation, letter writing or reverse role play to say what the child wished had been said.

Once the road blocks to grieving have been overcome the normal process can occur. Positive memories need to be identified and preserved. One can work with the child to create a memory book or box for pictures, photographs, keepsakes and stories. The child can consider asking others to contribute and thereby make it more of a family venture. You can write down or have pictures of the person's favourite clothes, habits, hobbies, best times together, expressions, and nicest things when someone dies.

Key issues for the parent–child combined session are that both parent and child need to receive praise for the effort and progress of their work. Each party needs to be debriefed after the joint session, and you need to evaluate whether further therapy is required. There are certain questions you can ask the child at the end of therapy to help them solidify what they have learned. (1) What would you tell another child who lost a parent, about what you learned? What would you want them to know? (2) What would you say if they thought therapy would be too hard? (3) What do you think about yourself now?

It is important to begin anticipating loss reminders, i.e. future special events and how one can cope. You also need to tell the child it is OK to feel sad at those times and to make sure that parents and other adults support this as well. Finally, 'Dream Programming' is a simple but important technique for dealing with nightmares. The child (or adult) tells him- or herself that the recurrent nightmare will turn out differently. For example, instead of the car crashing there will be a near miss. Instead of someone hurting him or her, a rescuer will appear in time to save them.

Treatment of adolescents

As children grow into adolescence their therapy increasingly resembles that of adults and play therapy is replaced by talking. The basic principles remain the same.

Central to starting any treatment is helping to shape the meaning of the event for the person. If someone sees (perceives) a disaster as a rare event unlikely to be repeated they will do much better than if they now believe that the world is a dangerous place. If the individual believes that they are weak or going crazy, they will do much less well than if they believe that they are having a normal reaction to a very abnormal situation. Correcting such perceptions and reassuring children about these issues can make an immediate difference. Helping the individual to reduce their overall stress and providing support from family and friends is also very important. Once this is done, the central part of therapy is to help the person decrease the pain attached to thinking about the traumatic event. The process of doing this is for the person to retell the story of the trauma. By going through it and seeing that they can handle it, the fear decreases. Some researchers suggest that you go through it a couple of times and then talk about how the experience has affected them (Resick et al. 1992, 2002).

Edna Foa's group has the patient go through the trauma many times and focuses overwhelmingly on the therapeutic aspect of retelling the story (Keene et al. 2004; Foa and Rothbaum 2004). Foa's technique involves having the person learn a relaxation technique and then tell the story with his or her eyes closed and using the present tense to speak about the event. This increases the intensity of the experience. If it is too intense the person is asked to keep their eyes open or use the past tense. Every minute or so the therapist ask the patient what their SUDs level (subjective units of distress) is. A scale from 0 to 100 is generally used. This helps the therapist know when to ask the person to take a moment to do deep breathing and relax and to know what aspects of the trauma are most painful to think about. They will review these 'hot spots' many times. Their experience is that most people get considerable benefit. Some people have a very hard time for the first two weeks, having an increase in symptoms. In the long run, however, they do just as well as those who experience an immediate reduction in symptoms.

References

Cloitre, M., Koenen K. C., Cohen, L. R. and Han, H. J. (2002) 'Skills training in affective and interpersonal regulation followed by exposure: a phase-based treatment for PTSD related to childhood abuse'. *Journal of Consulting and Clinical Psychology*, 70(5): 1067–74.

Cloitre, M., Chase Stovall-McClough, K., Miranda, R. and Chemtob, C. M. (2004) 'Therapeutic alliance, negative mood regulation, and treatment outcome in child abuse-related posttraumatic stress disorder'. *Journal of Consulting and Clinical Psychology*, 72(3): 411–16.

Cohen, J. A. (2002) *Treating Trauma in Children and Adolescents*. Newbury Park, CA: Sage.

Deblinger, E. and Heflin, A. H. (1996) *Treating Sexually Abused Children and Their Nonoffending Parents: a Cognitive Behavioural Approach*. Newbury Park, CA: Sage.

Foa, E. B. and Rothbaum, B. O. (2004) *Treating the Trauma of Rape: Cognitive-Behavioural Therapy for PTSD*. New York: Guilford Publications, Inc.

Freud, A. and Burlingham, D. (1943) *War and Children*. New York: Ernest Willard.

Friedberg, R. D., McClure, J. M. and McClure, Jessica (2002) *Clinical Practice of Cognitive Therapy with Children and Adolescents: the Nuts and Bolts*. New York: Guilford Press.

Grant, A., Mills, J., Mulhern, R. and Short, N. (2004) *Cogntive Behavioural Therapy in Mental Health Care*. London: Sage.

Janis, I. (1951) *Air War and Emotional Stress*. New York: McGraw-Hill.

Keane, M., Foa, E. and Friedman, M. J. (eds) (2004) *Effective Treatments for PTSD: Practice Guidelines from the International Society for Traumatic Stress Studies*. New York: Guilford Publications, Inc.

Laor, N., Wolmer, L., Mayes, L. C., Gershon, A., Weizman, R. and D. J. Cohen (1997). 'Israeli preschool children under Scuds: a 30-month follow-up'. *Journal of the American Academy of Child and Adolescent Psychiatry*, 36(3): 349–56.

Resick P. A. and Schnicke M. K. (1992) 'Cognitive processing therapy for sexual assault victims'. *Journal of Consulting and Clinical Psychology*, 60: 748–56.

Resick, P. A. and Schnicke, M. K. (1993) *Cognitive Processing Therapy for Rape Victims: a Treatment Manual*, Vol. 4. London: Sage.

Resick, P. A., Nishith, P., Weaver, T. L., Astin, M. C. and Feuer, C. A. (2002) 'A comparison of cognitive-processing therapy with prolonged exposure and a waiting condition for the treatment of chronic posttraumatic stress disorder in female rape victims'. *Journal of Consulting and Clinical Psychology*, 70(4): 867–79.

Resick, P. A., Nishith, P. and Griffin, M. G. (2003) 'How well does cognitive-behavioural therapy treat symptoms of complex PTSD? An examination of child sexual abuse survivors within a clinical trial'. *CNS Spectrums*, 8(5): 340–55.

Taylor, T. L. and Chemtob, C. M. (2004) 'Efficacy of treatment for child and adolescent traumatic stress'. *Archives of Pediatric Adolescent Medicine*, 158(8): 786–91.

Van der Kolk, B. A. (2003) 'The neurobiology of childhood trauma and abuse'. *Journal of the American Academy of Child and Adolescent Psychiatry*, 12(2): 293–317.

Van der Kolk, B. A., McFarlane, A. C. and Weisaeth, Lars (eds) (1996) *Traumatic Stress: the Effects of Overwhelming Experience on Mind, Body, and Society*. New York: Guilford Publications.

Ziv, A. and Israel, R. (1973) 'Effects of bombardment on the manifest anxiety level of children living in kibbutzim'. *Journal of Consulting and Clinical Psychology*, 40: 287–91.

7
Responding to Traumatized Children: a Psychopharmacological Focused Treatment Approach

Iyad Khreis and Rula Khreis

Introduction

This chapter will describe the current pharmacological treatment of Post-Traumatic Stress Disorder (PTSD) and the classes of pharmacologic agents used in such treatment. However, pharmacotherapy for PTSD with co-occurring psychiatric disorders will also be highlighted and discussed.

It has been suggested that multiple biological changes have been found among individuals diagnosed with full-blown PTSD. These include adrenergic hyper-responsiveness (Southwick et al. 1999), increased thyroid activity (Wang et al. 1995), increased levels of corticotrophin-releasing factor (Baker et al. 1999), and low cortisol levels with increased negative feedback sensitivity of the hypothalamic-pituitary-adrenal axis after the administration of low-dosage dexamethasone (Yehuda et al. 1993). The biological changes enhance memory over consolidation and classical conditioning of triggers, thereby influencing the development and perpetuation of PTSD (Orr et al. 2000). Here are some examples of pharmacotherapy used in PTSD.

Anti-psychotics

While conventional and atypical anti-psychotic agents have not been used to treat patients with PTSD, in cases where PTSD is co-occurring with psychosis, anti-psychotics have been proven to be useful. In extreme cases of PTSD, with disorganized behaviour and distinct dissociative symptoms, low doses of anti-psychotic drugs could be helpful. Anti-psychotics could also be useful in instances of rage, aggressive or violent behaviour. The three anti-psychotics that will be discussed are risperidone, olanzapine and quetiapine.

Risperidone is an anti-psychotic with D_2 and $5HT_2$ antagonism effects, and it was first noted to help with PTSD-associated flashbacks and nightmares (Schoenfeld et al. 2004; Krashin and Oates 1999). Monnelly et al. (2003) studied risperidone as an adjunctive treatment in a six-week double-blind controlled study of 15 patients with combat-related PTSD. The subjects received either risperidone (0.5 mg/day; N = 7) or matched placebo (n = 8) tablets during the first two weeks of the treatment period, with an increase of risperidone dosage up to 2.0 mg/day on the bases of response thereafter. The outcome measures used were the Patient Checklist of PTSD-Military Version (PCL-M) and the Overt Aggression Scale-Modified for Outpatients (OAS-M). There was significant improvement in irritability (OAS-M), total PTSD symptoms and intrusive thoughts (PCL-M). Risperidone has also been used among patients with PTSD and comorbid psychotic symptoms. In a five-week, prospective, randomized, double-blind, placebo-controlled trial, risperidone was prescribed as an adjunctive treatment among 40 combat veterans with PTSD (Hamner et al. 2003). This study used the Positive and Negative Syndrome Scale (PANSS). A reduction in PANSS scores was noted among those patients who had received risperidone, compared to those who had received the placebo. There was also a trend towards greater improvement relative to placebo. These studies on risperidone suggest that the drug could be helpful in treating some of the core symptoms of PTSD as well as associated psychotic symptoms.

In contrast, olanzapine as an atypical anti-psychotic with serotonergic properties was studied in an open clinical trial among 48 veterans with a diagnosis of combat-related PTSD (Petty et al. 2001). It was found that olanzapine was effective in alleviating all three symptom clusters of PTSD, demonstrating a 30 per cent reduction in the overall scores. In another study, Butterfield et al. (2001) found no differences between group and relief of PTSD symptoms. In this study, a high placebo-response rate was observed: symptom reduction rates from the active treatment group and placebo group were comparable to that in other active drug treatment trials. Stein et al. (2002) tested adjunctive olanzapine for SSRI-resistant combat-related PTSD in a double-blind placebo-controlled study. They found that olanzapine was associated with reduced PTSD symptoms when used as an adjunctive treatment for PTSD with associated depression and sleep problems that hadn't responded well to an SSRI previously. Olanzapine also improved depression and sleep disturbance.

In addition to its dopamine (D_2) blocking effect, quetiapine is an anti-psychotic that antagonizes α_1-adrenergic, 5-HT_{2A}, and histamine

(H_1). Such characteristics of quetiapine indicate that the drug could be helpful for PTSD sleep disturbances and overall PTSD symptoms. In a retrospective study on quetiapine for treatment of refractory symptoms of combat-related PTSD, 68 veterans were receiving low-dosage quetiapine as an adjunctive treatment after failure to respond to at least two psychotropic agents (Sokolski et al. 2003). The effectiveness of quetiapine was observed by the proportion of patients who were much or very much improved in one or more of the *DSM-IV* criterion symptoms of PTSD: criterion B for re-experiencing, 35 per cent; criterion C for avoidance/numbing, 28 per cent; and criterion D for arousal, 65 per cent of the study subjects. Low doses of quetiapine were associated with minimal side-effects. Such data, while retrospective, suggest that augmentative quetiapine could benefit some refractory symptoms of PTSD in combat veterans. For 62 per cent of the patients sleep disturbance improved, and nightmares improved among 25 per cent. In an open trial of adjunctive therapy, quetiapine was studied in a six-week open clinical trial among 20 veterans diagnosed with combat-related PTSD (Hamner et al. 2003). Studies of atypical anti-psychotic agents suggest that they are beneficial for patients with severe and treatment-resistant PTSD.

The selective serotonin re-uptake inhibitors or (SSRIs)

Anti-depressants are the pharmacologic treatment of choice for PTSD, mainly because of their effectiveness. Selective serotonin re-uptake inhibitors sertraline and paroxetine in large-scale, well-designed, placebo-controlled trials became the first medications to receive approval from the US Food and Drug Administration for the treatment of PTSD. Selective serotonin re-uptake inhibitors are the most carefully studied medications and are currently the most frequently prescribed agents for the treatment of PTSD. Open-label and double-blind trials of sertraline (Brady et al. 2000; Marshall et al. 2001; Zohar et al. 2002), paroxetine (Marshall et al. 2001), fluoxetine (Van der Kolk et al. 1994), fluvoxamine (Marmar et al. 1996), and citalopram (Seedat et al. 2002) have established SSRIs as the pharmacologic treatment of choice for PTSD. In an open trial Goddard et al. (1993) concluded that fluvoxamine was effective for treating core intrusion, avoidance and arousal symptoms of PTSD. The study of the 'Efficacy and safety of paroxetine treatment for chronic PTSD' carried out by Marshal and his group showed significantly greater improvement on primary outcome measures compared to placebo-treated patients. The study by Marshall et al.

Figure 7.1

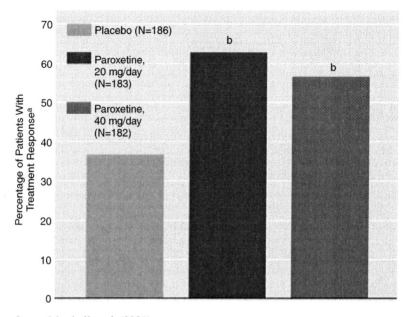

Source: Marshall et al. (2001).

(2001) concluded that doses of 20 and 40 mg/day of paroxetine are effective and well tolerated in the treatment of adults with chronic PTSD.

Figure 7.1 displays response to treatment of patients with chronic PTSD who were given either placebo or paroxetine, and a significant difference between 20 mg/day of paroxetine and placebo (χ^2=24.39, df=1, p<0.001) and 40 mg/day of paroxetine and placebo (χ^2=14.26, df=1, p<0.001).

Kathleen Brady and her group (2000) studied the efficacy and safety of sertraline treatment of PTSD in a randomized controlled trial. Patients studied were randomized to acute treatment with sertraline hydrochloride with flexible daily dosages of 50 to 200 mg/d, this following one week at 25 mg/d (n = 94); or placebo (n = 93). The main measures used were Impact of Event Scale total score (IES), and Clinical Global Impression-Severity (CGI-S), and CGI-Improvement (CGI-I) ratings, compared by treatment vs. placebo groups. Sertraline treatment yielded significantly greater improvement than placebo on three of the four primary outcome measures. The authors concluded that sertraline is a safe, well-tolerated and effective treatment for PTSD.

Tricyclic anti-depressants and monoamine oxidase inhibitors

The first anti-depressants used for the treatment of PTSD, tricyclic anti-depressants and monoamine oxidase inhibitors (MAOIs), have shown to have an anti-panic effect. It is their anti-panic affect and the parallel between such panic attacks and severe PTSD arousal responses that has increased the studies conducted. Amitriptyline, imipramine, and desipramine are all tricyclic anti-depressants that have been tested in controlled clinical trials using small samples. For the most part, there was a modest symptom improvement from imipramine, with an effect size of 0.25 (Frank et al. 1988). There was moderate improvement from amitriptyline (effect size, 0.64) (Davidson et al. 1990); however, no benefit from desipramine was reported (effect size, 0.05) (Reist et al. 1989). Tricyclic anti-depressants are not commonly used, mostly due to their ineffectiveness in reducing avoidance and numbing.

Like tricyclic anti-depressants, MAOIs have anti-panic activity and they have been successfully used to treat mixed states of anxiety and depression. Actually, in a review by Southwick et al. (1994), it was found that MAOIs were more effective when compared to tricyclics for the treatment of PTSD. Among all the MAOIs, phenelzine has been the most commonly studied and used. Because of their associated risk of hypertensive crisis, MAOIs must be used with caution. Reversible MAOIs have shown a smaller risk of hypertensive crisis. In an open-label trial, Neal et al. (1997) reported that moclobemide, a reversible MAO-A inhibitor, was associated with reduced symptoms in the three symptom categories that make up the PTSD diagnosis.

Novel anti-depressants

Nefazodone and trazodone both exhibit 5-HT_2 and α_1-adrenergic receptor antagonist activity. In a review of anti-depressant-induced sexual dysfunction, Gregorian and colleagues (2002) found that nefazodone, along with bupropion, appeared to be much less likely to cause sexual dysfunction. In a review of six open-label trials studying the effects of nefazodone on over 105 PTSD patients, the drug was found to reduce nightmares, generalized anxiety, as well as global ratings of PTSD (Hidalgo et al. 1999). Three different criteria were used for assessing response rates: the effect of nefazodone on each PTSD cluster, individually, and finally, variables that might predict response. On the basis of the criteria of a 30 per cent, 40 per cent, and 50 per cent drop in severity of symptoms, the following response rates were revealed: 46 per cent, 34 per cent, and 26 per cent respectively. As in the case with SSRIs, the response was better among patients who had experienced civilian trauma than those patients who had experienced combat-related trauma.

In a six-week study of 11 patients with PTSD, treatment with nefazodone suggested that it might be useful for PTSD-related sleep disturbance (Mellman et al. 1999). When treated with nefazodone, patients experienced an increased number of sleep hours and reduced intensity and qualitative features of dream recalls. The black box warning of nefazodone is due to its association with an increased risk of hepatotoxicity and even liver failure. Thus, nefazodone treatment shouldn't be initiated in cases of active liver disease or elevated serum transaminase concentrations. Because of its highly sedating strength, trazodone is difficult to tolerate at a full anti-depressant dosage. While trazodone has not proven to be significantly effective for treating core symptoms of PTSD (Herzberg et al. 1996), it can reverse insomnia that is sometimes caused by SSRIs such as fluoxetine and sertraline. Thus, an SSRI along with a lower dosage of trazodone at bedtime has become a widely used combination for treatment of chronic PTSD.

Venlafaxine, another novel anti-depressant, enhances the activity of serotonin, norepinehphrine, and, to a lesser extent, dopamine transmission. In an open clinical trial among Bosnian refugees, venlafaxine, sertraline and paroxetine were studied. Venlafaxine was associated with statistically significant improvement in total PTSD symptoms severity and Global Assessment of Functioning among five of the 13 patients (Smajkic et al. 2001). For major depression, venlafaxine did not improve symptoms significantly. Side-effects led to eight patients of the 13 dropping out of treatment. The patients who had received sertraline and paroxetine exhibited a more robust reduction in PTSD symptoms, and none of these patients dropped out of treatment. Interestingly, all of the study patients still met the diagnostic criteria at the end of the six-week study.

The novel anti-depressant mirtazapine enhances serotonin and noradrenergic neurotransmission. In a placebo-controlled double-blind pilot study, 29 patients were randomized to receive up to 45 mg/day of mirtazapine or placebo double-blind on a 2:1 ratio for a period of

8 weeks (Davidson et al. 2003; Butterfield et al. 2001). The primary PTSD outcome measure was the Short PTSD Rating Interview, in which much or very much improved was considered as a good response. The patients who had received mirtazapine had a 65 per cent response rate, compared with 22 per cent for those who received placebo. The treatment effect size for this study was at 0.49. Because of the small sample in this study though, the estimate of treatment effect is imprecise. Mirtazapine was found to be helpful for anxiety as measured by the Hospital Anxiety and Depression scale, with a strong effect size of 1.14. For the most part, mirtazapine was well tolerated. The drug shows promise as an effective form of treatment, especially for those patients with comorbid anxiety disorders.

While the mechanism of bupropion's anti-depressant effect has not yet been elucidated, it is perceived to have a weak norepinephrine re-uptake blocking effect and even come capacity to block the re-uptake of dopamine. In an open clinical six-week trial of bupropion among 17 combat veterans with PTSD (Canive et al. 1998), the blindly rated outcome measures included the following: the Clinician Administered PTSD Scale (CAPS), the Hamilton Rating Scale for Depression (HAM-D), the Hamilton Rating Scale for Anxiety (HAM-A) and the CGI-I. Fourteen of the original 17 patients completed the study. Among these, ten were rated as responders as measured by the CGI-I and the HAM-D. While there were reductions in CAPS and HAM-A, the changes were statistically insignificant. Symptoms of intrusion were noted to be unresponsive to bupropion in this study. These studies indicate that bupropion is well tolerated, but perhaps it is more helpful for depressive symptoms than PTSD symptoms.

Mood-stabilizing and anti-kindling agents

One theoretical model for explaining the development of PTSD is based on sensitization and kindling of the limbic system (Grillon et al. 1996). Sensitization is observed as an enhanced physiologic response after repeated exposure to a stimulus. This leads to kindling, a spontaneous discharge. The amygdale and hippocampus, both limbic structures, have a low threshold for sensitization and kindling. This decreased threshold leads to increased physiologic reactivity observed among patients with PTSD. Other symptoms of sensitization and kindling include spontaneous intrusive imagery and flashbacks.

Similar to anti-adrenergic medications, anti-kindling and mood-stabilizing agents have suggested a potential to prevent sensitization and kindling from developing in the hours and days immediately after exposure to a traumatic event. The following anti-adrenergic drugs have been used in clinical trials to treat PTSD: carbamazepine, valproate, topiramate, lamotrigine, lithium, and gabapentin.

Useful in treating seizure disorders of the temporal lobe, carbamazepine has strong anti-kindling qualities. In several studies, carbamazepine was associated with reductions in intrusive traumatic memories and flashbacks as well as improvements in insomnia, irritability, impulsivity, and violent behaviour (Lipper et al. 1986; Keck et al. 1992).

In terms of potency, valproate has a less potent anti-kindling action when compared to carbamazepine. An open clinical trial of valproate was studied in 16 Vietnam veterans diagnosed with combat-related PTSD. Of the 16 patients treated with valproate, ten showed significant improvement, especially in hyper-arousal/hyperactivity and avoidance symptoms but no improvement in intrusion (Fesler 1991). Topiramate is an anti-convulsant but with GABA enhancement as its mechanism of action. In an open trial of 35 patients with chronic PTSD who were unresponsive to previous pharmacology, Berlant and van Kammen found that topiramate administered alone or as adjunctive treatment was associated with reductions in PTSD symptoms including severe nightmares (Berlant and van Kammen 2002).

Gabapentin is an anti-convulsant that is structurally comparable to GABA; however, its mechanism of action is still unknown. Gabapentin doesn't appear to have a risk of serious side-effects and toxicity that is evident with other anti-kindling agents. In a review of gabapentin as adjunctive therapy for PTSD, the drug was found to be helpful for insomnia and reduced the frequency of nightmares (Hamner et al. 2001).

Lamotrigine is a glutamate-inhibiting anti-convulsant. In a three-month double-blind controlled trial among 15 PTSD patients, five of the ten prescribed with lamotrigine were treatment responders, while only one of the four placebo recipients responded to treatment (Hertzberg et al. 1999). In this study though, the small sample size makes the findings statistically insignificant. Furthermore, because of its association with risks of serious rashes, prescribing lamotrigine should be done cautiously.

Lithium is a mood stabilizer and it has a well-established efficacy for treating recurrent affective disorders. Its mechanism of action is complex and includes alteration of serotonin transport. In two small open trials, a total of 27 patients were treated for PTSD using lithium. Both trials showed an improvement in the arousal cluster symptoms (Van der Kolk, 1991; Kitchner and Greenstein 1983). Studies also suggest that adding lithium to a standard drug regimen could be helpful in reducing anger and irritability among patients with PTSD (Forster et al. 1995).

Adrenergic-inhibiting agents

Several studies have indicated that during sustained periods of increased adrenergic activity there is a greater risk for PTSD. The link between adrenergic agents such as norepinephrine and the over-consolidation of memories of a traumatic event has led researchers to find effective adrenergic-inhibiting agents for immediate treatment after a severe traumatic event (Pitman 1989). One such agent is propranolol.

In a pilot study of secondary prevention of PTSD, Pitman et al. assigned 41 trauma victims to a ten-day course of either propranolol or a placebo within six hours of a traumatic event (Pitman et al. 2002). This was a double-blind controlled trial. Within one month, 18 per cent of the patients who had received propranolol met the criteria for PTSD. On the other hand, 30 per cent of those patients who received a placebo met the criteria for PTSD. After a three-month period, no significant differences were observed between the two groups: 13 per cent of the patients who received propranolol and 11 per cent of those who received placebo met the criteria for PTSD. Also at three months, none of the patients who had received propranolol were physiologic responders to reminders of the trauma, while 43 per cent of those who had received placebo were physiologic responders.

In a non-randomized contrast group study by Vaiva et al., the efficacy of propranolol shortly after trauma exposure was tested (Vaiva et al. 2003). Eleven young adult trauma victims were given 40 mg of propranolol three times daily for one week, followed by a taper period of 8–12 days. These eleven patients were compared to eight patients who agreed to participate in the study, but refused propranolol. Both of these groups had similar demographics, exposure characteristics, physical injury severity, and peritraumatic emotional responses. Vaiva found that PTSD rates were higher in the group that refused propranolol (3/8) compared with those who had received propranolol. These results, as well as the results from the Pitman study, suggest that propranolol could be beneficial for mitigating PTSD symptoms and perhaps even preventing the development of PTSD.

By regulating adrenergic activity both at the central and peripheral level, adrenergic-inhibiting agents such as β-adrenergic blockers and α_2-

adrenergic agonists could reduce anxious arousal symptoms among patients with chronic PTSD. In a 1988 Harvard study, Famularo and colleagues tested 11 children with PTSD who had been physically abused or sexually abused or both and presented in an agitated, hyper-aroused state (Famularo et al. 1988). Treatment with propranolol was conducted in an off-on-off design of four-week blocks with a two-week drug taper between trials. During treatment, significant improvement was noted, while there was an increase in symptoms before and after treatment. Of the 11 children, eight experienced significantly reduced re-experiencing and arousal symptoms when they were taking propranolol compared with those periods when they were not taking propranolol.

The effects of propranolol on adults with PTSD was studied in two small trials. One of these studies showed a reduction in trauma-related nightmares, intrusive memories, hypervigilance, startle response, and expressions of anger in nine Vietnam veterans (Kolb et al. 1984). The other study though, reported that propranolol wasn't helpful in a sample of Cambodian refugees with PTSD (Kinzie 1998).

Clonidine and guanfacine, alpha2-adrenergic receptor agonists, act at noradrenergic autoreceptors, inhibiting the firing of cells in the locus ceruleus which effectively reduces the release of brain norepinephrine (Kaplan and Sadock 1998). In a study of nine severely traumatized Cambodian refugees with PTSD, it was found that the global symptoms of PTSD were reduced among six of the nine patients, and nightmares were reduced among seven when treatment consisted of a combination of clonidine and imipramine (Kinzie and Leung 1989). In other studies, clonidine showed an improvement in disturbed behaviour by reducing aggression, impulsivity, emotional outbursts, oppositionality, insomnia and nightmares (Harmon and Riggs, 1996).

Guanfacine produces less sedation than clonidine and therefore it could be better tolerated. In a case report, guanfacine reduced the trauma-related nightmares of a child with PTSD (Horrigan and Barnhill 1996). A recent randomized double-blind trial looking at veteran patients with chronic PTSD showed that augmentation with guanfacine (N = 29) was associated with no significant improvement in PTSD symptoms, mood, or subjective sleep quality when compared with placebo (N = 34).

Prazosin, alpha1-receptor antagonists was studied for its efficacy for treating PTSD among ten Vietnam combat veterans in a 20-week double-blind crossover protocol with a two-week drug washout to allow for return to baseline (Raskind et al. 2003). The primary outcome measures used were the Clinician Administered PTSD Scale (CAPS) and the Clinical Global Impressions-Change Scale (CGI-C). Prazosin was prescribed with a mean dose of 9.5 mg a day at bedtime and was superior to the placebo for the outcome measures. An improvement in re-experiencing, avoidance/numbing, and hyper-arousal was also noted. This study further supports the efficacy of prazosin for nightmares, sleep disturbance, and other PTSD symptoms.

Anti-anxiety agents

Benzodiazepines enhance the effects of γ-aminobutyric acid (GABA). The most common receptor in the brain which acts to inhibit activation of most neurons is the GABA-A receptor. Benzodiazepines act by reducing activity of the site of norepinephrine cell bodies in the brain, the central nucleus of the amygdale (the fear centre of the brain), as well as the locus ceruleus. Based on their structural functionality, it would seem that benzodiazepines would be a good choice for the treatment of PTSD, and often, these anti-anxiety agents are used for the treatment of PTSD. However, results of the few small studies on these agents suggest that there is limited value for treatment of the core symptoms of PTSD (Schoenfeld et al. 2004).

In a non-randomized prospective study on the treatment of recent trauma survivors with benzodiazepines it was found that the 13 patients who received benzodiazepine didn't experience fewer symptoms of PTSD compared to the 13 control subjects (Gelpin et al. 1996). After a period of six months, a follow-up indicated a trend towards higher rates of PTSD. One explanation for this is that benzodiazepines interfere with the normal ability to desensitize conditioned fear responses to trauma cues, this occurring by an alteration of optimal levels of working anxiety needed for desensitization or even by interfering with cognitive processing. For a more accurate analysis of the usefulness of benzodiazepines as an early treatment intervention, larger samples are needed.

In a randomized, double-blind crossover trial of 16 patients with chronic PTSD, the efficacy of alprazolam was tested (Braun et al. 1990). A two-week drug washout allowed for patients to return to baseline before entering the second phase of the study. The primary outcome measures in this study were: a 12-question PTSD scale, the Impact of Events sale, HAM-D, and the HAM-A. After five weeks of treatment, alprazolam was associated with a moderate effect on anxiety symptoms when compared to placebo (effect size, 0.7). Statistically significant reduction of intrusion or of numbing and avoidance was not observed.

This study also had a high dropout rate: three of the seven patients receiving alprazolam and three of the nine who received placebo did not complete the study.

Risse et al. found the presence of severe withdrawal symptoms after discontinuation of alprazolam in eight patients with combat-induced PTSD (Risse et al. 1990). All of the patients had a history of alcohol abuse or benzodiazepine dependence. The findings of this study support the concern of the risks of dependence with alprazolam. Perhaps sustained-released formulations using the drug would prove safer and more effective.

Buspirone acts as a 5-HT1A receptor against and is used to treat anxiety disorders. Buspirone has a low potential for abuse and withdrawal symptoms when compared to benzodiazepines. Furthermore, there are few studies looking at the efficacy of buspirone when treating patients with PTSD. In a small open trial looking at the efficacy of buspirone in the treatment of PTSD in eight Vietnam veterans, Duffy and Malloy (1994) found that buspirone was associated with significant improvements in re-experiencing, avoidance, and intrusion scores on the subscales of the Structured Interview for PTSD. While buspirone could be a safe and effective alternative to benzodiazepines in treating PTSD, its effectiveness remains to be established.

References

Baker, D. G., West, S. A., Nicholson, W. E. et al. (1999) 'Serial CSF corticotropin-releasing hormone levels and adrenocortical activity in combat veterans with posttraumatic stress disorder'. *American Journal of Psychiatry,* 156: 585–8.

Berlant, J. and van Kammen, D. P. (2002) 'Open-label topiramate as primary or adjunctive therapy in chronic civilian posttraumatic stress disorder: a preliminary report'. *Journal of Clinical Psychiatry,* 63: 15–20.

Brady, K., Pearlstein, T., Asnis, G. M. et al. (2000) 'Efficacy and safety of sertraline treatment of posttraumatic stress disorder: a randomized controlled trial'. *Journal of the American Medical Association,* 283: 1837–44.

Braun, P., Greenberg, D., Dasberg, H. et al. (1990) 'Core symptoms of posttraumatic stress disorder unimproved by alprazolam treatment'. *Journal of Clinical Psychiatry,* 51: 236–8.

Butterfield, M. I., Becker, M. E., Connor, K. M. et al. (2001) 'Olanzapine in the treatment of post-traumatic stress disorder: a pilot study'. *International Clinical Psychopharmacology,* 16: 197–203.

Canive, J. M., Clark, R. D., Calais, L. A. et al. (1998) 'Bupropion treatment in veterans with posttraumatic stress disorder: an open study'. *Journal of Clinical Psychopharmacology,* 18: 379–83.

Davidson, J. R., Kudler, H. S., Smith, R. et al. (1990) 'Treatment of posttraumatic stress disorder with amitriptyline and placebo'. *Archives of General Psychiatry,* 47: 259–66.

Davidson, J. R., Weisler, R. H., Butterfield, M. I. et al. (2003) 'Mirtazapine vs placebo in posttraumatic stress disorder: a pilot trial'. *Biological Psychiatry,* 53: 188–91.

Duffy, J. D. and Malloy, P. F. (1994) 'Efficacy of buspirone in the treatment of posttraumatic stress disorder: an open trial'. *Annals of Clinical Psychiatry,* 6: 33–7.

Famularo, R., Kinscherff, R. and Fenton, T. (1988) 'Propranolol treatment for childhood posttraumatic stress disorder, acute type: a pilot study'. *American Journal of Diseases of Children,* 142: 1244–7.

Fesler, F. A. (1991) 'Valproate in combat-related posttraumatic stress disorder'. *Journal of Clinical Psychiatry,* 52: 361–4.

Forster, P. L., Schoenfeld, F. B., Marmar, C. R. et al. (1995) 'Lithium for irritability in post-traumatic stress disorder'. *Journal of Traumatic Stress,* 8: 143–9.

Frank, J. B., Kosten, T., Giller, E. L. Jr et al. (1988) 'A randomized clinical trial of phenylzine and imipramine for posttraumatic stress disorder'. *American Journal of Psychiatry,* 145: 1289–91.

Gelpin, E., Bonne, O., Peri, T. et al. (1996) 'Treatment of recent trauma survivors with benzodiazepines: a prospective study'. *Journal of Clinical Psychiatry,* 57: 390–4.

Goddard, A. W., Woods, S. W., Sholomskas, D. E. et al. (1993) 'Effects of the serotonin reuptake inhibitor fluvoxamine on yohimbine-induced anxiety in panic disorder'. *Psychiatry Research,* 48: 119–33.

Gregorian, R. S., Golden, K. A., Bache, A. et al. (2002) 'Antidepressant-induced sexual dysfunction'. *Annals of Pharmacotherapy,* 36: 1577–89.

Grillon, C., Morgan, C. A., Southwick, S. M. et al. (1996) 'Baseline startle amplitude and prepulse inhibition in Vietnam veterans with posttraumatic stress disorder'. *Psychiatry Research,* 64: 169–78.

Hamner, M. B., Brodrick, P. S. and Labbate, L. A. (2001) 'Gabapentin in PTSD: a retrospective, clinical series of adjunctive therapy'. *Annals of Clinical Psychiatry,* 13: 141–6.

Hamner, M. B., Deitsch, S. E. and Brodrick, P. S. (2003) 'Quetiapine treatment in patients with posttraumatic stress disorder: an open adjunctive therapy'. *Journal of Clinical Psychopharmacology,* 23: 15–20.

Harmon, R. J. and Riggs, P. (1996) 'Clonidine for posttraumatic stress disorder in preschool children'. *Journal of the American Academy of Child and Adolescent Psychiatry,* 35: 1247–9.

Hertzberg, M. A., Butterfield, M. I., Feldman, M. E. et al. (1999) 'A preliminary study of lamotrigine for the treatment of posttraumatic stress disorder'. *Biological Psychiatry,* 45: 1226–9.

Hertzberg, M. A., Feldman, M. E., Beckham, J. C. et al. (1996) 'Trial of trazodone for posttraumatic stress disorder using a multiple baseline group design'. *Journal of Clinical Psychopharmacology,* 16: 294–8.

Hidalgo, R., Hertzberg, M. A., Mellman T. et al. (1999) 'Nefazodone in post-traumatic stress disorder: results from six open-label trials'. *International Clinical Psychopharmacology,* 14: 61–8.

Horrigan, J. P. and Barnhill, L. J. (1996) 'The suppression of nightmares with guanfacine'. *Journal of Clinical Psychiatry,* 57: 371.

Kaplan, H. I. and Sadock, B. (1998) *Synopsis of Psychiatry,* 8th edn. Baltimore: Lippincott Williams & Wilkins.

Keck, P. E. Jr, McElroy, S. L. and Friedman, L. M. (1992) 'Valproate and carbamazepine in the treatment of panic and posttraumatic stress disorders, withdrawal states, and behavioral dyscontrol syndrome'. *Journal of Clinical Psychopharmacology*, 12: 36S-41S.

Kinzie, J. D. (1998) 'Therapeutic approaches to traumatized Cambodian refugees'. *Journal of Traumatic Stress*, 2: 75–91.

Kinzie, J. D. and Leung, P. (1989) 'Clonidine in Cambodian patients with posttraumatic stress disorder'. *Journal of Nervous and Mental Disease*, 177: 546–50.

Kitchner, I. and Greenstein, R. (1983) 'Low-dose lithium carbonate in the treatment of posttraumatic stress disorder'. *Hospital and Community Psychiatry*, 34: 683–91.

Kolb, L. C., Burris, B. C. and Griffiths, S. (1984) 'Propranolol and clonidine in the treatment of the chronic post traumatic stress disorders of war', in *Post-Traumatic Stress Disorder: Psychological and Biological Sequelae*, ed, B. A. Van der Kolk. Washington DC: American Psychiatric Press.

Krashin, D. and Oates, E. W. (1999) 'Risperidone as an adjunct therapy for posttraumatic stress disorder'. *Military Medicine*, 164: 605–6.

Lipper, S., Davidson, J. R., Grady, T. A. et al. (1986) 'Preliminary study of carbamazepine in post-traumatic stress disorder'. *Psychosomatics*, 27: 849–54.

Marmar, C. R., Schoenfeld, F. B., Weiss, D. S. et al. (1996) 'Open trial of fluvoxamine treatment for combat-related posttraumatic stress disorder'. *Journal of Clinical Psychiatry*, 57(suppl. 8): 66–72.

Marshall, R. D., Beebe, K. L., Oldham, M. et al. (2001) 'Efficacy and safety of paroxetine treatment for chronic PTSD: a fixed-dose, placebo-controlled study'. *American Journal of Psychiatry*, 158: 1982–8.

Mellman, T. A., David, D. and Barza, L. (1999) 'Nefazodone treatment and dream reports in chronic PTSD'. *Depression and Anxiety*, 9: 146–8.

Monnelly, E. P., Ciraulo, D. A., Knapp, C. et al. (2003) 'Low-dose risperidone as adjunctive therapy for irritable aggression in posttraumatic stress disorder'. *Journal of Clinical Psychopharmacology*, 23: 193–6.

Neal, L. A., Shapland, W. and Fox, C. (1997) 'An open trial of moclobemide in the treatment of post-traumatic stress disorder'. *International Clinical Psychopharmacology*, 12: 231–7.

Orr, S. P., Metzger, L. J., Lasko, N. B. et al. (2000) 'De novo conditioning in trauma-exposed individuals with and without posttraumatic stress disorder'. *Journal of Abnormal Psychology*, 109: 290–8.

Petty, F., Brannan, S., Casada, J. et al. (2001) 'Olanzapine treatment for posttraumatic stress disorder: an open-label study'. *International Clinical Psychopharmacology*, 16: 331–7.

Pitman, R. K. (1989) 'Post-traumatic stress disorder, hormones, and memory'. *Biological Psychiatry*, 26: 221–3.

Pitman, R. K., Sanders, K. M., Zusman, R. M. et al. (2002) 'Pilot study of secondary prevention of posttraumatic stress disorder with propranolol'. *Biological Psychiatry*, 51: 189–92.

Raskind, M. A., Peskind, E. R., Kanter, E. D. et al. (2003) 'Reduction of nightmares and other PTSD symptoms in combat veterans by prazosin: a placebo controlled study'. *American Journal of Psychiatry*, 160: 371–3.

Reist, C., Kauffmann, C. D., Haier, R. J. et al. (1989) 'A controlled trial of desipramine in 18 men with posttraumatic stress disorder'. *American Journal of Psychiatry*, 146: 513–16.

Risse, S. C., Whitters, A., Burke, J. et al. (1990) 'Severe withdrawal symptoms after discontinuation of alprazolam in eight patients with combat-induced posttraumatic stress disorder'. *Journal of Clinical Psychiatry*, 51: 206–9.

Schoenfeld, F., Marmar, C. and Neylan, T. (2004) 'Current concepts in pharmacotherapy for posttraumatic stress disorder'. *Psychiatric Services*, 55: 519–31.

Seedat, S., Stein, D. J., Ziervogel, C. et al. (2002) 'Comparison of response to a selective serotonin reuptake inhibitor in children, adolescents, and adults with posttraumatic stress disorder'. *Journal of Child and Adolescent Psychopharmacology*, 12: 37–46.

Smajkic, A., Weine, S., Duric-Bijedic, Z. et al. (2001) 'Sertraline, paroxetine, and venlafaxine in refugee posttraumatic stress disorder with depression symptoms'. *Journal of Traumatic Stress*, 14: 445–52.

Sokolski, K. N., Denson, T. F., Lee, R. T. et al. (2003) 'Quetiapine for treatment of refractory symptoms of combat-related post-traumatic stress disorder'. *Military Medicine*, 168: 486–9.

Southwick, S., Paige, S., Morgan, C. et al. (1999) 'Neurotransmitter alterations in PTSD: catecholamines and serotonin'. *Seminars in Clinical Neuropsychiatry*, 4: 242–8.

Southwick, S. M., Yehuda, R., Giller, E. et al. (1994) 'Use of tricyclics and monoamine oxidase inhibitors in the treatment of post traumatic stress disorder: a quantitative review', in *Catecholamine Function in Post-Traumatic Stress Disorder: Emerging Concepts*, ed. M. M Murburg. Washington DC: American Psychiatric Press.

Stein, M. B., Kline, N. A. and Matloff, J. L. (2002) 'Adjunctive olanzapine for SSRI-resistant combat-related PTSD: a double-blind, placebo-controlled study'. *American Journal of Psychiatry*, 159: 1777–9.

Vaiva, G., Docrocq, F., Jezequel, K. et al. (1994) 'Immediate treatment with proparanolol decreases posttraumatic stress disorder two months after trauma'. *Biological Psychiatry*, 54: 947–9.

Van der Kolk, B. A. (1991) 'Psychopharmacological issues in posttraumatic stress disorder'. *American Journal of Psychiatry*, 148: 1086–7.

Van der Kolk, B. A. Dreyfuss, D., Michaels, M. et al. (1994) 'Fluoxetine in post-traumatic stress disorder'. *Journal of Clinical Psychiatry*, 55: 517–22.

Wang, S., Mason, J., Southwick, S. et al. (1995) 'Relationships between thyroid hormones and symptoms in combat-related posttraumatic stress disorder'. *Psychosomatic Medicine*, 57: 398–402.

Yehuda, R., Southwick, S. M., Krystal, J. H. et al. (1993) 'Enhanced suppression of cortisol following dexamethasone administration in posttraumatic stress disorder'. *American Journal of Psychiatry*, 150: 83–6.

Zohar, J., Amital, D., Miodownik, C. et al. (2002) 'Double-blind placebo-controlled pilot study of sertraline in military veterans with posttraumatic stress disorder'. *Journal of Clinical Psychopharmacology*, 22: 190–5.

8
Trauma, Resilience and Growth in Children and Adolescents

Stephen Joseph, Jacky Knibbs and Julie Hobbs

The topic of growth following trauma and adversity has become of increasing interest to researchers and practitioners in the last few years. In this chapter the research on growth in children and adolescents is reviewed. Growth has been observed following accidents, disasters, illness, and other trauma in children and adolescents. Trauma and adversity do not necessarily lead to a damaged life. There are important implications for the development of new positive psychology approaches to prevention, intervention and social policy.

A number of literatures, religions and philosophies throughout human history have conveyed the idea that suffering can provide a springboard to personal growth. However, it is only relatively recently that the topic of growth following trauma and adversity has become a focus for empirical research. The study of growth provides an alternative paradigm for the study of the effects of trauma on human functioning. This interest in growth is part of the wider movement in positive psychology. It is suggested by positive psychologists that in the past researchers and practitioners have overemphasized the understanding of psychological difficulties at the expense of understanding well-being and what makes life worth living. We should instead endeavour to understand the full spectrum of human experience. The study of growth following adversity provides a new positive psychological way of thinking about human response to trauma that is concerned with the full range of people's reactions to adversity.

The aims of the chapter are: first, to provide an overview of the field of growth following adversity; second, to review the empirical literature relating to children and adolescents; and third, to provide a theoretical discussion on the nature of growth in order to inform future research directions.

It is well established that many children in high risk environments achieve positive developmental outcomes despite adverse experiences (Garmezy 1984; Murphy and Moriarty 1976; Rutter 1979; Garmezy and Rutter 1983; Werner and Smith 1982). Individuals who achieve these better-than-expected outcomes have been labelled 'survivors', 'resilient', 'stress-resistant', and even 'invulnerable'. The study of resilience has emerged as a distinct domain of empirical and theoretical inquiry in developmental psychopathology (Sroufe and Rutter 1984; see Yates and Masten 2004 for a review). Although researchers in resilience emphasized the importance of strengths in individuals, families and communities, and ways of promoting positive psychological processes, the work was not as explicitly concerned with positive outcomes as opposed to the absence of negative outcomes as the new movement of positive psychology has espoused (Seligman and Csikszentmihalyi 2000). The topic of growth following adversity, however, is explicitly concerned with the development of positive functioning in relation to stress and trauma (Calhoun and Tedeschi 1999; Tedeschi and Calhoun 2004a; Tedeschi et al. 1998).

Growth following adversity

In the following section, we will provide a brief overview of the field of growth following adversity. Growth following trauma has been variously labelled as adversarial growth (Linley and Joseph 2004a), benefit-finding (Affleck and Tennen 1996; Tennen and Affleck 2002), flourishing (Ryff and Singer 1998), heightened existential awareness (Yalom and Lieberman 1991), perceived benefits (McMillen and Fisher 1998), positive by–products (McMillen and Cook 2003), positive changes (Joseph et al. 1993), positive meaning (Thompson 1985), post-traumatic growth (Tedeschi and Calhoun 1995 1996), quantum change (Miller and C'deBaca 1994), self-renewal (Jaffe 1985), stress-related growth (Park et al. 1996), thriving (Abraido-Lanza et al. 1998), and transformational coping (Aldwin 1994). These terms have been used interchangeably to refer to how stressful and traumatic events can sometimes serve as the impetus for a higher level of psychological functioning. Initially there was some debate over the validity of the concept of growth following adversity, with some commentators questioning whether it was anything more than positive illusion and self-deception. But there is now convincing empirical evidence that people often experience growth following trauma and adversity (see Linley and Joseph 2004a).

Three broad inter-related dimensions of growth have been discussed (Tedeschi and Calhoun 2004a; Tedeschi et al. 1998). First, relationships are enhanced in some way, for example, that people now value their friends and family more, and feel an increased compassion and altruism towards others. Second, people change their views of themselves in some way, for example, that they have a greater sense of personal resiliency, wisdom and strength, perhaps coupled with a greater acceptance of their vulnerabilities and limitations. Third, there are reports of changes in life philosophy, for example, finding a fresh appreciation for each new day, and renegotiating what really matters in the full realization that their life is finite, including possible changes in spiritual beliefs. There remains a need for factor analytic work in this area to confirm the structure of growth (see Joseph et al. 2005).

Prevalence varies between studies due to samples, contexts and methodological issues, but it would be expected that anywhere between 30 and 70 per cent of people may experience some aspect of growth following traumatic events (Linley and Joseph 2004a), although growth is not usually reported in the immediate aftermath but at some time later. Studies have reported benefits following a range of stressful and traumatic events, for example, bereavement, accidents and disasters, chronic and life-threatening illness, sexual, physical and emotional abuse in childhood, sexual assault, and war and conflict (see Linley and Joseph 2004a). Research has also begun to document the correlates and predictors of growth, with evidence pointing to the importance of stress-appraisal, coping and personality variables, with more optimistic, self-efficacious, extrovert and stable people, who use more spiritual, acceptant, and emotionally expressive and emotionally focused forms of coping being more likely to report benefits. Social support is thought to be important too (see Linley and Joseph 2004a, 2004b).

Also, growth may coexist with psychological distress. Statistical associations between measures of growth and distress can range from strongly positive to strongly negative. The relationship between growth and distress is complex. It has been suggested that the direction and strength of association between growth and distress depends on the extent to which the traumatic event has been emotionally processed. The prediction is that over time, as people emotionally process their experience, the direction of the association shifts from positive to negative. However, at this stage this suggestion remains speculative and a topic for further investigation, particularly using prospective studies (see Joseph et al. 2005a).

The above overview is based almost exclusively on work that has been conducted with adult populations. As interest in this topic of growth following adversity has developed, researchers have begun to ask whether what we know about growth also applies to children and adolescents (Aldwin and Sutton 1998). In the following section, the extant research with children and adolescents will be discussed.

Research with children and adolescents

There is much research documenting the negative effects of traumatic events on children and adolescents (see Yule et al. 1999). But it is not just highly traumatic events that can engender post-traumatic stress reactions in children and adolescents. Community research shows that around 80 per cent of adolescents experience at least one negative life-event, and of these around one-fifth develop moderate levels of post-traumatic stress (Joseph, Mynard and Mayall 2000). Thus, the negative effects of trauma and adversity are well documented.

But, as already mentioned, the idea that adversity in life can also serve as a springboard to greater personal growth is not new, and has been expressed throughout history by philosophers, poets and novelists. As the novelist Samuel Butler wrote in his semi-autiobiographical book, *The Way of All Flesh* (1984 [1903]: 327):

> In quiet, uneventful lives the changes internal and external are so small that there is little or no strain in the process of fusion and accommodation; in other lives there is great strain, but there is also great fusing and accommodating power; in others great strain with little accommodating power. A life will be successful or not according as the power of accommodation is equal to or unequal to the strain of the fusing and adjusting internal and external changes.

Research evidence supports the idea that it is often those whose lives are characterized by great strain that go on to success. It is established that trauma and adversity may provide the developmental antecedents of genius, creativity and leadership (Simonton 2000). For example, extensive empirical research on the eminent geniuses of history has shown them to have suffered much more troubled and traumatic experiences during their early childhood years (Simonton 1994), especially the loss of one or both parents (Eisenstadt 1978).

But it is only relatively recently that empirical studies have been published which focus specifically on the topic of growth in children and adolescents following trauma and adversity. Studies have reported growth following accidents (Salter and Stallard 2004), disaster (Cryder et al. in press), illness (Barakat et al. 2006), and other trauma (Horowitz et al. 1997; Milam et al. 2004). Thus, evidence is building that, as with adults, growth can occur in children and adolescents. But why is it that under adverse circumstances, some young people develop in a dysfunctional and damaged way, whereas others are able to thrive and to grow? We cannot yet answer this question authoritatively as research remains in its early stages, and there are three main directions for research.

First, there is a need to investigate whether growth is developmentally related. There is a need to investigate systematically growth across the age range. It is possible, as some have suggested, that growth following trauma may be developmentally related (Cohen et al. 1998). When age groups have been compared, there is the suggestion that older children are more likely to experience growth than younger children (Milam et al. 2004). This remains a topic for research, as do the factors that may serve to promote or impede the development of growth in children and adolescents.

Second, the relationship between growth and distress remains an important focus for investigation. Research with adolescents who survived cancer found that greater levels of post-traumatic stress were related to greater levels of growth (Barakat et al. 2005). Children affected by war who experienced greater post-traumatic stress scored higher on growth (Kuterovac Jagodic 2005). But, as noted above, there is a need for prospective studies. We might expect that in the short term there is a positive association between distress and growth, but how does this relationship evolve over time? We might predict that over time as growth develops, distress begins to diminish. We might also predict that greater levels of distress are predictive of greater levels of subsequent growth only up to a certain level of distress at which the person is overwhelmed by their experience and growth is impeded.

Third, there is a need to investigate the personality and social psychological factors that further impede or promote growth, and serve to mediate and moderate the relationship between distress and growth. It is likely that the factors that are known to foster resilience will also be important in predicting growth. For example: individual differences in locus of control and flexible coping strategies; warm, sensitive, and cohesive support from caregivers; nurturing teacher–child relationships, high quality educational environment; and a safe and protective community (see Yates and Masten 2004). It is likely that social resources are particularly important. Children affected by war who perceived themselves to have more social support scored higher on growth (Kuterovac Jagodic 2005). However, research is required to establish the role of these factors and their inter-relationship in predicting growth. Kilmer (2006) has described a model of growth in children which posits that the relationship between traumatic events and post-traumatic growth is mediated by perceived competency beliefs, appraisals, rumination and cognitive resources. Further theoretically driven research into the factors that promote and impede growth is necessary.

Growth in adults exposed to trauma in childhood and adolescence

A different line of investigation is whether events that are experienced in childhood and adolescence can serve as a springboard for growth in later life. Prospective studies are lacking, but retrospective accounts provide evidence that events that take place in childhood and adolescence can often be perceived by people as having provided the foundations for growth. Work has shown this with individuals who as children survived the Holocaust (Lev-Wiesel and Amir 2003), or who were abused emotionally or physically as children or adolescents (McMillen et al. 1995; Woodward and Joseph 2003).

The topic of growth is relatively new and for this reason idiographic approaches are useful. The study by Woodward and Joseph (2003) was a thematic analysis of transcripts obtained from 29 adults who had experienced sexual, physical or emotional abuse as children. The researchers were concerned with the turning points in peoples lives and how they were able to grow. Two important themes emerged.

First, Woodward and Joseph (2003) reported that respondents referred to or indicated some form of 'inner drive', which they felt was instrumental in enabling them to survive, seek meaning, and ultimately heal. For example, one participant had written:

> I know however much I wanted to die I had a massive will to live. Why else would I be alive after being sexually abused in every way possible ... why else could I be alive after being physically abused so often ... there was a part of me that they could never touch (Jane).

Second, participants had needs for validation, for liberation, for nurturance, for belonging, for mastery, for awakening and were able to make use of their life-experiences to meet their needs and to grow. Woodward and Joseph (2003) referred to these experiences as 'vehicles of change'. For example, Mary wrote about how having her own home had helped to nurture herself and to bring about change:

> Oh something else that has had a big impact is owning my own home. I bought my house about 18 months ago. It is a 3 bed mid-terrace with 3 floors (4 including the cellar) and a south facing yard at the back which produced some great sunflowers this summer! Having a home has given me a great sense of stability and security ... In a way I see it as a metaphor for my life. When I bought the property it was very run down and neglected. Every room needed total renovation ... It's while I'm fixing up my house. I'm fixing up myself too.

Whereas much of the empirical literature on growth focuses on dispositional aspects of the person, Woodward and Joseph's analyses also points towards the importance of the social environment. For Neil it was his wife and children who made such a difference first through their acceptance and then through their love:

> I was scared and I was alone. My ten feet concrete walls of hurt made sure no one ever came close enough to making me bleed pain again ... I was able to say to a friend 'I was abused'. I expected to be rejected but I was not ... She accepted me and did not reject me. I was able to trust and love someone else, she is the keystone that had been missing in my life. This keystone is the one crucial stone.

Qualitative studies are important in understanding the experience of growth from the perspective of the person themselves, and promise to be useful in the development of future constructs for empirical investigation. But there is also a need for further quantitative work in order to understand the correlates and predictors of growth. For example, does it make a difference in adults, such as those in the Woodward and Joseph study, at what age their trigger event was experienced? Again, the evidence is very limited. But, what the evidence suggests is that if the trigger event was experienced in adolescence compared to childhood, than growth is more likely (McMillen et al. 1995; Lev-Wiesel and Amir 2003; Oltjenbruns,1991). Social support appears to be important too (Lev-Wiesel and Amir 2003).

Theoretical development

Resilience researchers have often noted that self-righting tendencies are a central feature of all living organisms (see Yates and Masten 2004). Similarly, the person-centred approach to personality development suggests that there is a self-righting tendency, which is referred to as the 'actualizing tendency', and that this tendency will be facilitated or thwarted to the extent that the social environment is supportive. When this tendency is facilitated it will lead towards growth and optimal functioning (Rogers 1959 1963).

Drawing on person-centred personality theory, Joseph and Linley (2005) have proposed a theory of growth following adversity, 'organismic valuing theory', which states that human beings are active, growth-oriented organisms, and that they are naturally inclined to accommodate their psychological experiences into a unified sense of self, and realistic view of the world. Furthermore, cognitive accommodation processes require changes in meaning as significance, and this can be in either a negative or a positive direction. A person can accommodate new trauma-related information, for example, that random events happen in the world and that bad things can happen at any time, in one of two ways. This accommodation may be made in a negative direction (e.g. a depressogenic reaction of hopelessness and helplessness), or in a positive direction of meaning as significance (e.g. that life is to be lived more in the here and now). It is thought that it is human nature to be intrinsically motivated towards a positive accommodation of the new trauma-related information as opposed to a negative accommodation, insofar as an evolutionary psychology approach would suggest that this should be more adaptive (see Christopher 2004). However, although the theory says that people are intrinsically motivated towards positive accommodation, it requires the right social environment to support the process, otherwise the person is likely to negatively accommodate the experience instead.

As well as accommodation processes, which require the person to change their outlook on life in light of their experience, a more defensive reaction is cognitive assimilation. Cognitive assimilation is where the person appraises their experiences in such a way as to be consistent with their assumptive world. Thus, three cognitive outcomes to the psychological resolution of trauma-related difficulties are posited. First, that experiences can be assimilated (i.e. return to pre-trauma baseline), second, that experiences can be accommodated in a negative direction (i.e. psychopathology), and third, that experiences can be accommodated in a positive direction (i.e. growth). As an analogy, imagine a person is picking up the pieces of a shattered vase. He or she can attempt to put the vase back together exactly as it was (assimilation), but now the vase is more fragile, covered in fractures and held together with sticking tape. Alternatively, the pieces can be discarded and placed in the wastebin (negative accommodation) or used to build something new, perhaps part of a beautiful mosaic (positive accommodation). Growth, by definition, requires accommodation rather than assimilation.

The possibility of the three cognitive outcomes helps to resolve the question of why it is that previously traumatized people often appear to be more vulnerable rather than more resistant to the effects of future stressful and traumatic events. We expect that attempts at assimilation rather than accommodation are most common in practice. People who assimilate their experience thus maintain their pre-event assumptions despite the evidence to the contrary and thus would be expected to develop more rigid defences, which in turn leaves them at increased vulnerability for future development of post-traumatic stress. Accommodation, in contrast, is about a change in world-views in light of the new trauma-related information.

Although developed to provide a framework for understanding traumatic stress-related processes, organismic valuing theory might also provide a useful broader framework for understanding personality development. Organismic theory suggests that the assumptive world develops through a continual process of accommodation which, depending on the social environment, might be in a negative or a positive direction. For example, imagine a child exposed to repeated emotional abuse. Through gradual negative accommodation they could go on to develop personality problems, perhaps characterized by borderline personality disorder. Alternatively, through gradual positive accommodation, they could go on to become empathic and caring people. Theory suggests that it is the quality of the social environment that determines whether the child accommodates positive or negatively.

Thus, organismic valuing theory offers a way of understanding growth as a developmental process that is continuous, which is useful for understanding how some experiences affect the development of the assumptive world. However, it is also a theory of discontinuous change. The very young child is constantly needing to accommodate information in order to develop schematic structures to navigate the world. For most people, as the assumptive world becomes fixed, the person begins to engage with new person-environment encounters using the process of cognitive assimilation rather than cognitive accommodation. Thus, the assumptive world becomes fixed and rigid and prone to threat from incongruent information. Traumatic events can provide such incongruent information and thus serve to shatter the assumptive world, thus re-igniting the possibility of cognitive accommodation and the rebuilding of the assumptive world in either new positive or negative directions. Thus, growth can also appear as discontinuous, and as a result of a seismic shock.

This developmental perspective on growth requires empirical verification. In particular, there is a need to establish the theoretical premise that individuals are intrinsically motivated towards cognitive accommodation. There is also a need to establish the social-environmental conditions that influence the accommodation process to be in either a positive or negative direction.

Applications

Research in positive psychology is now beginning to focus on its applications (Linley and Joseph 2004b). The study of growth promises to have important applications for clinical, counselling and health psychologists (Calhoun and Tedeschi 1999; Tedeschi and Calhoun 2004b; Joseph and Linley, in press). The main implication of this work is simply that clinicians should be aware of the potential for positive change following stress and trauma. It is important to recognize that negative events in childhood and adolescence do not necessarily lead to a damaged life and that for some, their experiences can lead to positive change and growth. But it must also be recognized that adversity does not lead to positive change for everyone. Therefore clinicians need to be careful not to imply inadvertently that the person has in some way failed by not making more of their experience.

In recognizing the possibility of growth, we must be cautious not to imply to clients that there is anything inherently positive about their traumatic experiences. Calhoun and Tedeschi (1999: 366) suggest that in discussing growth with clients 'that it is important to use words that clearly locate the impetus for growth in the arena of struggle with the event, not the event itself'. Personal growth after trauma should be viewed as originating not from the event but from within the person themselves.

There remains a need for research into how to facilitate growth in young people. But, as community work into the effects of trauma on children and adolescents has shown, the experience of adversity is common and its effects more widespread than would be recognized just by consideration of those who come to the attention of health and social services. So, it is not just understanding how to foster resilience and facilitate growth in those already damaged that is important, there is also a need to develop the implications of this work into resilience and growth to wider social and community prevention programmes. The aim must be to ensure that society provides the right social environment to facilitate the self-righting tendency in children and adolescents in high risk environments and who have experienced adverse events.

Conclusion

The interest in growth following adversity can be seen as part of the wider positive psychology movement. Positive psychology is seen as a balance to mainstream psychology, which has been for too long overly concerned with the negative aspects of human experience. Alongside the resilience literature, the study of growth following adversity shows us that adverse experiences do not necessarily lead to a damaged life, but may serve as a springboard to a more fully functioning life. The recognition of this work promises to be important in trauma research and in the development of new positive psychology approaches to prevention, intervention and social policy.

References

Abraido-Lanza, A. F., Guier, C. and Colon, R. M. (1998) 'Psychological thriving among Latinas with chronic illness'. *Journal of Social Issues*, 5: 405–24.

Affleck, G. and Tennen, H. (1996) 'Construing benefits from adversity: adaptational significance and dispositional underpinnings'. *Journal of Personality*, 64: 899–922.

Aldwin, C. M. (1994) *Stress, Coping, and Development: an Integrative Perspective.* New York: Guilford.

Aldwin, C. M. and Sutton, K. J. (1988) 'A developmental perspective on posttraumatic growth', in R. G. Tedeschi, C. L. Park and L. G. Calhoun (eds), *Posttraumatic Growth: Positive Changes in the Aftermath of Crisis.* Mahwah, NJ: Lawrence Erlbaum, pp. 43–63.

Barakat, L. P., Alderfer, M. A. and Kazak, A. E. (2006) 'Posttraumatic growth in adolescent survivors of cancer and their mothers and fathers'. *Journal of Pediatric Psychology*, 31(4): 413–19.

Butler, S. (1984) *The Way of All Flesh.* Harmondsworth, UK: Penguin (Original work published 1903).

Calhoun, L. G. and Tedeschi, R. G. (1999) *Facilitating Posttraumatic Growth: a Clinician's Guide.* Mahwah, NJ: Lawrence Erlbaum.

Christopher, M. (2004) 'A broader view of trauma: a biopsychosocial-evolutionary view of the role of the traumatic stress response in the emergence of pathology and/or growth'. *Clinical Psychology Review*, 24: 75–98.

Cohen, L. H., Hettler, T. R. and Pane, N. (1998) 'Assessment of posttraumatic growth', in R. G. Tedeschi, C. L. Park and L. G. Calhoun (eds), *Posttraumatic Growth: Positive Changes in the Aftermath of Crisis*. Mahwah, NJ: Lawrence Erlbaum, pp, 23–42.

Cryder, C. H., Kilmer, R. P., Tedeschi, R. G. and Calhoun, L. G. (in press) 'An exploratory study of posttraumatic growth in children following a natural disaster'. *American Journal of Orthopsychiatry*.

Eisenstadt, J. M. (1978) 'Parental loss and genius'. *American Psychologist*, 33: 211–23.

Garmezy, N. (1984) 'Stress resistant children: the search for protective factors', in J. E. Stevenson (ed.), *Recent Research in Developmental Psychopathology*. Oxford: Pergamon Press, pp. 213–33.

Garmezy, N. (1994) 'Reflections and commentary on risk, resilience, and development', in R. Haggerty et al. (eds), *Stress, Risk and Resilience in Children and Adolescents: Processes, Mechanisms and Interventions*. New York: Cambridge University Press.

Garmezy, N. and Rutter, M. (1983) *Stress, Coping and Development in Children* New York: McGraw-Hill.

Horowitz, L. A., Loos, M. E. and Putnam, F. W. (1997) 'Perceived benefits of traumatic experiences in adolescent girls'. Paper presented at the 13th Annual meeting of the International Society for Traumatic Stress Studies, Montreal, Quebec, Canada.

Jaffe, D. T. (1985) 'Self-renewal: personal transformation following extreme trauma'. *Journal of Humanistic Psychology*, 25: 99–124.

Joseph, S. and Linley, P. A. (2005) 'Positive adjustment to threatening events: an organismic valuing theory of growth through adversity'. *Review of General Psychology*, 9: 262–80.

Joseph, S. and Linley, P. A. (in press) 'Growth following adversity: theoretical perspectives and implications for clinical practice'. *Clinical Psychology Review*.

Joseph, S., Linley, P. A., Andrews, L., Harris, G., Howle, B., Woodward, C. and Shevlin, M. (2005a) 'Assessing positive and negative changes in the aftermath of adversity: psychometric evaluation of the Changes in Outlook Questionnaire'. *Psychological Assessment*, 17: 70–80.

Joseph, S., Linley, P. A. and Harris, G. J. (2005) 'Understanding positive change following trauma and adversity: structural clarification'. *Journal of Loss and Trauma*, 10: 83–96.

Joseph, S., Mynard, H. and Mayall, M. (2000) 'Life-events and post-traumatic stress in a sample of English adolescents'. *Journal of Community and Applied Psychology*, 10: 475–82.

Joseph, S., Williams, R. and Yule, W. (1993) 'Changes in outlook following disaster: the preliminary development of a measure to assess positive and negative responses'. *Journal of Traumatic Stress,* 6: 271–9.

Kilmer, R. P. (2006) 'Resilience and posttraumatic growth in children', in L. G. Calhoun and R. G. Tedeschi (eds), *Handbook of Posttraumatic Growth: Research and Practice*. Mahwah, NJ: Lawrence Erlbaum Associates.

Kuterovac Jagodic, G. (2005) 'Posttraumatic attitudes, world assumptions and posttraumatic growth among war affected children'. Paper presented at 9th European conference on Traumatic Stress, Stockholm, 18–21 June.

Lev-Wiesel, R. and Amir, M. (2003) 'Posttrauamticgrowth among Holocaust child survivors'. *Journal of Loss and Trauma*, 8: 229–37.

Linley, P. A. and Joseph, S. (2004a) 'Positive change following trauma and adversity: a review'. *Journal of Traumatic Stress*, 17: 11–21.

Linley, P.A. and Joseph, S. (eds) (2004b) *Positive Psychology in Practice*. Hoboken, NJ: John Wiley & Sons, Inc.

McMillen, J. C. and Cook, C. L. (2003) 'The positive by-products of spinal cord injury and their correlates'. *Rehabilitation Psychology*, 48: 77–85.

McMillen, J. C. and Fisher, R. H. (1998) 'The perceived benefit scales: measuring perceived positive life changes after negative events'. *Social Work Research*, 22: 173–87.

McMillen, C., Zuravin, S. and Rideout, G. (1995) 'Perceived benefits from child sexual abuse'. *Journal of Consulting and Clinical Psychology*, 63: 1037–43.

Milam, J. E., Ritt-Olson, A. and Unger, J. (2004) 'Posttraumatic growth among adolescents'. *Journal of Adolescent Research*, 19: 192–204.

Miller, W. R. and C'deBaca, J. (1994) 'Quantum change: toward a psychology of transformation'. In T. F. Heatherton and J. L. Weinberger (eds), *Can Personality Change?*. Washington DC: American Psychological Association, pp. 253–81.

Murphy, L. B. and Moriarty, A. E. (1976) *Vulnerability, Coping and Growth: From Infancy to Adolescence*. New Haven, CT: Yale University Press.

O'Leary, V. E., Alday, C. S. and Ickovics, J. R. (1998) 'Models of life change and posttraumatic growth', in R. G. Tedeschi, C. L. Park and L. G. Calhoun (eds), *Posttraumatic Growth: Positive Changes in the Aftermath of Crisis*. Mahwah, NJ: Lawrence Erlbaum, pp. 127–51.

Oltjenbruns, K. A. (1991) 'Positive outcomes of adolescents' experiences with grief'. *Journal of Adolescent Research*, 6: 43–53.

Park, C. L., Cohen, L. H. and Murch, R. (1996) 'Assessment and prediction of stress-related growth'. *Journal of Personality*, 6: 71–105.

Rogers, C. R. (1959) 'A theory of therapy, personality, and interpersonal relationships as developed in the client-centered framework'. In S. Koch (ed.), *Psychology: a Study of a Science*, Vol. 3: *Formulations of the Person and the Social Context*. New York: McGraw-Hill, pp. 184–256.

Rogers, C. R. (1963) 'The actualizing tendency in relation to "motives" and to consciousness'. In M.R. Jones (ed.), *Nebraska Symposium on Motivation*, Vol. 11. Lincoln, NE: University of Nebraska Press, pp. 1–24.

Rutter, M. (1979) 'Protective factors in children's responses to stress and disadvantage'. In J. E. Rolf (ed.), *Primary Prevention of Psychopathology: Social Competence in Children*. Hanover, NH: University Press of New England, pp. 49–74.

Ryff, C. and Singer, B. (1998) 'The role of purpose in life and personal growth in positive human health'. In P. T. P. Wong and P. S. Fry (eds), *The Human Quest for Meaning: a Handbook of Psychological Research and Clinical Applications*. Mahwah, NJ: Lawrence Erlbaum Associates, pp. 213–35.

Salter, E. and Stallard, P. (2004) 'Posttraumatic growth in child survivors of a road traffic accident'. *Journal of Traumatic Stress*, 17: 335–40.

Seligman, M. E. P. and Csikszentmihalyi, M. (2000) 'Positive psychology: an introduction'. *American Psychologist*, 55: 5–14.

Simonton, D. K. (1994) *Greatness: Who Makes History and Why*. New York: Guilford Press.

Simonton, D. K. (2000) 'The positive repercussions of traumatic events and experiences: the life lessons of historic geniuses'. In P. A. Linley (ed.), *Psychological Trauma and its Positive Adaptations* [Student Members Group Special Bulletin, No. 1]. Leicester, UK: British Psychological Society, pp. 21–23.

Sroufe, L. A. and Rutter, M. (1984) 'The domain of developmental psychopathology'. *Child Development*, 55: 17–29.

Tedeschi, R. G. and Calhoun, L. G. (1995) *Trauma and Transformation: Growing in the Aftermath of Suffering*. Thousand Oaks, CA: Sage.

Tedeschi, R. G. and Calhoun, L. G. (1996) 'The Posttraumatic Growth Inventory: measuring the positive legacy of trauma'. *Journal of Traumatic Stress*, 9: 455–71.

Tedeschi, R. G. and Calhoun, L. G. (2004a) 'Posttraumatic growth: conceptual foundations and empirical evidence'. *Psychological Inquiry*, 15: 1–18.

Tedeschi, R. G. and Calhoun, L. G. (2004b) 'A clinical approach to posttraumatic growth', in P. A. Linley and S. Joseph (eds), *Positive Psychology in Practice* (pp. 405–19). Hoboken, NJ: Wiley.

Tedeschi, R. G., Park, C. L. and Calhoun, L. G. (eds) (1998) *Posttraumatic Growth: Positive Changes in the Aftermath of Crisis*. Mahwah, NJ: Lawrence Erlbaum.

Tennen, H. and Affleck, G. (2002) 'Benefit-finding and benefit-reminding'. In C. R. Snyder and S. J. Lopez (eds), *Handbook of Positive Psychology*. New York: Oxford University Press, pp. 584–97.

Thompson, S. C. (1985) 'Finding positive meaning in a stressful event and coping'. *Basic and Applied Social Psychology*, 6: 279–95.

Werner, E. E. and Smith, R. S. (1982) *Vulnerable but Invincible: a Longitudinal Study of Resilient Children and Youth*. New York: McGraw-Hill.

Woodward, C. and Joseph, S. (2003) 'Positive change processes and post-traumatic growth in people who have experienced childhood abuse: understanding vehicles of change'. *Psychology and Psychotherapy: Theory, Research and Practice*, 76: 267–83.

Yalom, I. D. and Lieberman, M. A. (1991) 'Bereavement and heightened existential awareness'. *Psychiatry*, 54: 334–45.

Yates, T. M. and Masten, A. S. (2004) 'Fostering the future: resilience theory and the practice of positive psychology'. In P. A. Linley and S. Joseph (eds), *Positive Psychology in Practice*. Hoboken: Wiley.

Yule, W., Perrin, S. and Smith, P. (1999) 'Post-traumatic stress reactions in children and adolescents'. In W. Yule (ed.), *Post-Traumatic Stress Disorders: Concepts and Therapy*. Chichester: Wiley.

9
Cultural Perspective of Healing Trauma

Roberto Dansie

As suggested throughout various chapters of this book (see Chapters 4, 5 and 13), culture sensitivity is becoming a significant variable in treatment and rehabilitation of traumatized children. Early work in this area, however, has been influenced by research on race, culture, migration and mental health (Murphy 1973, 1977; Ward et al. 2001; Fernando 2002). Indeed, some previous research work has faced design problems and has relied heavily on convenience cases and clinical samples (Brislin and Baumgardner 1971). However, the last four decades have witnessed a major shift from the medical model (Summerfield 1995; Timimi 2002; d'Ardenne and Mahtani 1989; Kareem and Littlewood 1992) towards the importance of culture influences on human behaviour. One aspect of this new orientation was the establishment of research and the foundation of the new disciplines such as cross-cultural psychology (Triandis 1980, 1994; Triandis et al. 1988; Lonner and Malpass 1994; Brislin 1993; Matsumoto and Juang 2004; Matsumoto 1994); trans-cultural psychiatry (Leff 1988; Bhugra 1993; Bhugra and Bhui 2001; Dwivedi 1996; de Silva 1999) and multi-cultural counselling (Pedersen 1985, 1991; Abramowitz and Murray 1983; Pomterotto and Casas 1991; Palmer and Laungani 1999). This emphasis has recently been extended to cultural awareness in nursing and health care (Holland and Hogg 2001). All these new fields now attract a multidisciplinary audience and address topics ranging from concepts of normality and abnormality across cultures and culture bound syndromes to other issues relevant to child-rearing practices across culture, acculturation, emotion across cultures, non-verbal communication and sensitivity to the values and beliefs of both minority groups and indigenous population during treatment and rehabilitation.

It should be emphasized here that these disciplines are studying variations in human behaviour as well as considering ways in which behaviour is influenced by cultural context. The new research in these disciplines has been also driven by the core propositions that sensitivity to culture can bring both better outcomes and avoid misdiagnosis and discontinuation of treatment (Abramowitz and Murray 1983). In fact, the patient's charter (DoH 1996) and the National Association of Health Authorities and Trust (NAHAT) in the UK are also taking this issue seriously. They have clearly stated in their guidelines, published in 1996, that the National Health Services (NHS) should respect both religion and cultural beliefs for all patients and families and avoid making assumptions about such needs. Further, John Cox (who served as President of the Royal College of Psychiatrists, UK) in his foreword statement (Bhugra and Bhui 2001) made the following remarks: '*the Royal College of Psychiatrists insists that training in* transcultural psychiatry and culture competence, for example, becomes a core requirement for trainees, as well as for consultants in continuing professional development'. Using a combination of cultural approaches alongside others seems to offer a better framework to help many troubled traumatized individuals.

Cultural psychology emerged and begun to grow during the 1960s as an independent discipline, evolving rapidly and led to several influential journals in the last four decades (Shiraev and Levy 2001; Berry et al. 1992). One of the most obvious goals of cross-cultural psychology is the testing of existing psychological knowledge and theories. Cross-cultural psychology also aims to improve our understanding of the diversity of human activity, and tries to understand the impact of culture on human behaviour. It also aims to look at emotional and behavioural characteristics of people and dismantle stereotypes and prejudices (Matsumoto and Juang 2004). In fact, many clinicians and therapists, when encountering a culturally diverse population, tend to use their own appraisal, i.e. applying their own individual standards and understanding when coming across different cultures. And the expected outcomes are therefore more likely to be inappropriate diagnosis and inappropriate management due to the fact that a psychologist here would be looking at a non-Western culture, through Western glasses, and failing to notice important aspects of the non-Western culture.

However, the idea behind introducing this chapter is to make clinicians and other mental health professionals start thinking seriously about differences and similarities across individuals and culture boundaries.

Focusing on culture and healing, the elements of earth, water, air and fire play a key role in the American Indian traditional healing. They have been known as the four suns of healing. However, I shall explain this using the narrative approach which is potentially helpful when discussing mental illness in relation to ethnicity and culture. According to Timimi (2002) the narrative approach emphasizes the importance of the stories and their influence on the development of psychopathology. Further, this approach tends to attribute meanings to the events of our lives and identities as told by influential figure(s). I shall take the four issues mentioned above in turn.

1. Land, the first sun

The first sun, the one of the 'Land' corresponds to the individual's relation to nature. It also refers to the individual finding his or her place in life, a sense of 'Destino' or purpose. The Mayas represented this purpose as a Quetzal (sacred bird) who lives in our heart. Those who follow its calling developed their true face (*rostro*); those who ignore it are never fully born, and this betrayal of self has physical and emotional consequences.

In the healing process, land represents the space that we create around our patient, which has to be a 'sacred space', a place of safety, nurturing and support. Sage and incense are often used and a ritual is followed to begin the healing session. The healer is in charge of bringing peace and trust into this space, and providing emotional, mental and spiritual support to the patient all along the healing journey.

2. Water, the second sun

Water is essential for life. Yet, too much of it, or too little of it, can have harmful consequences for the living being. To contain too many emotions is considered in Curanderismo as being 'ahogado', that is to 'drown in one's own water'. What is needed is 'des-ahogo' 'un-drowning', a process facilitated by breaking silence, talking from the heart, healing songs, 'mandas' (pilgrimage), visits to sacred sites, rituals or ceremonies. The characteristic of healthy water is its movement. Stagnant water is, just like stagnant air, 'toxic'. Flowing water is nurturing and life-giving, one of the key signs of ancient healers. The goal is to help the patient release his or her excess of water and restore the flow of emotions in their being, for water represents the emotions, which in trauma are viewed as stuck in the past.

3. Air, the third sun

It is common among the Latino population to speak of the 'air' of service providers of their community. The air can be 'buen-aire' (good air) and 'mal-aire' (bad air). Air is determined by the qualities of well-being or ill-being experienced by being around a particular person. It is believed in Curanderismo that the 'air' affects the blood of people. There are four basic types of blood. Light blood, meaning individuals with good air in their system, who bring forth healing energy wherever they may go. With them comes hope, inspiration, enthusiasm, well-being and clarity of mind. Heavy blood is characterized by toxic airs with no outlets that brings inner tension to the life of the individual. Bad blood, the third classification refers to the prolonged accumulation of toxic air that eventually blocks the living fire of the individual. Bleeder, is the fourth and last classification of the blood, and it consists of an overflow of negative energy, a contagious emotional virus whose consequences can be lethal. The healer is in charge of bringing good air to the healing encounter, and helping the patient release his or her bad air.

4. Fire, the fourth sun

When people are overflowed with water, there is no air. And with no air, there is no fire. Once water reaches a healthy level, air is restored to the individual. Now, the spark of life can be reignited, a process known since ancestral times as 'burning water'. And that fire is our own inner sun, the unfolding of the gifts that life has given us. Curanderos – traditional healers – tell us that the optimal sign of our health is us 'burning-up', releasing our sun to the universe. Fire is our life energy. When our energy is no longer trapped in the past, then our energy naturally rises, and we become more alive. We also become more balanced, less agitated, and more resourceful to meet the challenges of our present living situation. In traditional healing, trauma is overcome when patients reclaim their inner fire and have a system by which they can address their excess of water whenever they experience an emotional or psychological flooding.

In such tradition the human spirit is greatly resilient. Like the sunflower, it continues to seek the light of hope and meaning. And sometimes, beyond what all conditioning schools of psychology tell us, people can break free from the past and their environments and give birth to a life of unprecedented kindness and love. Like Victor Frankl before me, who had found the reality of the human soul in a Nazi concentration camp among his colleagues, I too found this human soul in all its magnificence among those who had survived the dark valley of human malignancy. This reality helped me take a stand and face trauma. Otherwise, I do believe, the darkness of depression and despair would have never released the grip they had taken of me. And like many who had had the courage to step into the field of trauma, I too wrestle from time to time with this dark demon and confront the gloom that it brings into our beloved world. Yet I have learned to transform painful knowledge into resolute action. It is passivity that sinks us in the moving sands of despair.

At times, I have marvelled at the clear heart that beats in me, fresh as the water that I drink of the mountain stream, or my mind, opened to experiences of goodness, like picking up coloured pebbles from the rock-bed of a river, with my youngest daughter, her smile as bright as the sun. My life has not been diminished by this awareness of human suffering. My heart has grown and has embraced all people. I have come to realize that those who inflict trauma or abuse on others do so by dehumanizing them in their mind first. With Gandhi, we can all say 'Hate sin, but love the sinner'. And there is still much work to be done, especially in the area of anger and rage towards the committed atrocities and towards those who committed them. I have seen different ways of coping with this need. In some cultures, the approach consists in 'active forgetting'. By focusing the entire energy in a vision of an attainable future, those embarking on this process decrease the turbulence of the psychological past and nurture current feelings of growth and well-being. In other cultures, particularly the ones of Western civilization, the task consists in revisiting the past and in bringing repressed experiences into the domain of consciousness. I have also seen some cultures conduct a blend of these two approaches, such as that practised by some Hmong members, which consists of making elabourate sowings that illustrate their personal journey into a healing present moment, depicting the inclemency that they have gone through in order to get there. When I asked one of their healers what was the purpose of those works of art, he responded with one of the traditional sayings of his culture: 'The best way to put the past behind you is by putting it in front of you.'

His answer brought back memories of my grandmother, who is following the ancient healing ways of the indigenous populations of the Americas used to treat certain types of trauma by having the survivor revisit physically or psychologically the place and time of their trauma. The trauma is known as 'Susto' which means soul-illness. It is believed that at the moment of trauma, a part of the soul leaves the body, and that afterwards the survivor loses part of his life-energy to a perpetual fear. In order to reclaim the survivor's lost part of the soul my grandmother would travel with the survivor to the land of suffering, a place where matters of the soul were still happening. There they were in 'heart time'. It was in this place where the survivor would reclaim his power and his heart. He was no longer avoiding this past, but facing it. Grandma, as a healer, would provide the support that survivors needed in order to come to terms with their past. I remember seeing the light of life return to the eyes of those who, having suffered 'Susto', would come to my Grandma.

'See that?' my Grandma would often tell me, referring to that mysterious light. 'That is the soul coming back to their bodies.' And that is what moved me to take the path of a healer: to share that moment, to see the light of life returning to the eyes of those in need.

Trauma and traditional healing

In Curanderismo, the Mexican traditional healing practice, we are told of a peculiar illness that disrupts our emotional and mental well-being. It is called 'Susto'. Susto is characterized by intense, prolonged, and highly uncontrollable bursts of fear, anger and anxiety. Susto also drains the psychic energy and dilutes the sense of life's meaning. Curanderos – traditional healers – maintain that even the composition of our body changes, a fact that is now being demonstrated by scientific researchers who found that traumatized individuals who suffered from Post-Traumatic Stress Disorder, after they were exposed to or had viewed relevant trauma cues, showed a pain sensitivity reduction as much as if they had received appropriate treatment (Yule 1991, 1992).

Individuals suffering from Post-Traumatic Stress Disorder pour a high number of natural pain-killers into their system at so little provocation that eventually they become addicted to their own internal narcotics. We can say with Curanderos that they are trapped in a circle of 'poisoning themselves'. In this case, the healing can only take place if there is a breaking of the poisoning circle. We have to keep in mind that the person afflicted by Susto is not living in the ordinary world. They are in the abyss, in a place of hopelessness. Dante in his book *The Divine Comedy* has a sign at the entrance of hell that reads 'Abandon hope all those who enter here.' And hope is what those who suffer from Susto leave behind. Hell is also characterized by absolute loneliness, a process by which one feels alienated from the world. That is why the circle of poison can begin to crack when another person enters it: the Curandero. This is someone willing to go to hell in order to reach another human being. The Curandero is willing to loan his centre of direction and well-being to the other individual who has lost his centre, and who is afflicted with ill-being. At times, the Curandero himself also sees the world that the other person is contemplating. And while this vision may be stressful and turbulent, the experience of having another person there with him, in that horrible place, has a healing effect in the person affected by Susto. Hell is for one person. With two, hell begins to give way. Just by entering hell the Curandero begins to change it.

Susto can also consist of one's inability to process a particular experience, one that is unbearable. Curanderos say that the head cracks in order to protect the heart from breaking. And yet, the heart is the only place where the suffering can exit the person. In this case the Curanderos assist the other person in seeing the truth, in facing the unbearable. It is in this stage that the pain descends from the head to the heart; the head comes together, the heart breaks. The Curandero knows that pain with no outlet causes ongoing suffering, the predicament of Susto. He also knows that healing begins by finding an outlet for pain. The Curandero knows this because his heart is also broken. He is a wounded healer. He also knows that the heart can come together. It comes together as we discover other human beings, as we build a community caring for one other. 'Corazon cura corazon' (heart heals heart) is a saying among Curanderos, and they should know for they do not hesitate to help others find their heart and process the experiences that life has set before them. Curanderos have a deeper message for all of us. They say, 'A broken heart has more room for love.'

Ancient healing system of the indigenous people of America

Curanderismo is the name that the Spanish gave to the traditional healing practices of the Indians of Mexico. Curanderismo is to modern medicine, what philosophy is to science. It is the origin and still its constant companion. On the other hand, the dichotomy between modern medicine and ancestral medicine is beginning to disappear even among mainstream populations of the industrialized nations.

Indeed, growing numbers of patients today are becoming more and more interested in traditional healing practices. This interest is not a fortuitous one. For all of the undeniable contributions of modern medicine, we are also becoming aware of the side-effects that the pharmacological revolution is causing in our patients. And in some circumstances we have gone full circle: the cure is becoming the disease. Curanderismo has been long practised, and seems to continue among various communities. Traditional healing continued to be one of the healing practices not only among the indigenous groups but also of the mix-blooded new populations. Western systems of healing had little or no classifications for healing properties of the herbs of the American continent, but the indigenous populations did. And part of this knowledge was preserved by popular traditions that went unnoticed by mainstream medicine. As time went by plants were given new names, but remained in use for the same healing purposes. Let us remember that for the ancient healers, the human soul covered the domains of the body, the heart, and the mind, each one of these areas being approachable with a wide variety of healing practices, the essential one being the healer's ability to search and assess the patient's soul. However, the Cartesian dichotomy between body and mind did not apply to the ancient healers, who viewed health as a continuum of energy in the human body. We owe to the ancestral healers the awareness that the emotional life and the physical life do not necessarily experience time and space in the same way. While it is in the nature of the physical body to be only in the present, that is, in one place and moment at a time, the emotional body can be in several places and moments at once. That is why it was represented as a sacred bird whose wings would allow the person to go beyond the boundaries of time and space. This defiance of physical limitations can also be done by our awareness body, for we can go from our individual consciousness, to the collective and Universal Consciousness, these last being experienced as 'visions' and 'prophecies' and other forms of enhanced perception.

It is this quality of transcendency that enables the emotional body to experience life from a much larger frame of reference than the ordinary one, the physical one. This transcendental peculiarity of the emotional body that grants humans an expanded sense of freedom, also makes us vulnerable to an equally intensified sense of oppression and fragmentation. Our emotional body, while it can take us to experience the essential oneness of life, can also have us experience the most extreme sense of desolation and despair. The dismemberment of the emotional body causes illness in the physical being. In this case, the healing of the body requires the integration of fragments of the emotional body, fragments that could be in different moments and places.

In order to address the human being in his totality, the Curanderos charted the world of the human soul. While some of the levels of the soul could not be reached by the ordinary people until they had left their body and experienced death, there were some extraordinary individuals who could reach such states while still being in the body. These last ones had either been born with this 'gift' or had come to develop it either by trauma, illness, initiation, or mystical experience. Curanderos then worked with the physical body, the emotional body, and the awareness body. The first question that they wanted answered was: 'Which part of the soul is being afflicted with this particular illness or wound?' If it was the one of the body, then ordinary remedies would be used in the healing process. These healing practices relied heavily on local herbs, places (such as natural sanctuaries), animal products, the use of cold and hot water, massages and sweat-lodges. However, if the affliction of the soul was at the level of the heart, or of the awareness body, then extraordinary psychospiritual procedures were set in motion.

The purpose of Curanderismo is to heal the wound at all of its levels, to facilitate the process of integration of the patient's soul to its essential unity within itself and with the Universal soul which the Aztec healers called 'ometeotl' (literally 'the one who is close and near'). Wholeness within the individual, and wholeness with nature and relations, is the essential paradigm of Curanderismo. The wound of the soul has to do with the 'shadow' or double, the part of our mind that is affected by our ordinary experiences, such as physical or emotional experiences. Oftentimes, it is this shadow that is trapped in the world of the mind, creating confusions and distortions (wounds) in our soul. The challenge of the Curandero is therefore two-fold. First, the task is to find the shadow of the afflicted individual. The second is to integrate this shadow to the soul who needs it as long as the soul is going to be encapsulated in the body. From the ancestral perspective, the shadow stores all of the experiences that the individual goes through. At times, the soul suffers because it refuses to integrate parts of the shadow to its being. In extreme cases, the individual fears his psychological shadow as if he was being persecuted by a separate entity.

During traumatic experiences, the soul leaves the physical body. It is with the aid of the shadow that the soul can be reintroduced to its physical being, a procedure used in the healing of 'Susto' (fright), or 'espanto' (freezing of the soul), spiritual wounds that are gradually overcome when the individual integrates the traumatic events into the field of his awareness, when his soul literally overcomes the 'fear'. The soul from the perspective of Curanderismo has physical, emotional, mental and spiritual dimensions. As such, it can reach lower and higher states of consciousness. The first ones are identified as the underworlds, and there are nine of them, each one of them with their own particular forces and characteristics. There are also specific emotional energies that fluctuate in each one of these domains. The Curandero, with his heart (who has been to every domain), can determine the location of the soul in any one of these worlds. And there are also thirteen overworlds, that can become harmful to the soul if the person does not learn how to descend from them and re-engage the ordinary world, an illness known as 'quedarse arriba', 'to get lost in the world of above'.

Curanderos assess not only the dwelling place of the soul (either underworlds or overworlds) but also the degree of absence or presence of the soul of which there are twenty stages, ten for the lower stages (belonging to the left side of the soul represented as the serpent-side), and ten for the higher stages (belonging to the right side of the soul, represented as the eagle-side). These stages have been used in the Aztec, Toltec, and even Mayan calendars, and were used also to name each one of the days of their month. Aside from the soul's predicament and location, there are four main elements that affect the soul, namely, land, water, air and fire. Each one of these elements has positive and negative qualities. Each one of the elements generates well-being when it reaches a level of balance or equilibrium, and illness when there is either too much or too little of it. And then there are the four main directions that the soul takes in its quest of realization (north, south, east, west), some of them that may not be appropriate, causing the individual a sense of confusion or fragmentation in life. Thus, the skilful Curandero is to determine: the level of energy of the soul in the physical body known as 'vitality'; the dominance of either soul or shadow in the person (mode); the area of the soul affected during a particular malady (either 'liver', 'heart', or 'head'); the direction of the soul (north, south, east or west); the active elements in the soul (earth, water, wind, fire); the stages of the soul (twenty of them); and the location of the soul (twenty-two of them).

Curanderismo addresses behaviour and consciousness as part of a larger paradigm, the one of the soul and the one of the community. As such, its domain is not limited to the areas of biology, health and illness, or even life, for Curanderos work within a paradigm of eternity and spirit. It is, by design, a system of wholeness. It works with the paradoxical predicament of human life (its mortality and eternity) and its energetic exchange with cosmic forces. Curanderismo remains the oldest and most widely used health system of the Americas as well as the least understood by the academic world.

Curanderos practise a 'therapist' centred healing, one where the healer takes responsibility for the energy, skills and processes that he or she brings to the healing encounter. The subject–object relation that modern mental health workers assume while addressing mental illness is absent in Curanderismo. In its place what we find is the essential skill of the Curandero to enter the world of the patient, a world whose validity is not questioned but acknowledged as real even when is not part of the ordinary world.

In the psychological paradigm of Curanderismo, the patient's subjectivity does not exist in isolation but in interaction with energetic forces. As such, it can be reached, influenced and guided by other subjectivities. The patient's energetic self may be fragmented and scattered across a wide range of realities and in need of integration, in which case the energy and awareness of the Curandero acts as medicine. The integrative personal experience of the Curandera gives her the ability to remain whole amidst fragmentation and skilled in working with the elements and forces of other planes of experience. The advance of Western civilization has deprived traditional communities of lifestyles and environmental resources that once supported the integration process of members afflicted with mental illness. Natural places of healing, time off, free mentors, as well as community uses of non-ordinary experiences, are now almost extinct practices, while the breakdowns of nature and community are overtaxing the role of the Curanderos, making them more vulnerable to succumb to the torments they attempt to heal.

Modern psychologists resemble some elementary practices of Curanderismo especially in their view and treatment of what they label 'spiritual emergence', a psychological process where there is a gradual unfolding of spiritual potential with minimal disruption in psychological, social and occupational functioning. On the other hand, when this process has significant disruptions and becomes a crisis, they call it 'spiritual emergency', and still try to support the individual in going through the experience instead of blocking or interrupting it. These and other more benign categories of 'mental illness' are now finding their way into different forms of psychotherapy and even to the main paradigm of the American Psychiatric Association, the *Diagnostic and Statistical Manual*. Some of the proponents of these changes are individuals who have undergone experiences that were or could have been labelled 'psychotic' but who addressed them through Curanderismo and emerged from them with a deeper understanding of the innerworld and more resourceful as they faced their ordinary life. In turn, they began to assist others undergoing similar experiences and providing alternative models to those who equate abnormality with pathology.

A multicultural world is giving us now the opportunity to see how experiences are greatly determined by the way they are viewed and treated, that a psychological crisis may be enhanced or managed by the way we approach it, and that experiences that have been void of meaning in one cultural context, can become significant and meaningful in another one. Cross-cultural experiences can provide us with a wide variety of tools to illuminate the inner life and come to its aid in times of need. And we can learn them by living and learning from each other, with respect. Our different ways can be an asset for us all. Perhaps it is now time to pause and to learn from each other. After all, while our past has been different, we all share the same future.

Traditional healing for the modern world

It is my opinion that there are common characteristics that most Native American Indians, as well as the farmworker community and other groups, share when it comes to healing and health. These include the following:

- Healing is due to the harmony between body, heart, mind, and soul.
- Our relationships are an essential component of our health.
- Life comes from the Great Spirit, and all healing begins with Him.
- Death is not our enemy, but a natural phenomenon of life.
- Disease is not only felt by the individual, but also by the family.
- Spirituality and emotions are just as important as the body and the mind.
- Mother Earth contains numerous remedies for our illnesses.
- Some healing practices have been preserved throughout the generations.
- Traditional healers can be either men or women, young or old.
- Illness is an opportunity to purify one's soul.

The use of magical herbs

There is an old Mexican song that says:

> Tell me, what you have given me
> Beautiful Dark Woman,
> Everything changes in life
> Only your love
> Has not changed at all.
> I believe you have given me
> A magical herb.

There may be something more than romanticism to this song. Now we know that some herbs can have powerful effects on our nervous system. There are some herbs that were held in high regard by the ancient Mexicans. Their usage is delicate and, at times, even dangerous. Some parts of these plants can be toxic, while other parts have healing properties. Several of these plants have a strong stimulating effect, which, like every other stimulant, have also an indirect depressive effect. This principle, known to many traditional healers, was used to retain a loved one. The herb was given in a drink and given to the loved one (who presumably was having an affair). Then, the potion will go into effect and he or she would go into a fever of love. This was a critical period for the person giving the herb, an ideal time for an intimate relation. Once the act of love was consummated, the depressive cycle of the herb would go into effect and the enchanter was given the instruction to find a way to send the loved one out of the house for three days. During this time, the depressive effects of the herb would be active and the loved one would not be able to perform their intimate functions. Most likely, the enchanted person would be with the lover and things would tend to fall apart between them. After three days, when the loved one returned home, the enchanter was instructed to take them in, and provide them with another potion of the herb, reliving the passion between them.

Herbs have been used as a powerful aid for the healing of psychological trauma. The use of these herbs is determined by the nature of the trauma and the personality type of the patient. 'Fire' children, for instance, are giving the 'three miracle' tea, made of spearmint, chamomile and anise star. Herbs indeed have been part of a millenary tradition to heal psychological trauma and remain constant in the practice of traditional healing.

The use of spiritual herbs

We live in a society prone to get involved in addictive behaviour. Thus, when a plant is known for its hallucinogenic properties growing numbers of people want to ingest these plants whenever they get a chance. There is a systematic knowledge in the cultures that surrounds these plants, knowledge that has been preserved in rituals, procedures, stories and traditions, knowledge that maximizes the healing properties of these plants while minimizing their negative effects. Before we ingest these plants, we had better listen to the people who have a millenary experience with their properties. After all, that is what we do with our physicians whose practices have been in existence only for a couple of centuries.

The use of spiritual plants has been reserved for treating some forms of psychological trauma; particularly those that have remained immune to previous healing interventions. And when used, they are part of rigorous preparations for both patient and healer, and often result in life-changing experiences for those who undertake them following the ancient traditions.

> *'The great error in the treatment of the human body is that physicians are ignorant of the whole. For the part can never be well unless the whole is well.'*

I confirmed the truth of this statement at an early age, when I was living in a small town in central Mexico. In my family's eyes, there were three professions that were 'sacred': priesthood, school teacher and medical doctor. It was during this time that one of my uncles had graduated from medical school and had decided to begin his medical practice in my grandmother's town. When my uncle got off the bus, all dressed in white, he was welcomed by the mayor, by the priest, by the nuns of my school, by the charro league, by most of the people of the town and even a musical band.

Weeks later, as my uncle began his practice, my grandmother decided to refer the people that came to see her to my uncle. My uncle did not have a nurse, or a receptionist, or an office manager, so he decided to train me in these affairs. When patients came in I would have to make a chart for each one of them, fill out several forms with their demographic information and then ask them about their reason for seeking medical help. Then, chart in hand, I would go and call my uncle, never addressing him as 'Uncle' but as 'Doctor'. My uncle said I needed to learn to be 'professional'. On one of the days I was on 'duty', helping the doctor, a middle-aged woman came to the house, asking to see my grandmother. I had been instructed to say that Grandma had retired from the healing practices, but that now, patients could be seen by a real doctor, my uncle. Reluctantly the lady agreed to see my uncle. When I had completed my part of the chart, I went to call the doctor. The lady had been complaining of stomach pains and, after a few questions, my uncle prescribed something for an ulcer.

The same lady came back a week later. She grabbed me by my shirt and told me 'this time I want to see your Grandma!' By the tone of her voice, I knew I was not going to be able to convince her otherwise, so

I went to get my grandmother. After I explained the whole incident to Grandma, she came out to see the lady. My Grandma opened her arms and looking at the lady in the eyes, she said, 'What happened to you my dear?' The woman broke down crying and just hugged Grandma. The lady cried for a while and Grandma, not saying a word, just held her. Later she would tell me that, most of the time, crying is good for the body. According to her, we can get rid of some pain and restore some of our energy when we cried.

Then she took the lady to a room where she had a candle perpetually burning. She asked the lady to sit there in silence, observing the light of the candle and breathing softly. Once she left the lady in the candle room, my Grandma prepared a tea with honey. Grandma said that accurate diagnosis could only be made when the patient was calmed. So, the first thing she would do was to help the patient achieve some kind of peace. Once the lady drank her tea, Grandma asked how her family was doing. Grandma said that a good woman is always more concerned with her family than with her own self, therefore, checking on her family was just as important as checking on her own heart. The lady said that her husband had left for the US almost three months before, and he said he was going to work and write and send money. It happened he had not done either one of these two things. 'You must be worrying a lot', Grandma said. The lady nodded in silence. Then Grandma asked how she was sleeping, if she was having head or stomach aches, and how she was eating. Once the lady responded, my Grandma said, 'I'll tell you what we are going to do my child. I'm going to write to one of my sons who is near where your husband was heading in the US and we will make him at least write you a note. Your kids will not go hungry, Roberto will go with you to the market once a week and will make sure you get enough food for your family. And for you, I'll give you one of my special remedies, so that you have enough energy to do the things you need to do, but you must eat well: You are not going to be of much help to your family if you get sick.'

The lady smiled and a few days later, came back with an entire new disposition. She was in good spirits and even smiled when she told me to call my grandmother. The lady hugged Grandma as she came to welcome her, and after exchanging a few words with her, she asked her to read a letter she had brought with her. It was a letter from her husband. The man said he had some problems getting a job, but that finally he had found some work harvesting peaches. He was going to have some work for a while. He even managed to send some money. At the end of the letter he added the following postscript: 'I have written to you and sent you some money, now please go and tell Dona Exiquia [my grandmother] to get off of my back.' The lady was delighted. She shared her joy with Grandma in the same way she had shared her pain. Grandma later told me 'Sometimes you have to get on the back of someone in order to heal the stomach of somebody else.'

Change and medicine

The sand paintings of the Native American Indians are medicine. They chart our inner world and help us find our way in life. The Navajo Indians have good reasons for making their paintings on sand. Much work goes into them, many details. Each one of them, like us, is unique. Yet, a moment later, the painting vanishes. Nothing remains but the sand. Why go through all of this work, if it is not going to last? One good reason: by making the painting, one reaches a unity with the moment. We step into timelessness, or as some indigenous groups prefer to call it, 'dream-time'. The painting lives for that moment, and like all life will move on. We get to see it take shape and return to the sand. It is life in motion, and in order to be alive it changes. There is no attachment to the painting. Its particles, one by one, rise and dance with the wind. No resistance. Only the flow. Then we see that the Grand Canyon in all of its majesty is nothing but a sand painting. Even the stars and the galaxies are a sand painting.

Most of us put the moment that we live into past experiences. The hands of life attempt to lay a sand painting on us, but we have frozen the painting of yesterday, we have not freed ourselves from the past, and we go forward, missing moment after moment. The older we get, the more our experiences keep us from meeting life. The sand that now shelters me as a body, how many mountains has it built in the past? How many trees? How many deer? And when I am gone, how many flowers will rise from this sand? For the paintings do not end with me. They go on. In a sand painting, there is no distinction between our environment and us. We are part of the same life. The sand of our environment is the same sand of our body. In this regard, to take care of rivers and lakes is to take care of our blood. To take care of the air is to take care of our lungs. To take care of the words that we put out there in the world is to take care of our heart. That is why most sand paintings are drawn in the form of a circle. We are connected to the world.

An elder lady of the Ute tribe, having drawn a circle on the ground told me: 'This is the way I greet each day. I make a circle. That is me.

Then I see the sun. Every day. And I say, "may I be like you throughout the day, with light in my heart for every one".' The elder lady told me that we all form circles around us. When we have fear or anger, our circles carry these emotions. But, strong as these emotions may be, the circles do not have a wide range. However, when we experience a strong feeling of love, then our circle can be as wide as to go beyond our world, all the way up to the sun. 'My grandfather,' said the elder lady 'said that many tribal members used to talk to the sun every morning. The love in their hearts was strong. Now few are the ones who can reach the sun. We need to change this. It is our destiny, as children of the Earth, to return light for light, small as we are, we can reach the sun every day of our lives.' And there is a second drum, this one beating much faster than the first one: our own heart. Both of them, the fast one and the slow one, make harmony. As we emerge from water into the world of air we preserve our ability to recognize not only the heartbeat of our mother, but the heartbeat of our loved ones as well, a phenomenon known in Spanish as 'Corazonada', which literally means 'a message from the heart'.

I remember the numerous occasions in which my Grandma would take her hands to her heart and exclaim 'una corazonada!' A while later we would be informed of an accident or sudden illness of a relative. At times, Grandma would even say the name of the afflicted person. Time and again, her corazonadas were accurate. After a while, I got to trust her heart. 'How come you can feel these things?' I once asked her. She looked at me and said 'How come you don't feel them?' I said that obviously my heart had nothing to tell me. Grandma laughed and shook her head. Then she said, 'Your heart talks to you too, but its voice is quieter than the one of your head. It talks to you with feelings, with images, like the ones you see in your dreams. When you love someone, their heart also speaks to you, it does not matter how far away they may be. You are likely to listen to a corazonada when you are not thinking too much, when you are calmed. Older people slow down, and find it easier to feel corazonadas, but in reality, everyone regardless of their age can feel them.'

Grandma said that we not only receive disturbing messages with the heart. We also receive pleasant ones too. Those were likely to happen when we found ourselves happy for no apparent reason. 'That is joy from far away,' she said. Years later, at the base of Mount Shasta, I found myself missing my two older kids, who were far away. A medicine man looked at me and asked me what was going in my heart. I told him. He nodded, and took out some sage from his bag. 'Let's sing,' he said as he burned some sage 'and we will have the song carry your love to your children.' And I sang, and poured my heart out to the song. And amazingly, at the exact moment when I got home, my oldest kids were calling me on the phone to tell me that they had just felt my presence and they wanted me to know how much they loved me! I have been fortunate to share with others a ritual of sending our 'heart energy' to our loved ones who are far away. This is often the case for those who are separated from their families and experience a chronic sense of depression and feelings of pain and guilt when they think of their loved ones.

Miraculous love: breaking inter-generational trauma

I am talking with a group of small kids and we are playing a game that they are really enjoying. It is called 'what would you like your Dad to tell you?' Fortunately for them, their parents are also attending the meeting, and they are in for a few surprises. One of the kids is particularly insistent. Patience, as you know, is a virtue that comes with age and these little ones are just starting in life. 'You!' I ask the most eager one. 'What would you like your Dad to tell you?' The kid jumps to his feet and tells me 'I want him to tell me "Pete, I love you very much"!' I look into his eyes, and I find the spark of excitement shining bright in this little one. 'Very well,' I say, and hear the commotion among the attendees. I then ask Pete if he would mind going and getting his dad. Pete takes off like a bullet. So much energy in such a little body.

A moment later, here he comes bringing this big man by the hand. The man looks nervously at me and takes a deep breath. I explain to him that we are giving children the words that they have been eager to hear from us, their parents. The man nods at me. 'So, what is it that you want your Dad to tell you?' I ask little Pete. The boy looks into his Dad and says, 'Pete, I love you very much!' The man holds his child's hand and forces a smile.

I ask him to get down to the eye level of his son. He does so, and the child smiles, saying 'nice to meet you Dad!'. The man looks at me and I see the mixture of anger and pain in his eyes. I ask him, 'Did your dad ever tell you that he loved you?' The man silently and slowly shakes his head. 'Your son is waiting,' I tell him, 'for words that you never heard. This is one of those times when you can give that which you never received. I call it miraculous love, precisely because it comes from those who never received it. Look into those eyes, find out what they awaken in you.' And there is Pete, waiting to see his dad come into life. I put my hand on the shoulders of this big man. He clears his throat, keeps his eyes on his son for a long time – the little one waits for him, confident that his Dad will come through – and then some broken words come out of him. 'Pe-te ... I ... Love you!' And tears come out with these words. This is like a second birth: tears, the embrace, and fresh air coming into his life. Pete is immensely happy to see and feel this love of his dad, as if knowing that we are fully alive only when we love. When the man stands up, there are no remains of nervousness or tension. He is at home in his body because his heart and soul are in it. His eyes warmly smile at me; those same eyes where moments before I had seen anger and pain. Now these eyes have solid love all the way through them. And the child takes his father home. Forever.

The healing power of the sweat-lodge

A couple of friendly dogs came my way as I arrived at Angel's house in Big Bend. The fire was going strong and several volcanic rocks were heating in it. Abraham was tightening some old blankets over the Sweat-Lodge, making sure no light came through them. The time finally came for all of us to go in.

Radley gave a few words as to the purpose of the gathering and the specific healing request of a family who was attending. We offered some tobacco to the fire. We got in line and Radley used a long feather to do some passes on us as we entered the Sweat. I was asked to sit in the inner circle, right in front of the centre where the volcanic rocks were to be laid. 'I am a bear dancer,' Angel said, 'and a man prayed for me to receive my Bear. Now, the only way for me to keep him, is to work with the people, and to go through life in a good way.' The rocks were brought in and the heat immediately took over the Sweat. The first round consisted of four songs. It was a round of purification. The songs were a relief and one effective way to endure the heat. I thought to myself that with such heat, anyone could sing and do it wholeheartedly.

We were tempted to sing faster and faster, increasing our rhythm with the rising temperature of the Sweat. Then, one of the elders sang, and did it slowly. After a while of listening to his song, his rhythm made sense to me. It was a matter of slowing our minds as we were enduring the heat, and I marvelled at the command that this old man had over himself. As he took the heat, he was neither impatient nor agitated. His song was calm and steady even when the heat was rising.

Here I was finding refuge in the calmness and sweetness of this song as waves of steam were rising from the fire-red rocks.

Intense heat always makes anger a temptation. And one can give oneself to anger for a while, but eventually one becomes depleted of energy. Anger consumes a lot of energy. The ceremony of the Sweat seems designed to help us move from anger into other emotions as we endure the heat. As we sweat, we rid ourselves of toxins and tensions. The negativity that has accumulated in our bodies, our emotions, and even in our thoughts, rises to the surface and is taken away by the Sweat. In a few minutes, we miss the fresh air. A while later we feel as if we have been without water for days and without food for weeks. How precious the fresh air is. How precious water and food are. Basic simple things, the Sweat puts us in touch with our needs. Nevertheless, it is good to go without things. It is good to let go of things and get in touch with our essential nature, the one reached when there is nothing left in us. There, in the darkness, with the stones glowing with their heat, and the steam impregnating the Lodge with sweet sage, one has nowhere to go but within.

Each round is characterized by bringing new heated rocks into the Sweat. The more rounds we go together, the fewer layers we have between us and the life that lives all around us. During the second round, once purified, we ask for goodness for others, particularly for those living in the Ancestral Land. We may think of particular individuals, but we ask for the elders, the adults, the youth, the children. One of the elders tells us that what we ask for – like the layout of the Sweat-Lodge – always goes in a circle. Eventually what we give is what we receive.

We are encouraged to ask for what we need and not for what we want. I ask for water. I am told that one of the lessons of the Sweat for me may be to be without water for a while so that I may experience the world of those who are in need. Then I am offered a cup full of water. I hold it in my hands, but I do not drink it. Not even a sip. I begin to understand with my mind, my heart and my body, the world of those in need. I tell myself that I am gong to listen better to others, that I am going to be kinder to others.

The round goes by, the heat becoming almost unbearable. It is then that Angel sings the Bear Song. We all join him. I let his singing guide me. The tone tells me if I have to go high, or low, if I have to use intensity, or if I have to fade almost to silence. The song somehow gives us the same feeling. The song is perfected with every repetition. Towards the end of the song, we are giving the same intonations, the highs and lows, the rising and lowering of the voice, just as if there is only one of us singing this song.

The Bear Song gives us a sense of unity and harmony. It is not only a human harmony; it is a cosmic harmony. Then we are told that we, humans, are the most pitiful of all creatures of the earth. All other beings know their place and their purpose. We are the only ones in need of so many reminders to find our way in life. It is because of us losing our way that the rest of the creatures of the earth are suffering the consequences of our ignorance and our arrogance. We have become bad medicine to the earth. The harmony of the Sweat brings us closer to the flow of life, the silent life that goes on underneath our ordinary consciousness, the same one that flows throughout all of the other living beings.

For the third round, one of the elders sings a youth song. The man sings with a strong voice and we hear him go beyond the point of exhaustion. We feel he is making an extraordinary effort and gradually the young ones are moved to sing with him. Their voices give the song a new strength. The Sweat-Lodge affirms us to our Being.

By the time we reach the fourth and final round, we have nothing left but our inner being right in the surface of our body, our heart, our mind. We have been humbled to the point that we all have our faces to the ground. We have gone beyond our discomfort and our pain, beyond our individuality. We have also gone beyond our humanity. For a moment, we have become life-centred. And from here we entered the fourth round, appropriately called the round of thankfulness.

We feel this overwhelming gratitude towards life. The pain is somewhere down there, no longer reaching us. The heat is there, but it no longer burns us, there is no one there left to be burned. We have finally become one with the volcanic rocks. The steam is in us and we have become like those rocks that produced this heat. There is nothing left between us. There is communion with the rocks. We know them from within. Our journey has been completed.

De Silva (1999: 131) who cited Wilson (1989: 44) has provided an account on the main findings of the Sweat-Lodge purification ritual and experiment (*inipi onikare*) of the Native Americans. It was suggested that this religious ceremony of thanksgiving and forgiveness is typically conducted by a 'medicine person' in the tribe and includes extreme heat, signing, self-disclosure and a sense of collectiveness. And it is regarded as a process of purification and a serious and sacred occasion, which contributes to spiritual insights, relief of disturbing symptoms or trauma, personal growth and physical and emotional healing and well-being (see also de Silva and Samarasinghe 1998).

Wilson (1989) and Johnson et al. (1995) pointed out that historically, in many cultures and societies, rituals and ceremonies were performed to heal trauma and help trauma victims to reintegrate and go back to their normal routines. However, the question of whether or not cultural ceremonies and rituals can be usefully incorporated into the PTSD treatment approaches and used with trauma victims in different cultures is an open question. It has been suggested that the evidence is not yet conclusive and further empirical research work is needed (see de Silva 1999; Lloyd and Bhugra 1993).

Finally, Van der Veer (1992), whose work was focused on traumatized refugees in the Netherlands, noted that psychological therapy could be used with dissimilar groups if the patients perceive it as appropriate and in harmony with their beliefs. Turner et al. (2003) also suggested that treatment approaches for trauma victims should be unintrusive and sensitive.

References

Abramowitz, S. I. and Murray, J. (1983) 'Race effects in psychotherapy', in J. Murray and P. R. Abramson (eds), *Bias in Psychotherapy*. New York: Praeger.

Berry, J. W. (1992) *Cross–cultural Psychology: Research and Applications* 2nd edn. Cambridge: Cambridge University Press.

Bhugra, D. (ed.) (1993) *Cross-cultural Psychiatry: Special Issue of International Review of Psychiatry*, 5(2–3).

Bhugra, D. and Bhui, K. (2001). *Cross-cultural Psychiatry: a Practical Guide*. London: Arnold.

Brislin, R. (1993) *Culture's Influence On Behaviour*. New York: Harcourt Brace Publishers.

Brislin, R. and Baumgardner, S. (1971) 'Non-random sampling of individuals in cross-cultural psychology'. *Journal of Cross-cultural Psychology*, 2: 397–400.

d'Ardenne, P. and Mahtani, A. (1989) *Transcultural Counselling in Action*. London: Sage.

de Silva, P. (1999). 'Cultural aspects of post-traumatic stress disorder', in William Yule (ed.), *Post Traumatic Stress Disorders: Concepts and Thera*py. New York and Chichester: Wiley.

de Silva, P. and Samarasinghe, D. (1998) 'Behaviour therapy in Sri Lanka'. In T. P. S. Oei (ed.), *Behaviour Therapy and Cognitive Therapy in Asia*. Glebe, NSW: Edumedia.

Department of Health (1996) *The Patient's Charter and You*. London: HMSO.

Dwivedi, K. N. (1996) 'Culture and personality', in K. N. Dwivedi and V. P. Varma (eds), *Meeting the Needs of Ethnic Minority Children*. London: Jessica Kingsley Publishers.

Fernando, S. (2002) *Mental Health, Race and Culture*. Basingstoke: Palgrave Macmillan.

Holland, K. and Hogg, C. (2001) *Cultural Awareness in Nursing and Health Care*. London: Arnold.

Johnson, D. R., Feldman, S. C., Lubin, H. and Southwick, S. M. (1995) 'The therapeutic use of ritual and ceremony in the treatment of post-traumatic stress disorder'. *Journal of Traumatic Stress*, 8: 283–98.

Kareem, J. and Littlewood, R. (1992). *Intercultural Therapy: Theory and Practice*. Oxford: Blackwell.

Leff, J. (1988) *Psychiatry Around the Globe: a Transcultural View*, 2nd edn. London: Gaskell.

Lloyd, K. and Bhugra, D. (1993) 'Cross-cultural aspects of psychotherapy'. *International Review of Psychiatry*, 5: 291–304.

Lonner, W. and Malpass, R. (1994) *Psychology and Culture*. Harlow: Allyn & Bacon.

Matsumoto, D. (1994) *People: Psychology from a Cultural Perspective*. Pacific Grove, CA: Brooks/Cole Publishing.

Matsumoto, D. and Juang, L. (2004) *Culture and Psychology*. Thomson/Wadsworth.

Murphy, H. B. (1973) 'Migration and major mental disorders: a reappraisal'. In C. Swingmann and M. Pfister-Ammende (eds), *Uprooting and After*. New York: Springer-Verlag, pp. 221–31.

Murphy, H. B. (1977) 'Migration, culture and mental health'. *Psychological Medince*, 7: 677–84.

National Association of Health Authorities and Trusts (1996) *Spiritual Care in the NHGS: a Guide to Purchasers & Providers*. Birmingham: NAHAT.

Palmer, S. and Laungani, P. (1999) *Counselling in a Multicultural Society*. London: Sage.

Pedersen, P. B. (1985) *Handbook of Cross-cultural Counselling and Psychotherapy*. New York: Praeger.

Pedersen, P. B. (1991) 'Introduction to spcial issues on multiculturalism as a fourth force in counselling'. *Journal of Counselling and Development*, 70: 4.

Pomterotto, J. G. and Casas, J. M. (1991) *Handbook of Racial/Ethnic Minority Counselling Research*. Springfield, IL: Chalres C. Thomas.

Shiraev, E. and Levy, D. (2001) *Introduction to Cross-cultural Psychology: Critical Thinking and Contemporary Applications*. Boston, MA: Allyn and Bacon.

Summerfield, D. (1995) 'Addressing human response to war and atrocity: major challenges in research and practices and the limitations of Western psychiatric models'. In R. J. Kleber, C. R. Figley and B. P. R. Gersons (eds), *Beyond Trauma: Cultural and Societal Dynamics*. New York: Plenum Press.

Timimi, S. (2002) *Pathological Child Psychiatry and the Medicalization of Childhood*. London: Brunner, Routledge.

Traindis, H. C. (1980) *Handbook of Cross-cultural Psychology*. Harlow: Allyn & Bacon.

Triandis, H. (1994) *Culture and Social Behaviour*. New York: McGraw-Hill, Inc.

Triands, H., Brislin, R. and Hui, C. (1988) 'Cross-cultural training across the invidulaism-collectivism divide'. *International Journal of Intercultural Relations*, 12: 269–89.

Turner, S., Bowie, C., Dunn, G., Shapo, L. and Yule, W. (2003) 'Mental health of Kosovan refugees in the UK'. *British Journal of Psychiatry*, 182: 444–8.

Van der Veer, G. (1992). *Counselling and Therapy with Refugees*. New York. Wiley (2nd edn, Philadelphia and Hove, East Sussex: Routledge).

Ward, C., Bochner, S. and Farnham, A. (2001) *The Psychology of Culture Shock.* London: Routledge.

Wilson, K. P. (1989) *Trauma, Transformation and Healing: an Integrative Approach to Theory, Research and Post-traumatic Therapy.* New York: Brunner/Mazel.

Yule, W. (1991) 'Work with children following disasters'. In M. Herbert (ed.), *Clinical Child Psychology: Social Learning, Development and Behaviour.* Chichester: Wiley, pp. 349–63.

Yule, W. (1992) 'Post-traumatic stress disorder in child survivors of shipping disasters: the sinking of the *Jupiter*', *Psychotherapy and Psychosomatic,* 57: 200–5.

10
Caring for the Carers: Preventing and Managing Secondary Traumatic Stress

Kate Cairns

Four hundred years ago William Shakespeare (*Macbeth*, Act V, scene 3) provided a vivid description of what we would now call Post-Traumatic Stress Disorder, as Macbeth begged the doctor to provide some relief for the suffering of his wife, Lady Macbeth:

> Can'st thou not minister to a mind diseas'd
> *Pluck from the memory a rooted sorrow*
> Raze out the written troubles of the brain
> *And with some sweet oblivious antidote*
> *Cleanse the stuff'd bosom of that perilous stuff*
> *Which weighs upon the heart?*

Shakespeare clearly recognized the signs and indicators of a mind disordered after overwhelming experience. His description of her disorder would satisfy our current research-based understanding of the effects of horrifying or life-threatening experience on victims of trauma. For what we now call traumatic stress does leave us with rooted sorrows that are written on the very fabric of the brain, and emotional trauma is indeed perilous stuff which weighs upon the heart. Recent developments in research and clinical understanding on this topic have also enabled us to offer considerably more to those who have lived through such terror than the response of Macbeth's doctor – 'therein the patient must minister unto himself'.

Lady Macbeth was, of course, the source of her own horrors through her part in the murder of the king. Most people who live through horrifying experience are victims rather than perpetrators of the terror that disintegrates their lives. And children who survive horrific events are most vulnerable to the destructive effects of overwhelming terror. It is a moral obligation on the adult community to ensure that child victims of terror are cared for, and not left with the bleak task of ministering unto themselves. Yet as our understanding of the impact of emotional trauma has grown, so it has become clear that caring for victims of trauma has an impact of its own. We cannot discharge our obligation to care unless we recognize and willingly accept the consequences of caring.

Surviving primary emotional trauma

Living through horrifying experience or overwhelming threat changes people. The imperative of survival in life-threatening situations results in the human body instantly transforming into an organism with only one focus and purpose, the undivided intention to survive. Any function that would distract from the urgent task of staying alive is automatically switched off.

Human beings are a complex mix of physical, emotional, intellectual, social and spiritual functions. All these are vital components of day-to-day human life. But when confronted with real threat to life or personal integrity, most of these functions are redundant. Feelings, ideas, values, creativity, all the glory of human potential is sacrificed in the cause of survival.

As research has increased our understanding of the way the human brain works (see, for example, Van der Kolk et al. 1996: 293–4), it is clear that the automatic changes that improve the chances of survival in the face of overwhelming threat have greatest impact on the brain. Areas of the brain that deal with complex functions of language, thought, belief and the processing of feelings are instantly deprived of oxygen through reduction in blood supply. Brain function under extreme threat becomes much quicker but also much more primitive.

In adults these changes are superimposed on a brain already working at full functionality. In children the changes brought about by horrifying events are more complex, since they affect brains that are still developing. People who survive traumatic events have to recover the use of brain function through creating new connections and pathways to replace those that have been damaged. Such spontaneous recovery requires:

- Safety: We cannot recover from traumatic stress until we feel safe enough to allow the stress arousal to reduce.
- Supportive social networks with secure attachment relationships: We need other people, people in whom we have complete trust,

who will help us process the traumatic events safely, so that we do not become further overwhelmed by the stress of recall.
- The ability to express what has happened: Processing the traumatic experience through language converts it from a persistent state of high arousal in the present to a memory of a terrifying event that happened in the past.

If people are unable to recover in this way from traumatic events they may be able to encapsulate the trauma, tucking it away out of conscious experience as though it were locked in a box. This can allow us to get on with life, but it is an unstable condition. The trauma box tends to leak, spilling emotional turmoil into everyday life, and altering behaviour in ways inexplicable to the person who cannot remember the cause of the turmoil.

And if we do not recover from or encapsulate the trauma, then individuals are likely to develop various symptoms of a Post-Traumatic Stress Disorder. Such disorders are the result of a persistent state of high stress arousal, and affect every aspect of our functioning (Joseph et al. 1997). Most people, most of the time, survive emotional trauma transformed but not diminished. Indeed the process of recovering from trauma can strengthen us as individuals and as supportive communities (Tedeschi and Calhoun 1995). Where the outcome of living through the horror of overwhelming threat is more destructive, however, survival may leave us with lasting areas of vulnerability in relation to the unprocessed trauma, or actively struggling with disorders of thought, feeling and behaviour.

Human beings can recover from extreme trauma, but there are traumatic events so horrible that most people will be marked by having lived through them. Genocide, the torture of those we love, organized and persistent sexual and emotional degradation, and other such profound distortions of our human relatedness will leave scars in the mind of the most resilient. At the other end of the scale, some people are so vulnerable that they will find it difficult to recover from traumatic events that others will put safely behind them. And vulnerability and resilience fluctuate, so that the outcome of any particular traumatic experience is always uncertain. The outcome of surviving horrific events depends upon a complex interaction between the nature of the trauma we have endured, our own vulnerability and resilience at the time of the trauma, and the capacity of the community that supports us to enable and encourage us to recover from the trauma.

Attachment, empathy and recovery from trauma

Traumatic stress disintegrates key structures of human personality. Whatever complex cognitive structures have been built through our childhood immersion in a network of human interaction, these functions are more or less stripped away by being subject to overwhelming threat. The key to recovery from trauma lies in relationships. We humans have the capacity to form affective bonds that allow us to be patterns and templates for the forming and reforming of cognition in others. Our young depend upon our ability to relate to them in this way. Through the first year of life the human infant has barely enough brain function to survive, and certainly not enough to survive without being dependent on others. But babies can rely on the adults who care for them not only to provide the physical care they need in order to survive, but also to provide their own functioning brains as a template for the developing brain of the infant. This is the process which we call infant attachment. And this ability to act as a pattern against which a non-functioning brain can build itself is the true antidote to the perilous stuff of trauma.

The mechanism for this patterning is empathy. Our ability to harmonize or attune with others, so that we can appreciate their inner world because it echoes in our own person, is central to our ability to survive as a species. And our ability to enable each other to use this attunement to create or repair brain function is central to our ability to survive as individuals and as human groups.

When someone we love, someone with whom we have an attachment relationship, lives through emotional trauma, we make ourselves available to enable them to recover. They will have lost the capacity to regulate stress, so we soothe them. They may have lost the capacity to connect to their own sensory experience, so we engage their attention and reconnect them to the world of their own senses. They will probably have lost some of their ability to be articulate, so we talk and listen and encourage them to communicate. They are likely to have lost the ability to express their feelings, so we prompt them, and guide them, and hold them safe as feelings return and they relive the terrors. They may have lost their ability to regulate and manage their own impulses, so we remind them of their rationality and encourage them to think and plan and take control of their own lives again. We continue to use our functioning brains to support, and protect, and prompt, and encourage them until their own injured brain recovers. And we do all this because we can connect to their inner world through empathy.

Empathy and secondary trauma

Emotional trauma is a social phenomenon. It occurs to individuals and groups in a social context, and recovery from it requires the support of a social network that includes well-formed attachment relationships. Empathy, the pathway to recovery, is also a social phenomenon. It occurs between persons, a complex process of physiological attunement allowing us to function as highly adaptive groups and groupings.

Attunement automatically adjusts our physiology in the direction of the physiology of the person to whom we are relating. It allows us to enter a shared emotional space, aligning our brain and body function so that we can operate as a single unit, a human group. But just as this physiological harmonizing enables the traumatized person to recover, it also has a cost for the attachment figure. The process of attunement regulates the stress response in the victim of trauma, but moves the dyad of victim and carer in the direction of dysregulation. Traumatic stress is contagious.

This stress response, caused by caring for or about someone who has been traumatized, is known as secondary trauma or vicarious trauma. It can produce profound changes in physiology, leading to changes in functioning similar to those created by primary trauma. So people who have not themselves lived through the primary trauma can be affected as though they had lived through the terrifying event. Charles Figley (2002, for example) has produced significant research over many years in this field, and has shown the benefits of using this as a model to support the work of a range of people exposed to risk of secondary trauma. The concept of secondary trauma has proved immensely helpful over the past few years for people caring for traumatized children in the UK who have come across it and applied it as a model to make sense of their experience and inform their working practice.

Vulnerability and resilience when exposed to trauma

It is clear that everyone who works with traumatized children is exposed to trauma. Most of these people most of the time are highly resilient, this being a field of work that generally attracts healthy, positively motivated and resilient individuals. People who choose to work with traumatized children will usually be people who have a considerable capacity to continue their life development healthily even under adverse conditions. They will be people who tend to bounce back from adversity.

Resilience is not static, however. We are differently resilient under different conditions. Some of the factors that influence our resilience are individual, and some are social and cultural. People who are and remain socially competent and autonomous in the situation in which they find themselves, able to apply thinking skills and problem solving ability creatively, and able to maintain a sense of perspective and humour are more likely to be resilient in the face of trauma. If we can retain a sense of overarching moral order, of meaning and purpose, and of spiritual values, we are more able to stay centred and healthy when exposed to the disintegrative chaos of traumatic stress. And people who are held in a network of close, confiding, intimate relationships with positive and secure attachments are much more resilient in the face of potentially overwhelming stress.

Everyone who is exposed to trauma is vulnerable to the effects of secondary traumatic stress, and, since resilience fluctuates, everyone is also potentially vulnerable to being unable to bounce back or recover spontaneously from such stress. Anyone who works with traumatized children may develop a secondary stress disorder (Cairns and Stanway 2004).

Signs and indicators of developing disorder

There are a number of common themes that emerge from our work with carers and social workers that are consistent with the research of Charles Figley and Beth Hudnall Stamm. These themes were also apparent in the lives of the many people that the author of this chapter interviewed when preparing *Surviving Paedophilia* (1999). In working, and supporting work, with traumatized children it is important to be alert for changes in functioning that may affect anyone involved with the work. Such changes may be indicators that the worker is becoming overwhelmed, and that they will need help to prevent disorder developing.

- Increase in distressing emotions:
  - Anger, irritability or rage in otherwise equable people
  - Tearfulness or sadness in otherwise sanguine people
  - Fearfulness or generalized anxiety in otherwise tranquil people
- Otherwise unexplained changes in health:
  - Altered sleep patterns
    - Finding it difficult to get to sleep
    - Waking often
    - Waking early
    - Sleeping longer and more heavily

- ○ Altered patterns of consumption – eating, drinking, smoking
  - ■ Changes in appetite
  - ■ Craving stimulant or soothing foods and drinks
  - ■ Using mood altering substances such as tobacco or alcohol
- ○ Stress-related physical illnesses not present, or noticeably less intense, before the work
  - ■ Migraine or tension headaches
  - ■ Mouth and throat problems related to reduced saliva
  - ■ Respiratory problems such as asthma
  - ■ Digestive disorders
  - ■ Sexual dysfunction
  - ■ Skin disorders
  - ■ Tension in the long muscles leading to aches and pains
- Persistent physiological arousal:
  - ○ Exaggerated startle response, jumpiness
  - ○ Nightmares – dreams with traumatic content
  - ○ Hypervigilance
    - ■ Diminished concentration
    - ■ Reduced attention span
    - ■ Impaired short-term memory
- Avoidance of working with traumatic material:
  - ○ Unable to enter emotional space of child, or over-identified with child and sharing child's avoidance of the trauma
- Impairment of day-to-day functioning, leading to behavioural changes:
  - ○ Decreased use of support networks
    - ■ Gradual loss of language function, especially in relation to speaking feelings, leads to inability to make use of support and withdrawal from existing networks of support and supervision
  - ○ Missed or cancelled appointments
    - ■ Unconscious avoidance of exposing impaired ability to communicate can lead to missing appointments where the child would be discussed
  - ○ Diminished self-organization
    - ■ Being late
    - ■ Reduced self-care
  - ○ Increased feelings of isolation, alienation and lack of appreciation
    - ■ 'No one understand what it's like working with this child'
    - ■ 'No one appreciates my situation'

Once we begin to suffer from secondary traumatic stress disorders there will be changes in our work performance. We may simply be unable to do as much work in the time available, or we may work even harder but much less effectively, so that there is a change in both the quantity and quality of work. We are likely to make more mistakes. We may become avoidant of certain specific tasks, such as report writing, or particular areas of direct work with the traumatized child. People in this situation often develop work habits that seem obsessive or perfectionist to colleagues, usually over trivial matters that in other circumstances would not engage their interest. As the disorder persists people inevitably become exhausted. At that point, having lost energy, motivation and perspective they will become risky workers who can no longer handle the responsibility of the work.

There is a similar progressive deterioration in morale. We become less confident as brain function diminishes under the impact of the secondary stress. The reduced function in areas of the brain that regulate stress also leads to impairment of the capacity to experience joy, so that there is a growing sense of apathy. The loss of joy can also lead to a loss of optimism, and a bleak negativity that stifles creative and constructive action. People often experience a generalized sense of dissatisfaction and feelings of incompleteness, as though some core part of the self had vanished, which indeed is the case in that core brain functions have diminished. And finally, in this dreary progression, the person loses touch with their own core sense of identity, and becomes completely subsumed in the work and detached from the roots of their own being. At this stage, paradoxically, the worker can be seen as utterly dedicated to their work, although sadly ineffective individually and as a member of the team.

The impact of secondary traumatic stress on the whole network

This destructive dynamic can afflict anyone and everyone involved in working with traumatized children. Emotional trauma, especially when it affects children as the primary victims, spreads like blast from a bomb. It affects people apparently at random, so that someone relatively close to the centre of the traumatic event may emerge unscathed, but someone apparently much more distant is completely knocked out by it and may be seriously wounded.

The consequences of such destructiveness can be grave. Just at a time when we most need to work together as a cohesive team, we withdraw from one another, protecting ourselves from the splitting and disintegrative effects of trauma by allowing ourselves to be split apart, and unable to see the splitting because the causes of it lie in the closing down of our own functionality. We lose our ability to appreciate and even to respect one another. Individuals and groups can enter into a perverse trauma dynamic of neediness and blame, perceiving others as inadequate, or as hostile and persecutory. Professional colleagues who should be providing multidisciplinary services can find themselves enmeshed in conflict instead of sharing a genuine collaborative effort.

Disruptions of emotional functioning can lead to irritability and impatience between colleagues. And disruptions in cognitive function can seriously impair communication. Individuals may become less able to communicate accurately or constructively with other individuals, and whole organizational and inter-agency communications strategies can be shattered.

As the disintegrative effects of trauma begin to affect the functioning of individuals and teams, the management response can be controlling or punitive, with managers attempting to hold off the encroaching chaos by trying to impose structures that appear to them to be clear, but in the environment of threat engendered by trauma are often perceived by others as rigid and punitive. Then an adversarial situation can arise, and issues of discipline and compliance or non-compliance replace the creative give and take of a healthy functioning team or organization.

Prevention of secondary traumatic stress disorder

In our work with people caring for traumatized children three key areas have emerged as vital in creating strategies to prevent secondary traumatic stress disorder: training, supervision and social support. These findings are in line with research such as that discussed by Ursano and colleagues (Van der Kolk et al. 1996: Chapter 19), and the work of Charles Figley and of Beth Hudnall Stamm (Figley 2002; and Hudnall Stamm 1995). These three essential strands of prevention policy can together do a great deal to reduce the impact of exposure to trauma, and to enhance the resilience of trauma exposed individuals and groups.

Training

People are more resilient, and less vulnerable to developing disorder, while caring for traumatized children if they have an understanding of the impact of traumatic stress in general, and the impact of secondary traumatic stress in particular. They need to know what happens to traumatized children when they try to live day by day with the long-term effects of trauma, and they need to know what happens to adults who live and work with traumatized children.

Other types of training can also build resilience. Learning new skills in stress management can provide an enhanced repertoire of responses to exposure to stressors. Training that leads to recognized professional development promotes an enhanced sense of identity separate from the traumatized child, as does any training that leads to substantive personal development.

Hudnall Stamm (1995) addressed the fact that people who work with victims of trauma can be isolated both geographically and socially. Her work on the development of telemedicine, establishing virtual communities for mutual learning, support and supervision, has inspired us to produce training and qualifications online for people who work with traumatized children, providing information, the opportunity to acquire and practise new skills and professional development through gaining a qualification. The evidence so far from this project is that it is showing benefits to the carers and workers, and to the traumatized children with whom they work.

Supervision

People working with traumatized children need to do so within a safe professional structure. The tendency for secondary trauma to lead to distortions and impairments of thought, feelings and behaviour can lead to errors of professional judgement as well as to diminished health and self-care in workers. Supervision of the work and the worker therefore needs to be structured and regular, with the agency clearly taking responsibility for the nature and quality of the work. Supervisors will need to be able to provide 'grief leadership' (Van der Kolk et al. 1996: 452), paying attention to and containment for the strong feelings involved, as well as task-centred and practical management of the work.

Above all, supervisors should be working from a knowledge base that includes a clear understanding of the dynamics of trauma work. They will then play their part in developing and maintaining a whole team and whole organization approach to working with trauma that ensures that the splitting and disintegrative impact of trauma does not destroy the work.

Social support

The quality and resilience of the social network supporting a trauma worker is a key factor in preventing stress disorders. And conversely, exposure to trauma, especially in work with traumatized children, can produce such changes in people that key relationships are diminished or may disintegrate entirely (Cairns 1999: 110–11). Partners and families can become caretakers, distorting the usual pattern of these close intimate relationships and putting strain on everyone involved. Yet if partners and families can become aware of the issues of secondary trauma they can become the most powerful preventive factor, keeping the person they love safe from harm despite the demands of their work with traumatized children. Information and training aimed at the network of social support around those who work with traumatized children will help to maintain the health of both the worker and the network, and so effectively contribute to preventing secondary traumatic stress disorder.

Colleagues are also a vital source of support, provided that they understand the issues and are not themselves affected by disorder. In addition to informal collegiate support, teams and organizations can establish formal structures of peer support that can have a powerful preventive effect. Peer groups set up to address issues of professional and personal self-care when exposed to trauma, and mentoring systems in which experienced workers provide targeted support for those less experienced, are both effective support structures within teams, across organizations, and across disciplines. At times of particular difficulty, telephone or email helplines between peers may also be useful support mechanisms.

Treatment of secondary traumatic stress disorder

It is not possible always to prevent secondary stress disorders. No one can be constantly resilient, and work with traumatized children presents constant levels of exposure whilst vulnerability to being injured by that exposure shifts. People who do develop stress disorders as a result of working with traumatized children, however, can generally recover quickly if offered treatment that genuinely addresses their condition (Figley 2002).

The first step to treatment is for the person to recover physiological self-management so that they are no longer persistently hyper-aroused or dissociated. To do so, the person affected must recognize the need for treatment. This will require the help of a trusted challenger, someone who will take responsibility for overcoming the fear of disorder and neediness, and encourage the person to accept the help they need, and they will also need medical supervision of their recovery process.

Then the individual will be encouraged to notice the changes in their own functioning, especially in relation to stress regulation, relaxation and pleasure responses. They will need to commit themselves to practise activities that should produce relaxation and pleasure, and to notice the absence of their accustomed responses. Often this is enough in itself to produce the first signs of change, and they can be encouraged to notice this resurrection of tranquillity and joy in their lives, making sure that they record their progress as fully as possible in spoken words, written words, and other symbols that promote recovery of brain function. If this programme is enough to produce the desired recovery, they will then need to develop with their supervisor or therapist strategies to prevent recurrence and maintain health and wellbeing.

Sometimes the hyper-arousal is too entrenched for such methods to be effective, and people need temporary medication prescribed by a doctor with specialist knowledge of the treatment of trauma. Work with traumatized children may also produce profound cognitive distortions, leaving workers ruminating ceaselessly on images of catastrophe, or unable to form structures of meaning and purpose. They may then need some sort of cognitive therapy to enable them to rebuild healthy cognitive function. When descending into stress disorder people may develop adverse patterns of behaviour in an attempt to manage the increasingly out of control stress. Behavioural patterns such as smoking, heavy drinking, overeating, gambling, excessive physical exercise, and so on may start as maladaptive responses to the stress but become habits which the individual needs help to overcome after they have recovered from the stress disorder.

Working with traumatized children may also trigger unresolved traumas from the past history of the workers themselves. These traumatic events may be quite different from the traumas suffered by the children with whom they are working, but the exposure to trauma is the trigger breaking open the encapsulated past event. Workers triggered in this way will need help to resolve their own previous trauma safely. Couple relationships anywhere in the network supporting traumatized children are also potentially at risk as trauma has a splitting effect. This splitting may divide partners, but can also affect any dyad relationships such as pairs of colleagues, or friends. It is vital for traumatized children that dyad relationships in the network remain intact and strong, and it is also essential for the workers that they are able to maintain, and if necessary have help to restore, their close and intimate relationships. Whole groups can also be split by trauma, including care teams and care families. Group therapy, or family therapy, may be needed to restore the strong relationship patterns that are so vital for the health of the network. Such therapy should always be provided by therapists who thoroughly understand the issues and dynamics involved in working with trauma.

Agency responsibility for prevention and treatment

The recognition, prevention and treatment of secondary traumatic stress disorder are a matter of health and safety for every organization providing services to traumatized children. Agencies have a responsibility to recognize hazards to workers, including any hazards arising from occupational stress. They need to assess the risks associated with such hazards, and to have strategies in place to reduce and to manage risk.

This is not just a matter of responsibility and liability, however. There are clear benefits to agencies in dealing appropriately with secondary traumatic stress. Organizations that put in place strategies to prevent and treat secondary traumatic stress are likely to find that they reduce absenteeism and stress-related sickness, increase efficiency and effectiveness in the workforce, reduce workplace and interagency conflict, increase collaborative working practices, and increase job satisfaction. These are rich rewards for relatively little outlay. To gain these benefits the organization will need to ensure that there is an understanding of the hazards and risks of secondary stress throughout the entire organizational structure, with integrated whole organization policies and procedures.

Concluding remarks and key messages

Finally, a few key messages drawn from the work of Figley and colleagues (2002). People who live and work with traumatized children are caregivers, and the evidence is that such people do not readily take to being recipients of care. They need to be enabled and empowered to accept and benefit from the care that they require in order to maintain health and well-being when engaged in toxic work. It is vital that any workplace delivering services to traumatized children is based on respect. This sounds trite, but in reality genuine respect is one of the first casualties of secondary stress, since others in the network begin to be perceived as malign persecutors or pathetic victims instead of respected colleagues. So establishing and maintaining an environment of respect is work requiring dedication and energy when working with trauma. It is also vital to recognize that every human being is equal in the face of trauma. We are all vulnerable, and we are all in need of mutual support and encouragement.

The world needs people who are willing to work with traumatized children. They carry much of our hope for the future. It must be the responsibility of the rest of the community to ensure that those who devote themselves to the well-being of vulnerable and wounded children are supported and sustained in their work, so that their own health and well-being are maintained and strengthened.

References

Cairns, K. (1999) *Surviving Paedophilia: Traumatic Stress after Organized and Network Child Sexual Abuse*. Stoke on Trent: Trentham Books.

Cairns, K. and Stanway, C. (2004) *Learn the Child: Helping Looked-after Children to Learn: a Good Practice Guide for Social Workers, Carers and Teachers*. London: British Association for Adoption and Fostering.

Figley, C. (ed.) (1995) *Compassion Fatigue: Coping with Secondary Traumatic Stress Disorder in Those who Live with the Traumatized*. Reading, CT: Brunner Mazel.

Figley, C. (ed.) (2002) *Treating Compassion Fatigue*. Reading, CT: Brunner-Routledge.

Joseph, S., Williams, R. and Yule, W. (1997) *Understanding Post-Traumatic Stress: a Psychosocial Perspective on PTSD and Treatment*. Chichester: Wiley.

Stamm, B. H. (ed.) (1995) *Secondary Traumatic Stress: Self-care Issues for Clinicians, Researchers and Educators*. Towson, MD: Sidran Press.

Tedeschi, R. G. and Calhoun, G. C. (1995) *Trauma and Transformation: Growing in the Aftermath of Suffering*. Thousand Oaks, CA: Sage.

Van der Kolk, B. A., McFarlane, A. C. and Weisaeth, L. (eds) (1996) *Traumatic Stress: the Effects of Overwhelming Experience on Mind, Body and Society*. New York: Guilford Press.

Part II

Applied Context of Trauma Psychology

11
Responding to the Protection Needs of Traumatized and Sexually Abused Children

Liz Davies

Child sexual abuse[1] has been described as soul murder due to the serious and lasting damage to the child's emotional, neurological and physiological development that results from the overwhelming impact of trauma which includes both fear and pain (Strong 1998: 65). However, the word 'trauma' comes from the Greek word meaning 'to pierce' which Bentovim explains as a piercing of the protective layers of the mind (1992: 24). Victims of such overwhelming trauma tend to live in a world of continual and unpredictable danger, alone and powerless without means of escape. Van der Kolk (cited in Strong 1998: 95) equates the abuse as more pernicious than that affecting prisoners of war in that the abusers are often the people who are supposed to protect and nurture the child. Frampton (2004: 218) in a graphic account of his childhood in residential care noted that the gleam had gone from a child's eyes when they had suffered abuse at the hands of those employed to care for them. He described trying to reach out to his abused friend: 'We all peered inside but the watchman's lamp had gone out.' Like him I 'pay tribute and marvel at how out of so little, so many children are able to shape reasonable lives as adults' (2004: 290). Therefore this chapter aims to highlight both the extent of the suffering of sexually abused children and the nature of such trauma.

Understanding the extent of child sexual abuse

To understand the incidence of abuse, it has been suggested that one should imagine three victims of child sexual abuse for every car on the road (Survivors Swindon 2005). Children from all cultures and ethnicities are sexually abused at all age levels by men, women and other young people. The abuse is generally repeated and lasting in 50 per cent of cases between the ages of 2 and 18 years, and in 67 per cent of cases beginning before the age of 11 years (National Commission of Inquiry, 1996). More than 80 per cent of the victims of sexual abuse know their abuser and most abuse takes place in the home of the child or the abuser (Cawson et al. 2000; Grubin 1998). Disabled children are 3.1 times more likely to suffer sexual abuse than non-disabled children (Sullivan 2000). Other statistics confirm that 6 per cent of child abductions are sexually motivated (Newiss and Fairbrother 2004). It also seems that children are commonly victimized by more than one abuser (APRI 2004: 70).

The extent of child sexual abuse is underestimated given the low level of child and adult reporting. Children may deny abuse, not understand that it is wrong, or their reaction to it may be significantly delayed sometimes due to the lack of recall of the abuse. The more extreme the level of abuse the more likely it will be shielded from the child's consciousness (Briere and Conte 1993; Briere and Elliott 1994; Finkelhor 1979; Summit 1988). The focus on the 'false memory' debate detracts from the reality of the abuse recollections by children (APRI 2004: 35). In a study of ten young adults who were sexually exploited as children through abusive images, none had told freely of the events in 28 years. This provides a very different view to the idea that children make false allegations (Svedin and Bach 1996). An NSPCC[2] study concluded that 72 per cent of sexually abused children stated that they were too frightened to tell anyone at the time of the abuse and 31 per cent still had not told anyone by early adulthood (Cawson et al. 2000). It must be understood that to speak of abuse is a deeply painful task for a child or adult. A young man aged 14 years spent interview after interview telling the author of this chapter about the many types of bottle on a shelf, their colours and contents and types of lid. After one excruciating 20 minutes of silence he finally said these were used by the abuser to prepare him for rape.

The abuser's insistence on secrecy with direct or indirect threats is a powerful influence (APRI 2004: 35). Mudaly and Goddard (2001: 228) noted that 'the abuser like a terrorist utilises a state of fear in the victim to obtain compliance ... the victim is a need satisfying object'. Survival strategies assisting a child to cope with continuing maltreatment may include the child abuse accommodation syndrome including reactions of secrecy, helplessness, entrapment, delayed unconvincing disclosure and retraction (Summit 1983). One of the most vivid accounts of being a child and unable to speak about sexual abuse is that of Mary Bell who killed two children when she was 11 years old. At the age of 40 she looked back on a childhood where her mother exposed her to abuse by numbers of men. 'I was so frightened because she says if I ever told anything I would be locked up. You know I told you about the sentry box on the Tyne bridge? That's where she said I would go and she said nobody would believe me. And anyway, I think I must have thought it was my fault. I had done wrong and was being punished ... I felt so dirty' (Sereny 1999: 335). Many child victims only disclose much later in life commonly when they wish to prevent other children being abused by the same perpetrator. Detective Chief Inspector Spindler commented that out of over 2000 child sexual abuse investigations in London each year over 30 per cent are 'historic', i.e. cases of adults who were sexually abused as children (Fairhurst and Spindler 2005).

There is concern that as much as 95 per cent of sexual crime against children is unreported (NCIS 2003). The low level of adult reporting of serious crimes against children was raised during the review of the West case (Bridge 1996) and also by Chief Inspector Stoodley at the time of Operation Orchid, an investigation of the abduction and murder of young boys in London and the south east, who stated that children had vanished without trace without anyone caring or having looked for them. 'The bodies of young boys were being carried about the Kingsmead Estate in broad daylight' (Oliver and Smith 1993: 275). Cawson et al. (2000) reported the incidence of child sexual abuse as 21 per cent of girls and 11 per cent of boys when defined as acts to which they had not consented or where consensual activity had occurred with someone five years or more older and the child was 12 years or less. Yet when placed within a context of knowledge about the offending patterns of child sex abusers (NSPCC 2005a), child trafficking for sexual exploitation (Metropolitan Police 2003), the marketing of abusive images of children (Renold et al. 2003) and the entire globalized industry of child sexual exploitation, it is extraordinary that so few children's names are on the UK child protection registers under the category of child sexual abuse – only 2700 in 2003, a considerable reduction compared with 6600 in 1999 (NSPCC 2005b). Multi-agency community prevention programmes aimed at increasing public awareness to ensure appropriate reporting of suspicion and knowledge of child sexual abuse must be in place if children are to access the investigative, protective processes (Davies 2004). However, the main focus of this chapter is the professional response both pre- and post-referral.

The pathologization of child victims of sexual abuse

Frampton (2004: 290) noted that 'society pays for its neglect – children become adults'. Yet instead of focusing protective systems on the child victims of abuse, current policy pathologizes children as potential criminals and threats to the social order. Children whose lives have been damaged by neglect and abuse are the very children who occupy the juvenile remand wings of prisons (Goldson 2002: 5.1). Further, it is estimated that one-third of women and one in twenty men in prison have suffered child sexual abuse. A prison inspection report states that 'many or most children in locked establishments have suffered neglect, ill treatment and violence but few have received the treatment that is their right' (Children's Rights Alliance 2002). Children negatively described as 'feral' – a term for a forgotten underclass of children that roam inner cities, and claimed by a police commissioner to be a threat second only to terrorism – have typically been sexually assaulted whilst in care. Homeless children have commonly been sexually abused (Townsend 2004). Hence, punitively stigmatizing these children as criminals diverts attention from the importance of child protection investigation and the targeting of child abusers – it is a crude dynamic of blaming the victim.

Professionals are key messengers between the child and the state and as such bear a major responsibility for listening to the child's voice and representing the right of children to be free from abuse (UNCRC 1990: Articles 3, 19, 34 and 39). The Children Act 1989 is unequivocal in requiring the protection of children from actual or likely significant harm (1989 s. 47) but it is a far from simple task. Monahon (1993) compares the traumatic effect to a childhood wound that is often invisible, internal and where there are no X rays to define the damage (cited in Hutchinson 2005: 7). The following sections will describe the enormity of the professional task of recognizing and understanding the trauma of child abuse, of rigorously investigating allegations of abuse and of seeking justice for the child victims through the identification and prosecution of perpetrators.

It's hard to tell

The subject of this poem was a 15-year-old girl who was being sexually and physically abused by her father:

> I wonder how a child
> Who is being tortured day and night
> Who's body aches and pains
> Can sing Or laugh Or anything?

How can such a child
Play in the playground
And pretend
So perfectly?
There is no feeling
That's how it's done.

She hung her head and Spoke
In soft, dull tone
One word blended with
the next in a stream of
Unspecific sorrow
Sometimes, she said, a male voice was in her head.
She waited hour on hour
to see someone, anyone.
'What's she here for?' They said.
'She's here again'
'Not again'
'there's no dialogue.
What's the point?'

Some persisted
Reaching out within the pain
Entering inside the enigma
and barely holding on.

Still she came
She was so young.
He trapped her every day.
Six times.
She could not fight.
He gave her drugs.
He pinned her down.
Her inner voice kept her sane.
The phantom male loved her while
her father stole her body
and tore her mind.

Now she can – now and then
look me in the eye
for one small fleeting moment only.

As a professional social worker, I had a problem. I was guessing. She presented in my office almost daily after school for no apparent reason and in a way unseen by other agencies. At school she was the model child but I would see her muttering to herself. Very slowly I gained her trust. Not by questioning and pressurizing but by listening, often in silence, feeling her pain and waiting patiently until she was ready to tell. At any stage it would have been easy to wreck this delicate process. Each time I reassured her that if she needed me to make her safe I would do so – because that was my job. I also spoke with her about my police colleague whom I trusted and who would be willing to meet her. The joint police and social work investigation waited in the wings until one day she made the decision that her need for her only parent to give her love was not as great as her need to escape his sexual abuse and violence.

This was the London Borough of Islington in 1992. It was just one of the many cases where young people came to trust social workers in a small local neighbourhood office. The young people demonstrated Factor X. An unknown. A gap in professional knowledge leading to the all important hypothesis about what the child's experience might be given small pieces of available information about drug and alcohol misuse, petty crime, mental ill health and attempted suicide often in a context of parental neglect and abuse.

The hypothesis that a high number of young people were being sexually exploited in the locality had to be tested. This was achieved through a number of strategies. It became obvious that the nervous, disorientated, secretive and frightened young people would not provide the evidence – it was only later that the social workers learned of the abusers' threats to 'bury them alive' or 'knife them if they told'. Whilst social workers befriended the young people individually and tried to gain their trust, the strategy did not depend on the child's account as sole evidence. The children needed no added pressure. They were suffering enough and it is clearly an adult responsibility to protect children.

Police and social workers worked with all other agencies in the area and local community representatives to collate information. This was mapped and analysed together with the many clues provided by the children and their families such as places, names, car and telephone numbers. The joint investigation strategy focused on gathering intelligence about the child abusers and targeted them through proactive surveillance and profiling. As children were protected by their families or through child protection procedures and civil proceedings the abusers simply drew more young people from the pool of vulnerable children so constantly available to them in this disadvantaged area of the city. It later became known that the network of abusers extended throughout the children's homes – the places where as social workers we had placed them for safety. Demetrius Panton, a survivor of the Islington child abuse scandal, spoke of a healing that needed to take place within him that couldn't begin until someone had apologized to him (Blitz 1996).

Perpetrator focused strategies and seeking justice for children

Enabling and empowering children to speak of their experiences in their own time and at their own pace in child-centred environments to professionals trained in specialist child interview skills is one key component of a child protection investigation. However, to effectively protect children there must be risk assessments of the abusers and where necessary the abuser must be removed from the child's environment. Child protection procedures must include a dual strategy – work with the child and the non-abusive family to respond to the child's need for safety as well as investigative work to identify and target the child abuser. Sarah Nelson states in her research of women survivors of child sexual abuse: 'the survivors felt strongly that they should have been protected at an early age and that the perpetrators should have faced legal justice many years before' (Nelson 2001). Seeking justice is an important aspect of the healing process for children, and whilst going to court may be stressful for children it can also help the child gain a sense of empowerment (Vieth in APRI 2004: 36).

For the relatively small numbers of children who seek justice through the courts there is a low rate of prosecution and conviction. A recent study suggests only one in 50 sex offences against children result in conviction (Stuart and Baines 2004). One in three children who report child sexual abuse are under the age of 8 years and yet a study of four police authorities found that prosecutions are extremely rare for this group. There is much concern that children with disabilities and children for whom English is not their first language are not sufficiently represented among the cases that proceed to trial (Utting 1997: 20.10).

One graphic example is that raised by the QC to the Waterhouse Inquiry. 'Police interviewed 2500 people leading to the investigation of 500 complaints of physical or sexual abuse and arising out of this inquiry 8 individuals were prosecuted. On the face of it this appears an extremely small number. Only 6 were convicted' (G. Elias, QC to the Tribunal cited in Utting 1997: 20.4). When child sex abusers are convicted it is not uncommon for there to be a long history of previous incidents of abuse allegations which had not led to prosecution. The review which examined the history of thirteen cases of sexually abusive incidents in the Ian Huntley case stated that, 'even this is almost certainly not a complete list of the young women' (Kelly 2004: 32). Abusers commonly evade investigation for years before finally being brought to court.

There are 24 721 sex offenders on the Sex Offenders Register in England and Wales. This statistic includes offences against adults and children and only accounts for sexual crime convictions post-1997 (Home Office 2004). Suspected and known child sex abusers are monitored by the Multi Agency Public Protection Panels (MAPPP) in each authority which consider the current circumstances of registered sex offenders and potentially dangerous adults in the community and develop a multi agency risk management strategy to reduce the risk of further offending and protect the public (Home Office 2003). Concerns about a child sex abuser should be reported to the panel either to the chair or through one's own agency representative on the panel.

The process of criminal proceedings may itself be abusive to children. The court is an adult arena and is guided by the principles of criminal justice rather than the Children Act 1989. Some 16 out of 50 children interviewed in a recent study described the experience as extremely negative (Plotnikoff and Woolfson 2004). Whilst the investigative interview of the child using the Achieving Best Evidence Guidance (Home Office 2002) is favourably described by children as a child-centred process, the court appearance itself may be traumatic as children are frequently discredited as witnesses and they often have to undergo lengthy and harsh cross-examination (Davies and Westcott 1999: 28). Increased attention to the obtaining of forensic evidence and the identification of adult witnesses – such as former victims of the same alleged abuser or witnesses to the abuse – would take the onus of proof off the child and also assist in providing supportive corroborative evidence.

An evaluation of child protection policies and procedures

Although few child sexual abuse cases progress to criminal proceedings in the UK, children do gain protection through civil legislation and child protection procedures under the balance of probabilities standard of proof. Since 1945 child abuse inquiries have provided a vast knowledge base for protecting children through the formal processes of professionals working together. The statutory guidance 'Working Together to Safeguard Children' (DfES 2006) provides the formal framework for good practice known to be effective in protecting children and very few children who die from abuse are subject to child protection procedures such as the Child Protection Register (Reder et al. 1994; Munro 2002). The guidance is implemented through local child protection procedures under the scrutiny of the Local Safeguarding Children Boards.

There is a myth that failure to protect children derives mainly from miscommunication between agencies. The picture is instead commonly one of a great deal of inter-agency communication but absence of analysis and non-compliance with statutory guidance. The key reason for such professional failure is staff employed within unsafe working environments, lacking in supervision, good management and training and overwhelmed with high workloads (CST 2005; Munro 2005).

Indeed, a considerable number of traumatized abused children do not gain access to protective child protection strategies. *Messages from Research* (DoH 1995) began a policy shift which emphasized that too many children were entering the child protection net. It was also suggested that the threshold defining child protection was set too high. This viewpoint continues to steer government policy away from proactive child protection intervention and towards universal policies which focus on prevention and involve a focus on all children and inter-familial child 'concerns' rather than the significant harm criteria defined in the Children Act 1989. This perspective is seriously flawed as child sexual abuse does not correlate with social and economic disadvantage and strategies which aim at an end to social exclusion and will not resolve the protection issues for children at risk of abuse which occurs in all social classes (Munro 2005; Munro and Calder 2005). The Green Paper *Every Child Matters* (ECM) (The Treasury 2003) and the subsequent Children Act 2004 define risk as children at risk of social exclusion, which moves professionals further away from the investigation of children at risk of child abuse. Strategies focusing on perpetrators, particularly those located outside the immediate family, are noticeably omitted – probation, the key agency with knowledge about child abusers, is absent from the hub of agencies described in ECM as needed to network in the interests of the child. During the 1980s and early 1990s agencies working together worked well to produce hundreds of child protection investigations achieving justice for children. A backlash led to steady erosion of the child protection system and the language of child protection has become lost. Instead of a focus on child abuse, significant harm, risk, investigation and protection the words used are concern, need, inquiry and safeguarding.

Laming emphasized the importance of social workers being involved in investigation and analysis (Laming 2003: 9.593), yet since the introduction of *The Framework of Assessment for Children in Need and their Families* (DoH 2000) social workers conduct assessments to strict timescales in a conveyor belt approach with fast turnover of cases (see also Reder et al. 1993; Reder and Duncan 1999). Government targets drive managers to close cases prematurely and keep the numbers on the Child Protection Register low. This trend was noted in a recent inspection report: 'councils have unusually high thresholds for responding to child protection referrals and in taking action to protect children' (CSCI 2005: 2.7). The threshold for Section 47 intervention is actually low: 'reasonable cause to suspect actual or likely significant harm' (Chidren Act 1989: 47). Haringey social work managers pursued a family support model of social work, emphasizing the needs of Victoria Climbie's carers as a refugee family for housing and financial support rather than a child protection investigative approach. When Victoria Climbie's aunt alleged sexual abuse of Victoria by Carl Manning, the referral did not result in formal child protection processes. There was no joint investigation with police, formal interview of the child, paediatric assessment or a child protection conference. Yet Victoria told the social worker, 'I'm not lying. I must tell you more. It's true' (Laming 2003: 6.395). It was thought that the referrer was using the allegations as a ruse to obtain housing and the child was unheard. Victoria did not achieve the status of being defined as a child in need of protection. 'She was labelled from the outset as a child in need' (Reder et al. 2004: 95).

Locating intervention within the needs of the child and family distracts attention from the abuse of children by organized networks of child abusers through trafficking, abusive images and sexual exploitation. A recent critique of the professional response to child sexual abuse was that of the inspection into the care and protection of children in Eilean Siar (SWIA 2005). Although no criminal prosecutions achieved convictions the review made a finding that three children were repeatedly sexually abused and concluded that there was an 'unhelpful imbalance in the weight given to the rights and duties of parents as against the needs and rights of the children'. Professionals had been over-optimistic about the capacity of the parents to protect the children, and large amounts of information had been logged and shared as part of assessment but there had not been any analysis of the meaning of that information or proper debate among professionals enabling tough decisions to be made.

Laming recommended a police focus on investigation of crime 'completely and exclusively' (Laming 2003: 14–57). This has led police to withdraw from the joint investigation of actual or likely significant harm unless there is clearly an offence which has been committed. Social workers are now often left alone to conduct assessments and unless they find 'evidence of abuse' little proactive joint work takes place. The polarization of the two statutory agency responsibilities – the police focus on crime and the social work focus on assessment – 'leaves a gap in the statutory response to child sexual abuse which will lead to vulnerable children slipping through the protective net' (Davies and Jarman 2005: 814). One example of this approach is the statutory response to the accessing of abusive images of children. Detective Chief Inspector McLachlan, former head of Scotland Yard's Paedophile Unit has commented that the police focus on inter-familial sexual crime led to a lack of investigation of predatory child sex abusers (McLachlan 2003). In 2002 he had found abusive pictures of 13 000 young people and only 175 of the child victims were identified due to lack of police resources and cases not progressing to joint investigation or organized abuse procedures (DfES 2006: 6–8; Home Office 2002; ALG 2003: Ch. 11). 'The victims of these horrendous crimes – the children themselves – are not being found and helped' (Carr 2005). The police child abuse investigation teams only respond to cases of abuse within the family or by carers. There are very few police resources dedicated to the investigation of organized abuse of children.

Listening to children – making a referral

Sexually abused children come to the attention of professionals in a number of ways. There may be a direct disclosure, signs and indicators of child sexual abuse, admission by a known offender, discovery of abusive images of the child, or medical and/or forensic evidence. Children's disclosures are frequently met with disbelief as adults mirror the child abuse accommodation syndrome (Summit 1983) and excuse, minimize or deny the allegation. In one study half of 124 adults who had suffered child sexual abuse and spoken out at the time had not been believed (Mullen et al. 1996). The few children who do speak about child sexual abuse may present as tearful and depressed but equally they may drip feed the information slowly over time constantly testing the response of the adult they have chosen to trust. Children do not wish to harm a positive relationship with an adult and will need to reassure themselves that the horror or the trauma of the disclosure will not frighten the adult away. Some children speak in a joking or matter of fact manner about the abuse which may lead the professionals mistakenly to question the validity of the disclosure. One girl wrote the allegation on the classroom whiteboard in a lunchtime with explicit diagrams of the abuse. A small boy shouted out in class 'I have some news – he puts his willy in my bum.' These children knew no other way. The manner of disclosure is an important factor to inform the investigators about the abuse. If the sexual abuse has been repeated over time it may be that the child's defence is to normalize the abuse and speak of it with lack of emotion. In a serious case review the author of this chapter conducted about Aliyah – a child of 13 years who died following sexual exploitation – it was clear that her presentation as a sparkling and bubbly child diverted professional attention from her desperation (Payne 1999). Children may report at seemingly inopportune times or for what appear suspect motives such as when they have misbehaved at school, or when parents are in conflict. 'The very problems that have developed in an effort to cope with the abuse are then seen as reasons to discount the reports' (APRI 2004: 35).

The first point of a child's disclosure is very important evidentially and constitutes evidence of early complaint in criminal proceedings. The knowledge that children frequently retract allegations (Summit 1983; APRI 2004: 35) makes it very important for the investigator to retain a perspective based on evaluation of the first disclosure. Professionals who are not in the role of investigators should respond to a disclosure through probing just sufficiently to allow them to be certain of the need to make a referral at the threshold of 'reasonable cause to suspect actual or likely significant harm' (Children Act 1989: 47). This is achieved primarily through the use of open questions such as 'tell me what happened', 'explain/describe to me' without presupposing what has actually happened to the child. It is important not to corrupt the child's innocence by implying abuse by someone who may be innocent (Sturge 1997).

The one assumption that may be made is that the child will blame themselves in some way for the abuse. Clarifying from the beginning that they are not responsible will enable the child to disclose further. Children may ask for the disclosure to remain secret. This presents a dilemma for the professional wishing to provide the child with maximum support. However, there must be no collusion with the secrecy of child sexual abuse and the child must be reassured about the importance of their safety and the need to make the referral. It may of course be that the child then decides to say no more at that stage. A girl aged five repeatedly came to the author during supervised contact visits with a parcel. She demanded more and more sticky tape, brown paper and string and the parcel was made bigger each week. This was a secret she couldn't tell. After two years in a safe foster placement she told all. Children may speak of feeling dirty, contaminated by the abuse or abnormal. Such feelings must be acknowledged and not dismissed. Feelings are so powerful: children may resort to obsessional hand washing, showering or drinking bleach to 'cleanse' their bodies.

The initial disclosure must be recorded contemporaneously for evidential purposes. The interviewer's responses must be stated as well as the child's account in their own words. The interviewer may well not understand the meaning of the detail of the disclosure. In one case a child spoke to me of 'white pee'. It was only later in the investigation that it was realized he was referring to abuse by the abuser urinating on him. Another referred to the 'goliards' with a high level of anxiety. It took two years before the investigators realized he meant the 'followers of Goliath' in a Davidian religious cult. The context of the disclosure must also be recorded. Children commonly disclose after talks by the police in their class about Yes and No touches; such a context adds to the validity of the child's statement. Repetition and consistency in the child's statement and the addition of sensory detail also add validity. A child who spoke of digital penetration by her grandfather at the age of 13 had spoken in exactly the same detail at the age of 4. This had been recorded on file and was a strong test of validity over time. A child describing the smell of alcohol or tobacco on the abuser's breath or the sticky, gluey feel of semen is telling of direct sensory perceptions such as could not be said to have been obtained from viewing a video or having heard a 'story'.

The first point of disclosure may be through observed sexualized behaviour. Mary Bell describes visiting an old man and touching his genitals. She thought this was acceptable behaviour. As a report to social services this might have been the first indication that this child was being sexually exploited (Sereny 1999). Sexually abusive behaviour by young people should lead to child protection procedures which need to be organized in parallel to any criminal prosecution (ALG 2003: 152–8). The question that always has to be asked is 'how did the child learn this behaviour?'

The professional response post-referral

On receiving a referral social services will make checks with relevant agencies to see if the child is known and a strategy discussion will be held with the police (DfES 2006: 5.54). A decision will be made as to whether any intervention is required immediately to protect the child. An assessment may have to be swiftly made as to whether or not there is a non-abusive carer who can be a proactive protector of the child. Attempts will always be made to secure the child within their home environment. Social services can fund the alleged perpetrator to be rehoused temporarily away from the home. However, it may be necessary to remove the child from the household temporarily to allow time for the investigation to take place. This might involve the use of police powers of protection to remove the child to a place of safety or social services obtaining an Emergency Protection Order (EPO). A key omission in the Victoria Climbie case was that the child was not made safe prior to investigation. It was unsurprising then that the child did not communicate about the abuse to the police officer and social worker (Laming 2003: 6.253). An excellent and creative account of the sexually abused child's need to be safe prior to interview is the account of a 3-year-old girl called Tracey who needs a policeman in uniform in the interview room before she can speak of the abuse (Bray 1997: 50–66). An Emergency Protection Order can be sought with conditions such as for a medical assessment, a formal interview of the child or to prevent the alleged abuser having contact with the child. A decision will be made as to whether Section 47 inquiries are required and whether these will be conducted by a single or joint agency. Following inquiries a strategy meeting will be convened. This is chaired by a social services manager and attended by police and other relevant agencies (DfES 2006: 5.60). It is at this professionals' meeting that decisions are made as to whether the child should be formally interviewed, a child protection conference should be convened, a paediatric assessment is indicated and what plans need to be made to inform the parents of the strategy unless to do so would place the child at risk of harm. A paediatric assessment cannot be conducted without the child's consent, unless it is a life and limb situation; however, children will often be more willing to attend a paediatric consultation which enables then to gain an understanding of what would be involved in an examination and provides an opportunity for them to pose questions. The child protection doctor in each locality will make a decision about who should conduct any examination to ensure that it is correctly carried out and to lesson the possibility of further examinations being required for evidential purposes.

The implementation of the above procedures has become confused since the introduction of the Framework of Assessment (DoH 2000; Calder and Hackett 2003: 3–60). The initial assessment of seven days tends to overshadow the decision to provide the child with safety and does not provide a risk assessment tool. The timescales are not relevant to investigation of child sexual abuse which may take many weeks or months but because of performance targets cases are closed after the initial assessment if there is no clear evidence to progress the case further along the route of child protection. There is a clear distinction to be made between investigation and assessment. A core assessment under the Framework focuses on the child and family and their needs and is now deemed to be an essential component of a Section 47 investigation subject to performance targets. In fact a child protection investigation may include a component of assessment but also involves evaluation of risk and focus on the alleged or known perpetrator. It is a different but parallel process. This was a key confusion in the Climbie case. Laming commented that he had 'heard no evidence of what I would term a Section 47 inquiry ever having been carried out by Haringey social services' (Laming 2003: 6.217).

The child protection conference is the most important tool in child protection. It brings together all key professionals with the parents to make a decision about whether or not the child's name should be placed on the Child Protection Register and under which category (DfES 2006: 5.80). The abuse must be defined as of continuing concern. If the child has already been made safe there may not be a need for a conference. Children may attend but the experience may add to the child's trauma. It is a decision for the independent chair as to whether the child wishes to attend for all or part of the meeting and whether the conference can be child-centred. It may be inappropriate for children to be exposed to details of forensic and medical examinations or information about the parental histories. If the child's name is placed on the Register then a protection plan outlines what is required for the child to be made safe and a key worker is appointed to coordinate all aspects of the case working with a core group of professionals and non-abusive carers. The plan is reviewed initially at three months and after six monthly intervals until deregistration when the child is deemed to be safe.

The formal interview of the child by police and social workers according to the Achieving Best Evidence (ABE) Guidance (Home Office 2002) is primarily to collect evidence for criminal proceedings although the video may also be released for civil proceedings. The aim of the interview is to identify sources and levels of risk and to assist the investigation in relation to the need to protect the child. It is conducted according to the phased interview approach in a dedicated child-centred suite and essentially provides a child-focused environment to facilitate the child being confident to speak about what has happened. Children who have provided evidence on tape are found to be more relaxed than those testifying live in court (Davies 1995). The use of video would be usual unless it was known that the child had been filmed as part of the abuse. The decision to interview a child formally has to include consideration of the ability of the child to undergo cross examination in court though children as young as 4 years old have been deemed capable (Davies and Westcott 1999). Children with communication difficulties or where English is not the first language must be given every opportunity to provide evidence through the use of interpreters and intermediaries. Whilst the support of the non-abusive carer is vital they do not attend the interview. Following consultation with the child the interviewers will communicate with the carer after the process. The interviewers make use of drawing and toys to assist in the interview process (Wilhelmy and Bull 1999). If the strategy meeting does not advise a formal interview consideration may be given to a facilitative interview (Bentovim 1995). This provides a specialist assessment by a child psychiatrist or psychologist and is conducted as part of the joint investigation process to ensure that the information obtained could be used as evidence if indicated. It may or may not then lead on to an ABE interview. Such an assessment interview would be appropriate when a young child has a medical only presentation where sexual abuse is suspected but there may be an innocent explanation, where there are solely behavioural indicators of sexual abuse, where a young person has a psychiatric disorder or where there are specific issues relating to fear or intimidation. In such cases clarification may also be sought through the use of books such as *My Body My Book* (Peake and Rouf 1995) or the *Anti-Colouring Book* (Striker and Kimmel 1979) which allow the child to work with a trusted adult in exploring 'yes' and 'no' touches and be given open-ended opportunities to express feelings. Both during and after the investigative process professionals need to consider the therapeutic needs of the child. The Home Office provides guidance on the provision of therapy prior to trial (Home Office 2002) and methods such as storytelling can be simple non-interpretive mechanisms to provide healing to the child (Davis 1990).

The impact of child sexual abuse

Around 80 per cent of all child victims of sexual abuse experience Post-Traumatic Stress Disorder (Briere and Elliott 1994). PTSD may be caused by critical and shocking events that are a threat to life and the psychological well-being of the victims. The key symptoms are disturbed sleep patterns, experience of flashbacks, phobias, anxiety attacks, lack of trust, lack of social activities, depression, self-harm, addiction and suicidal ideations (Guy 2004). A proportion of medical complaints are also often thought to represent somatic equivalents of anxiety arising from the experience of abuse, unexplained symptoms being the body's response to stress (Putnam 1997). However, Nelson challenges this and compares physical disorders to accounts of child sexual abuse by adult survivors as well as to the physical effects of torture and child marriage (Nelson 2002: 52–3). She refers to violent repeated assaults on developing bodies untreated through lack of care or the desire to conceal the evidence. Attention is drawn to the impact on a child's back or pelvis of being crushed by a large man, of shoulders and necks bent back during oral abuse and throat rape leading to infections and difficulty in swallowing and breathing.

According to Strong (1998), a history of child sexual abuse was found in 50 per cent of eating disorder cases, 90 per cent of dissociative disorders and between 50–90 per cent of those who self-harm. Research conducted in adult male prisons also revealed that suicide and self-harm were more prevalent if prisoners had suffered child sexual abuse (Liebling and Krarup 1993). Van der Kolk observed immune system abnormalities in women with a history of child sexual abuse (cited in Strong 2005: 99) and 46 per cent of chronically hospitalized psychotic women were identified as having a history of child sexual abuse (Beck 1987). Mason-John describes in her novel about her experience of sexual abuse whilst a child in care, the many invisible friends she created to protect herself and how whilst suffering abuse she held her breath and squeezed herself out of her body and flew up onto the ceiling (Mason-John 2005: 34). The impact of child sexual abuse is known to be exacerbated if the abuser is in a close relationship with the child as the sense of betrayal is increased. Physical contact, abuse at a younger age, the use of force and threats as coercion and whether or not they were believed and supported are key factors affecting the impact on the child. In this context it is important to mention sexually abused children who have suffered female genital cutting and their need for specialist medical services such as those provided by the

African well women clinics. A detailed account of a girl's experience in modern-day slavery which covers the subject of rape of a child who had suffered the practice of female genital cutting is provided by Mende Nazer (2004).

Sexually abused children (victims) demonstrating PTSD need stability, therapy, secure social attachments and the possibility of joy (Cairns 2000: 144). Following Aliyah's death (Payne 1999) the author of this chapter had the chance to interview many of her friends, within the network of victims of the abuse, who said they needed safe houses, drop-ins and locally based helplines. Children being sexually exploited need exit strategies and places to find safety and be nourished. Nelson (2001: 41) writes of survivors valuing a 'listening ear', a person to offer 'warmth, respect, understanding, kindness and honesty'. Children who feel betrayed by the abuse of their parents may not wish to be placed in a family situation. The case for small group homes has to be made to provide a therapeutic environment where healing can begin. The Sexual Abuse Consultancy Service provides residential care and a valuable resource for children with therapeutic needs (www.saccs.org.uk).

However, the reality for child victims is that children once removed from their families are often passed from one placement to another. Aliyah (Payne 1999) had moved placement 68 times in her short life of thirteen years. Frampton (2004) claims this is not unusual. In a study of 3500 looked after children almost all noted they would rather have continued to have been abused than have experienced endless placement disruptions (Walsh 2005). As a further indictment of the system there is now a performance target to ensure children are placed within 20 miles of their localities. The result of this target is that authorities are moving children out of stable placements causing them further disruption (Smith 2005). For those on the streets the risk of sexual abuse is estimated as one in nine children (Biehal et al. 2003: 32) and for those fleeing abuse there is only one safe house in the country.

The adequacy of service and therapeutic facilities

Children who have been neglected or abused should get special help to get back their confidence and self-respect (UNCRC 1990: 39). The United Nations (2002) recommended that state parties provide for the care, recovery and integration of victims of child sexual abuse. Children need help to rebuild their sense of trust in adults. One boy, known to the author, could only envisage his future as a long distance lorry driver where his sense of isolation would find a place. The 'damaged goods syndrome' is described by child victims as the feeling that they carry on them a sign showing the world that they have been abused. Children need reassurance about who does know about the abuse, particularly within the school environment, and to increase their self-esteem they need help to learn assertiveness and self-protection skills. Feelings of guilt for disclosing the abuse, disrupting the family or harming the perpetrator may exacerbate a sense of shame and children may state that they just wanted the abuse to stop and not for their entire world to change. Sexually abused children may have been introduced to adult activities such as drugs, alcohol and sexual practices as part of the abuse. Therapy is needed to restore the child's world and for the child to gain a sense of themselves as a child once again. One young woman, known to the author, mourned the loss of the 'best' year of her life spent within a sexually exploitative network. She had defined the experience as positive. Enjoyment of the feelings aroused as a result of the abuse has to be acknowledged and not denied and the child supported in redefining the experience as abusive. Anger may sometimes be directed not only towards the abuser/s but to the non-abusive carer for their lack of protection and the child needs help to disentangle the emotional confusion.

In the large majority of studies of group, individual and behavioural therapy, children's symptoms of distress and psychological disturbance following child sexual abuse decrease following therapeutic intervention. In research relating to girls, significant reductions were noted in depression and separation anxiety, and PTSD (Trowell 1998). The consistent support of the non-abusive carer and social work support, with integration of the therapy into wider case management, are both key factors in the therapeutic process being of sustained value to the child. The child's safety and the continuance of therapy over time are also important factors if a child is to benefit from therapy (Jones and Ramchandani 1999: 55). The most effective treatment seems to be cognitive-behavioural in achieving improvement of symptoms (Jones and Ramchandani 1999: 57) but it may be appropriate for the therapy not to focus solely on symptoms but to address the particular experience of sexual abuse. Group work can be particularly effective in reducing stigma and isolation and in normalizing feelings with peer support. However, about 25 per cent of child victims deteriorate following psychological treatment and the reason for this is not understood (Jones and Ramchandani 1999: 58). One study noted that for both children and families there was a 'web of conflicting emotions' about therapy and that whereas some children found it helpful to talk about the abuse others said it was much too painful. Encouraging children to write down their experiences was seen to be helpful (Taylor 1994). The author's experience is of young people dictating into a cassette recorder in the quiet of their rooms often in the middle of the night. An innovative project in Lancashire offered a safe haven to children and families where they could talk at their own pace, at any time around the clock whilst knowing they were on neutral ground (Mapp 1995).

Despite the undoubted importance of therapy, one-fifth of children referred to the Child and Adult Mental Health Services (CAMHS) are refused a service and in 2003 a Department of Health briefing paper stated that there is a considerable shortage of any type of therapeutic facilities (cited in Corby 2004)

In a sample of 41 sexually exploited young people most said they had insurmountable problems with no one to turn to (Taylor-Browne 2002). A study by Young Minds (2000) exposed long delays in children accessing CAMHS services with a national shortage of child psychiatrists and in-patient provision. Often adult psychiatric beds are used for children; or children are left in police custody, secure accommodation or respite care. Parents are often under pressure to cope. There is lack of provision for 16–18-year-olds, it was common for children to have to wait between six months and a year for an appointment and access was particularly fraught for children from black and ethnic minority groups. Many children only accessed help after an emergency situation (Young Minds 2000). The Safeguards Review similarly highlighted that the help and treatment for abused children is still inadequate and one recommendation was for major improvements in the CAMHS system (Stuart and Baines 2004).

For child victims living in detention centres such as asylum seekers who may have suffered sexual abuse before entry into the country there is a concern at the lack of specialist mental health provision. 'CAMHS providers report that there is a lack of capacity and research evidence on which to base assessment and provision for victims ... with specific care needs including gynaecological problems following sexual abuse or rape' (CSCI 2005: 7.25). 'The lack of effective guidance and procedures agreed between the Immigration and Nationality Directorate and Local Safeguarding Children's Boards on child protection is of considerable concern. Such guidance should include immediate and continuing independent social services assessments, education and care plans and child protection team strategy conferences, which should inform decisions about continuing detention' (CSCI 2005: 7.39).

This chapter has been an attempt to assist those who dare to enter the world of the sexually abused child and provide an effective child-centred protective and therapeutic response by hearing the child's voice. One person who hears the child's voice can make a difference. This takes courage and persistence. It is, as Madge Bray says, a daunting task: 'When we enter this world we may find things which deeply disturb us. A child having sexual knowledge and experience clashes sharply with our belief in childhood innocence and our emotions are likely to be those of shock, horror and disgust. The discovery may make us want to beat a hasty retreat and slam the door shut' (Bray 1997: xv). If this chapter helps to keep that door open to the child victims of sexual abuse it will have achieved its purpose.

Notes

1. Sexual abuse involves forcing or enticing a child or young person to take part in sexual activities, including prostitution, whether or not the child is aware of what is happening. The activities may involve physical abuse, including penetrative (e.g. rape or buggery) or non-penetrative acts. They may include non-contact activities, such as involving children in looking at, or in the production of pornographic material or watching sexual activities, or encouraging children to behave in sexually inappropriate ways (DfES 2006: 1.32).
2. National Society for the Prevention of Cruelty to Children, UK.

References

Advisory Council for the Misuse of Drugs (2003) *Hidden Harm*. London: Home Office.

American Prosecutors Research Institute (APRI) (2004) *Investigation and Prosecution of Child Abuse*. London: Sage.

Association of London Government (ALG) (2003) *All London Child Protection Procedures*. London Child Protection Committee.

Beck, J. and Van der Kolk, B. (1987) 'Reports of childhood incest and current behaviour of chronically hosiptalised psychotic women'. *American Journal of Psychiatry*, 144(11): 1474–6.

Bentovim, A. (1992) *Trauma Organised Systems: Physical and Sexual Abuse in Families*. London: Karnac Books.

Bentovim, A. (1995) 'Facilitating interviews with children who may have been sexually abused'. *Child Abuse Review*, 4: 246–62.

Biehal, N., Mitchell, F. and Wade, J. (2003) *Lost from View: Missing Persons in the UK*. Bristol: Policy Press.

Blitz, R. (1996) 'One man's fight for a simple apology'. *Hamstead and Highgate Express*, 29 March.

Bray, M. (1997) *Poppies on the Rubbish Heap. Sexually Abused Children: the Child's Voice*. London: Jessica Kingsley Publishers.

Bridge Child Care Development Service and Gloucester Social Services Department (1996) *In Care Contacts. The West Case.* London: The Bridge NCH.

Briere, J. and Conte, J. (1993) 'Self reported amnesia for abuse in adults molested as children'. *Journal of Traumatic Stress*, 6(1): 21–31.

Briere, J. and Elliott, D. (1994) 'Immediate and long term impacts of child sexual abuse'. *The Future of Children*, 4(2): 54–69.

Cairns, K. (2006) *Surviving Paedophilia: Traumatic Stress after Organised and Network Child Sexual Abuse.* Gloucester: Akamas.

Calder, M. and Hackett, M. (2003) *Assessment in Child Care.* Dorset: Russell House Publishing.

Care Standards Tribunal (CST) (2005) *Lisa Arthurworrey v Secretary of State.* www.carestandardstribunal.gov.uk.

Carr, J. (2005) *No Funds to Tackle Child Porn.* www.policeoracle.com/news/detail.h2f?id=5634.

Cawson, P., Wattam, C., Brooker, S. and Kelly, G. (2000) *Child Maltreatment in the UK.* London: NSPCC.

Childhood Matters National Commission of Inquiry into the Prevention of Child Abuse (1997) London: NSPCC.

Children Act (1989). Available at http://www.opsi.gov.uk/acts/acts1989/UKpga_19890041_en_1.htm

Children Act (2004).

Children's Rights Alliance (2002) *Rethinking Child Imprisonment: a Report on Young Offender Institutions.* London: Children's Rights Alliance for England.

Corby, B. (2004) 'Putting a price on health'. *Community Care*, 15 January, pp. 34–5.

CSCI (2005) *Safeguarding Children.* The Second Joint Chief Inspector's Report on Arrangements to Safeguard Children. London: CSCI.

Davies, G. (1995) *Videoing Children's Evidence: an Evaluation.* London: Home Office.

Davies, G. and Westcott, H. (1999) 'Interviewing child witnesses under the Memorandum of Good Practice: a research review'. *Police Research Series.* Paper 115. London: Home Office.

Davies, L. (2004) 'The difference between child abuse and child protection could be you: creating a community network of protective adults'. *Child Abuse Review*, 13: 426–32.

Davies, L. (1997) 'The investigation of organised abuse'. In H. Westcott and J. Jones (eds), *Perspectives on the Memorandum.* Hants: Arena.

Davies, L. and Jarman, M. (2005) 'Social workers' professional practice after Climbie'. *Family Law*, 35: 814–19.

Davis, N. (1990) *Once Upon a Time: Therapeutic Stories.* Psychological Associates.

Department for Education and Skills (DfES) (2006) *Working Together to Safeguard Children. A Guide to Inter-Agency Working to Safeguard and Promote the Welfare of Children.* London: Stationery Office.

Department of Health (1995) *Messages from Research.* London: HMSO.

Department of Health (2000) *The Framework of Assessment for Children in Need and their Families.* London: HMSO.

Department of Health (2003) *Costs and Outcomes of Different Interventions for Sexually Abused Children in Costs and Effectiveness of Services for Children in Need.* Briefing Paper 2. London: HMSO.

Fairhurst, D. and Spindler, P. (2005) 'Are the police failing victims of child sexual abuse?' BBC Radio 4 *Woman's Hour*. 2 November.

Frampton, P. (2004) *Golly in the Cupboard*. Manchester: Tamic.

Finkelhor, D. (1979) *Sexually Victimised Children*. New York: Free Press.

Goldson, B. (2002) *Vulnerable Inside*. London: The Children's Society.

Grubin, D. (1998) *Sex Offending Against Children: Understanding the Risk*. Police Research Series. Paper 99. London: Home Office.

Guy, N. (2004) 'Trauma out of a crisis'. *Community Care*, 2–8 December.

Home Office (2002) *Achieving Best Evidence in Criminal Proceedings. Guidance for Vulnerable and Intimidated Witnesses Including Children*. London: Home Office.

Home Office (2003) MAPPA Guidance available from website: www.dfes.gov.uk/childrenandfamilies/docs/MAPPA%20&%20DTC%20summary%20Nov%2003%20-%202.doc

Home Office (2004) *Public Protection from Dangerous Offenders Better than Ever*. Home Office press release, 28 July.

Home Office and DoH (2002) *Complex Child Abuse Investigation – Inter Agency Issues*. London: Home Office.

Hutchinson, S. (2005) *Effects of and Interventions for Childhood Trauma from Infancy Through Adolescence: Pain Unspeakable*. New York: Haworth Press.

Jones, D. and Ramchandani, P. (1999) *Child Sexual Abuse: Informing Practice from Research*. Oxford: Radcliffe Medical Press.

Kelly, Christopher (Sir) (2004) *Serious Case Review 'Ian Huntley'*. For North Lincolnshire Area Child Protection Committee, 21 July.

Laming, H. (2003) *The Victoria Climbie Inquiry. Report of an Inquiry by Lord Laming*. London: HMSO.

Liebling, A. and Krarup, H. (1993) 'Suicide attempts in male prisons'. *London Home Office Research Bulletin*, 36: 23–9.

Mapp, S. (1995) 'In the interval'. *Community Care*, 30 March 1995, 21.

Mason-John, V. (2005) *Borrowed Body*. London: Serpentstail Books.

McLachlan, B. (2003) 'Slipping through the net'. *Sunday Herald*, 19 January. www.sundayherald.com/print30756

Metropolitan Police (2003) *Operation Paladin Child. A Partnership Study of Child Migration into the UK Via London Heathrow*.

Monahon, C. (1993). *Children and Trauma: a Guide for Parents and Professionals*. San Francisco: Jossey-Bass.

Mudaly, N. and Goddard, C. (2001) 'The child abuse victim as a hostage: Scorpion's story'. *Child Abuse Review*, 10: 428–39.

Mullen, P., Martin, J. L., Anderson, J. C., Romans, S. E. and Herbison, G. P. (1996) 'The long term impact of the physical, emotional and sexual abuse of children: a community study'. *Child Abuse and Neglect*, 20: 7–22.

Munro, E. (2002) *Effective Child Protection*. London: Sage.

Munro, E. (2005) 'A systems approach to investigating child abuse deaths'. *British Journal of Social Work*, 35(4): 531–46.

Munro, E. and Calder, M. (2005) 'Where has child protection gone?' *Political Quarterly*, 76(3). Oxford: Blackwell.

National Commission of Inquiry into the Prevention of Child Abuse (1996) *Childhood Matters: Report of the National Commission of Enquiry into the Prevention of Child Abuse*. NSPCC.

Nazer, M. (2004) *Slave*. London: Virago.

NCIS (National Criminal Intelligence Service) (2003) 'UK threat assessment of serious and organised crime. Sex offences against children including online abuse'. www.ncis.org.uk.

Nelson, S. (2001) *Beyond Trauma: Mental Health Care Needs of Women who Survived Childhood Sexual Abuse*. Edinburgh: Health in Mind (EAMH).

Nelson, S. (2002) 'Physical symptoms in sexually abused women: somatisation or undetected injury?' *Child Abuse Review*, 11: 51–64.

Newiss, G. and Fairbrother, L. (2004) 'Child abduction: understanding police recorded crime statistics'. *Home Office Research Findings 225*. London: Home Office.

NSPCC (2005a) http://www.nspcc.org.uk/inform/Statistics/KeyCPstats/12.asp.

NSPCC (2005b) http://www.nspcc.org.uk/inform/Statistics/CPR.asp.

Oliver, T. and Smith, R. (1993) *Lambs to the Slaughter*. London: Warner Books.

Payne, S. (1999) 'Tragic Aliyah: ten years of abuse'. London: *Evening Standard*, 12 October.

Peake, A. and Rouf, K. (1995) *My Body My Book*. London: The Children's Society.

Plotnikoff, J. and Woolfson, R. (2004) *In Their Own Words: the Experiences of 50 Young Witnesses in Criminal Proceedings*. London: NSPCC and Victim Support.

Putnam, F. (1997) *Dissociation in Children and Adolescents: a Developmental Perspective*. New York: Guilford Press.

Reder, P., Duncan, M. and Gray, M. (1993) *Beyond Blame. Child Abuse Tragedies Revisited. A Summary of 35 Inquires since 1973*. London: Routledge.

Reder, P. and Duncan, S. (1999) *Lost Innocents: a Follow-Up Study of Fatal Child Abuse*. London: Routledge.

Reder, P. and Duncan, S. (2004) 'Making the most of the Victoria Climbie inquiry report'. *Child Abuse Review*, 13: 95–114.

Renold, E. and Creighton, S. with Atkinson, C. and Carr, J. (2003) *Images of Abuse: a Review of the Evidence on Child Pornography,* London: NSPCC.

Sereny, G. (1999) *Cries Unheard: the Story of Mary Bell*. London Macmillan.

Smith, R. (2005) 'Looked after children, drive to cut distant placements not in child's best interests'. *Children Now*, 31 August.

Striker, S. and Kimmel, E. (1979) *The Anti-Colouring Book*. London: Scholastic Press.

Strong, M. (1998) *A Bright Red Scream: Self Mutilation and the Language of Pain*. London: Virago.

Stuart, M. and Baines, C. (2004) 'Safeguards for vulnerable children: three studies on abusers, disabled children and children in prison. Progress on safeguards for children living away from home'. *A Review of Actions since the People Like Us Review*. York: Joseph Rowntree Foundation.

Sturge, C. (1997) 'Investigative interviewing in child sexual abuse: minimising the tainting of evidence and the corruption of children'. *Practitioner's Child Law Bulletin*, 10(2).

Sullivan, A. (2000) cited on NSPCC Inform website: http://www.nspcc.org.uk/Inform/OnlineResources/InformationBriefings/Disabled_asp_ifega26019.html

Summit, R. (1983) 'The child abuse accommodation syndrome'. *Child Abuse and Neglect*, 7: 177–93.

Summit, R. (1988) 'Hidden victims, hidden pain'. In G. Wyatt and G. Powell (eds), *Lasting Effects of Child Sexual Abuse*. New York: Sage, pp. 34–66.

Survivors Swindon website accessed November (2005): http://www.survivors swindon.com/stats.htm.

Svedin, C. and Bach, K. (1996) *Children Who Don't Speak Out about Children Being Used in Child Pornography*. Sweden: Radda Barnen.

SWIA (2005) Report by Social Work Agency Inspection into the care and protection of children in the Western Isles. August. Scottish Executive/Astrone.

Taylor, C. (1994) 'Speaking Out'. *Community Care*, 3 March, pp. 18–19.

Taylor-Browne, J. (2002) *Voicing our Views*. Ecpat. www.ecpat.org.uk/voicing%20 our%20views.pdf

The Treasury (2003) *Every Child Matters*. London: HMSO.

Townsend, M. (2004) 'Trapped in a teenage wasteland'. *The Observer*, 18 July·

Trowell, J. (1998) *Psychotherapy Outcome Study for Sexually Abused Girls* (Report submitted to the Department of Health).

UNICEF (1990) *Convention on the Rights of the Child*. Full text available at http://www.unicef.org/ccrc/fulltext.htm.

United Nations (2002) *Report of the 31st Session of the Committee on the Rights of the Child*.

Utting, W. (1997) *People Like Us*. The Report of the Review of Safeguards of Children Living Away from Home. London: TSO.

Walsh, M. (2005) 'Care system more harmful than abuse'. *Community Care*, 17–3 March.

Wilhelmy, R. and Bull, R. (1999) 'Drawing to remember: using visual aids to interview child witnesses'. *Practitioners Child Law Journal*, 12(6).

Young Minds (2000) *Minority Voices*. www.youngminds.org.uk/minorityvoices/

Young Minds (2000) *Whose Crisis?* www.youngminds.org.uk/whosecrisis/ summary/

12
Legacies of Conflict: Children in Northern Ireland

Eve Binks and Neil Ferguson

Introduction

For children in many countries, political violence has been a defining characteristic of their lives (Jones 2002). In a recent review of the literature on children, war and trauma, Barenbaum et al. (2004) claim that children are a highly vulnerable and voiceless population during war, and more needs to be done to understand the impact of exposure to conflict on mental health and to bring this to public attention. Northern Ireland has, for the past 35 years, been a country characterized by political violence and societal instability and it has a relatively youthful population (Cairns 1987). Therefore it would be pertinent to review over three decades of research exploring the legacies and impacts of exposure to political conflict on child mental health conducted in Northern Ireland.

It has been estimated that the Troubles in Northern Ireland are directly responsible for in excess of 3700 deaths, and injuries to over 40 000 people (Smyth and Hamilton 2004). In addition to this, it has been estimated that 10 per cent of the population have had relatives killed as a result of the Troubles, while 50 per cent of people know someone who has been killed (Smith 1987). These records of fatalities and injuries due to 'the security situation in Northern Ireland', as the Police Service of Northern Ireland (PSNI) euphemistically call 35 years of violence, are not the only consequences of the conflict. In addition to this physical suffering, the conflict has created economic costs, increased community division, and had a psychological impact on those affected, directly or indirectly, by the conflict. Economically, Northern Ireland has had to deal with the costs of rebuilding the damage caused by thousands of explosions, maintaining a large security force presence, the emigration of the skilled and/or educated population as well as coping with a lack of inward investment and tourism due to the violence (Cairns and Darby 1998). On top of these costs, Northern Ireland is one of the least affluent regions of Western Europe with higher levels of unemployment and lower average incomes than the rest of the UK (Cairns et al. 1995). The violence has also led to forced migration within Northern Ireland, often due to intimidation (Cairns and Darby 1998). This migration has led to Northern Ireland's two ethno-religious communities living relatively separate lives. The communities are largely geographically segregated (Boal 1978) and the persistent violence since 1969 has led to the communities becoming more segregated than at any time in the past (Shirlow 2003). However, this segregation runs deeper than pure geography; it manifests itself in all spheres of Northern Irish society. Catholics and Protestants are divided in housing, employment, their leisure pursuits, and in which newspapers they read. It was also suggested that they build friendships predominantly within their own community and rates of endogamy are high (Ferguson and Cairns 1996).

The third consequence of this prolonged political violence is the psychological impact it has on the Northern Irish population. Since the early 1970s, psychologists, psychiatrists and other mental health professionals have been concerned about the psychological effects of living with the conflict (Fields 1976; Fraser 1973). In particular the unpredictable and random nature of the violence and the resulting stress caused has been viewed as a source of significant emotional stress, especially for children (Cairns et al. 1995).

The impact of the Troubles on children in Northern Ireland

Since the onset of the Troubles in 1969, the Northern Irish conflict has been one of the most intensely reported. Despite this, it has been difficult to know with any degree of certainty exactly how many child victims there have been (Cairns 1987). Some estimates have indicated that a possible 8 per cent of all victims have been children (Murray 1982) while other estimates place the number higher than this (Cairns 1987), with Smyth and Hamilton (2004) suggesting as many as 1 in 6 victims are aged 19 or under. In addition to these direct victims, Cairns (1987) believes there are many more who have undoubtedly felt that their lives were in danger, while many hundreds, indeed, maybe thousands, have been indirect victims of the political violence. Muldoon and Trew's (2000) study of 689 8–11-year-olds in greater

Belfast supports Cairns' (1987) fears. Muldoon and Trew found that 24 per cent of children reported having witnessed rioting, 23 per cent had witnessed shooting, 14 per cent had been picked up by the police, 54 per cent had been stopped at security force checkpoints, 60 per cent had been in a bomb scare, while 70 per cent had seen soldiers on the streets of Belfast. Similar findings from an earlier decade (McGrath and Wilson 1985) reported that almost 20 per cent of a randomly selected sample of 10 and 11-year-old children from across the province had been in or near a bomb explosion, while 20 per cent also had a friend or relative killed or injured, and 12 per cent felt that where they lived was not a safe place.

These statistics and estimates suggest that children in the province are affected by the political violence that is so prevalent (e.g. Cairns and Wilson 1989), and it has consequently been suggested (Wilson and Cairns 1992: 247) that as a result of the strong community ties that exist in Northern Ireland, the psychological effects of violence 'extend far beyond the immediate relatives of the victims'. Accordingly, it is possible that most, if not all, individuals in Northern Ireland are affected psychologically by the Troubles and by the societal instability in the province (Wilson and Cairns 1996). However, it must be remembered that not all children are exposed to the same levels of violence. Firstly, the violence in Northern Ireland is not static – it is dynamic and fluid (Cairns 1987). There are differences over time, as the level of violence fluctuates from year to year; there are spatial differences, with some areas having high levels of ethno-political violence, while others have not witnessed violence; also the form of violence has qualitative differences, with one-to-one assignations, rioting, car bombs, mortar attacks, sniper attacks, etc., impacting on individuals, families and communities in different ways. Therefore some children have astonishing experiences of violence, as illustrated by McAuley and Kremmer (1990), while others have only witnessed the conflict through the nightly television news (Cairns 1990; Cairns et al. 1980). Secondly, psychosocial factors such as age, gender, social class and religious affiliation modify levels of exposure to the conflict in Northern Ireland (Cairns 1996; Muldoon et al. 2000). Age is related to the amount and nature of exposure to political violence. In Northern Ireland older children report the greatest exposure to conflict related incidents (Mercer and Bunting 1980). Anyone who has watched a riot on the streets of Belfast on their television screens will know only too well that children are not always passive victims; many are vigorous participants in an activity that is seen as fun and recreational in some areas of Northern

Ireland (Jarman and O'Halloran 2001), but one that heightens their risk of serious injury and incarceration. Also since the beginning of the Troubles it has been suggested that the child's age mediates how they react to the same violent events. Fraser (1973) pioneered this work in Northern Ireland and determined that a child under 8 years of age is likely not to fully understand the threat of the political violence, and this lack of understanding protects the child from the full impact of the traumatic experience. Fraser also asserts that children in the adolescent age bracket do tend to understand the danger associated with the incident of political violence, but are able to employ the fight or flight response and deal with that danger accordingly. However, children aged between 8 years and adolescence tend to be the worst affected by the political violence (Fraser 1973).

Research into the psychological impact of exposure to violence in children, however, has identified that Post-Traumatic Stress Disorder (PTSD) does occur in school age children and Almqvist and Brandell-Forsberg (1997) have suggested that exposure to organized violence is related to PTSD diagnoses in children under the age of 5 years. Almqvist and Brandell-Forsberg continue that although these diagnoses of PTSD in children are evident, parents have a tendency to either underestimate or deny these reactions in the hope that their children will 'forget' about the traumatic experience whereas the children themselves have a tendency not to address the situation as a way of protecting their parents.

With regard to the treatment approaches employed to help the most vulnerable children, and particularly those who show signs of PTSD, several methods have been suggested and numerous recommendations have been made. Cohen (1998) suggests that the major recommendations made for treating vulnerable children, particularly those with PTSD, include the use of clinical interviewing, and although there is limited empirical support for the treatment approaches for children, Cohen claims that the use of Cognitive Behavioural Therapy (CBT) has received the most support. The main consensus regarding the treatment of traumatized children is that there needs to be, at a clinical level, a direct exploration of the traumatic event(s), the employment of relative and specific stress management techniques, and exploration and correction of inaccurate attributions about the event. There is also a need for the inclusion of the parents/caregiver in the treatment process. The direct exploration of the event should allow the child to achieve a sense of control over their situation and, as such, this feeling of control should allow the child to explore their feelings without becoming overwhelmed by them. There is also research evidence to demonstrate that the emotional reaction of parents to the traumatic stressor and the subsequent parental support of the child are significant mediators of a child's PTSD symptomatology. As such, Cohen (1998) suggests that parents should be involved in any treatment approaches in order that they are able (a) to monitor the child's situation and (b) learn appropriate behaviour management strategies.

Almqvist and Brandell-Forsberg (1997) suggest that, in terms of PTSD symptomatology in both adults and children, exposure to traumatic stressors is of paramount importance. This research suggests specifically that children who witness an assault on either of their parents, or who are within 50 metres of an explosion, such as a bomb, develop PTSD on a significantly more frequent basis than children who are not exposed in these ways to these stressors. However, what Almqvist and Brandell-Forsberg also maintain, is that the children included in their investigation that had been exposed to these, and other, traumatic stressors also had parents who have been exposed to these traumatic stressors and suggest that if these 'traumatized ... children generally belong to "traumatized families", their parents' capacity and the family cohesion are changed in negative ways' (Almqvist and Brandell-Forsberg 1997: 363). Connolly and Healy (2004) have built on this work by documenting attitudes towards the Troubles. They suggest that children aged 3–4 spend 'very little' time focusing on the conflict, but are beginning to obtain an appreciation of the attitudes that underscore the sectarian beliefs that exist in Northern Ireland. By 7 years of age, Connolly and Healy suggest that they are now explicitly aware of the threat posed to them not only by the political violence, but also by the 'other side'. By the time children in Northern Ireland reach 10 or 11 years old they have advanced experience of living in a society in conflict, are able to talk at length about the activities of paramilitary groups, and apply a more detailed historical knowledge to the current state of political unrest and associated violence in the province. A child's gender can alter their exposure to the conflict in Northern Ireland, with boys reporting significantly more exposure to conflict related incidents than girls (McGrath and Wilson 1985; Muldoon and Trew 2000). As the conflict in Northern Ireland is much more intense in economically disadvantaged locations, and these areas also tend to be heavily populated by Catholics (Smyth and Hamilton 2004), it is of no surprise that children from lower socio-economic status (SES) and/ or a Catholic background have more experiences of conflict related events (Muldoon and Trew 2000).

Political violence and child mental health in Northern Ireland

Research from countries other than Northern Ireland has tended to confirm the common theory that when children are exposed to political violence, they will suffer some serious psychological consequence (Barenbaum et al. 2004; Cairns 1996). Research by Cairns and Wilson (1993) seems to confirm this and indicates that in societies in conflict, a possible 10 per cent of children may suffer these consequences – compared with a possible 6 per cent in societies free from this conflict. However, although these suggestions have been made, Liddell et al. (1993) continue to note that even in those countries characterized by political violence, only 50 per cent of the children exposed to the most acute stressors are psychologically affected, while the other 50 per cent appear to be highly resilient. Similar research by McAuley and Troy (1983) found that psychiatric referral rates were less in years characterized by high levels of violence than in other, less violent years. As Cairns (1987) attests, this could simply be due to a change in the referral practices in the early 1970s or to the fact that not all children in need of specialist help were referred to a psychiatrist – some will have been referred to other agencies and support networks and as such will not have been included in McAuley and Troy's numbers. Alternatively, Cairns continues, it could be that child psychiatric referral rates in these years fell into line with those of adults and that there actually was no increase in psychiatric referrals at this time. There have also been a number of surveys of child mental health in Northern Ireland which have explored the impact of exposure to violence. Fee (1980 1983), for example, conducted the first two studies in 1975 and 1981, with 5000 and 7000 Belfast school pupils. Fee's research probed for cases of emotionally disturbed children with the Rutter Teacher Rating Questionnaire (Rutter et al. 1975), and the survey indicated that the rates were 15 per cent in 1975 and 9 per cent in 1981. Fee compared the Belfast sample with a London sample and found that levels of behaviour disturbance in children in Northern Ireland were comparable with those of children in London, concluding that the exposure to political violence in Northern Ireland does not have an increasingly detrimental effect on children's behaviour.

A third study by McWhirter (1983) compared 1000 children from high violence and low violence areas to 210 children from Manchester. Her results indicated that the Northern Irish children did not report higher levels of anxiety than either the English children or British and

American norms, irrespective of where they lived. However, the children did report higher levels of psychoticism, especially the children living in more violent areas. The fourth survey, conducted by McGrath and Wilson (1985) and measuring depression and manifest anxiety, employed the Rutter scale and measured exposure to violent incidents, with a random sample of 10 and 11-year-old children from across Northern Ireland. Their findings suggested a slight increase in levels of depression in comparison to other British samples, but this was not associated with exposure to violence. Exposure to conflict-related incidents was associated with increased symptoms of anxiety. McGrath and Wilson's findings also showed similarity to the three previous studies in that the children demonstrated elevated anti-social behaviour, acting out behaviour, and conduct disorder. This finding was also hinted at by Fraser (1973) in one of the earliest studies of children's responses to the unfolding conflict in Northern Ireland, where purposeless excitement and 'ill-directed nervous energy', such as shouting, were noted (1993: 83).

Donnelly (1995) explored levels of depression among a stratified random sample of 887 11–15-year-olds from the north west of Northern Ireland and did not find any higher rates for severe depression; however, there were higher rates for mild depression, but these higher rates were significantly associated with social class. Donnelly was encouraged by the results and concluded that most children were coping well and were not depressed.

Overall these surveys make two important points: that the experiences of emotional disturbances and depression are not related to violence, but that these experiences are contributing to externalizing behaviour such as conduct disorders, anti-social behaviour and possible anxiety. However, it should be remembered that as exposure to conflict is related to socio-economic disadvantage (Muldoon and Trew 2000) it is difficult to disentangle the impact of violence and deprivation (Wilson and Cairns 1992). Muldoon et al. (2000) also point out that the studies suggesting increased acting-out behaviour (Fee 1980 1983; McGrath and Wilson 1985; McWhirter 1983; Muldoon and Trew 2000) are based on psychometric profiles and not on incidence of anti-social or delinquent behaviour, thus these findings require a cautious interpretation.

Anti-social behaviour and moral development

As mentioned above, previous research employing psychometric measures of acting-out behaviour and psychoticism suggests that exposure to sustained conflict and witnessing violent incidents is related to externalizing anti-social or delinquent behaviour. This suggestion is commonly made (Cairns 1996; Elbedour et al. 1997), and has been a source of debate within Northern Ireland since the beginning of the conflict (Cairns 1987; Ferguson and Cairns 1996). Fraser (1972) suggested that Northern Irish children could become delinquent and develop into amoral adults, while Fields (1976) believed she could already detect this process, and predictions were also made that this amoral society would even outlast the conflict (Lyons 1973). A number of approaches have been employed to study the link between the conflict and anti-social behaviour and/or moral reasoning. A series of studies reviewed the moral behaviour of children through the levels of school absenteeism, self-reported delinquency and juvenile crime, in comparison with other areas in Great Britain, the Republic of Ireland, Europe and North America, to assess actual moral behaviour.

McKeown (1973) examined how Northern Irish children actually behaved via a survey of secondary school teachers from 150 schools. Half of the schools replied that there had been a growing lack of respect for the authority of the class teacher over the past three years. Although half of the schools reported this trend, Catholic schools and schools located in high violence areas were over-represented. One-third also reported increased vandalism, and a majority recorded an increase in the amount of expletives used by the children. In relation to levels of absenteeism, 6 per cent reported that there had been a large negative effect, while 52 per cent reported no effect at all due to political conflict. The Department of Education conducted two studies into persistent absenteeism in Northern Ireland in 1977 and 1982. The percentage of persistent absenteeism in Northern Ireland in 1977 was running at 4.2 per cent of children absent for reasons other than physical illness. Yet in 1982 the survey showed a decrease from 4.2 per cent to 2 per cent. Cautious interpretation of these results indicates that although in the early 1970s levels of absenteeism may have risen with the increased turmoil caused by the Troubles, the prediction that this level would increase, with successive generations acting out the amoral behaviour of older siblings, did not follow and the level of school absenteeism actually reduced over time (Fields 1976; Fraser 1973; Lyons 1973).

Research on juvenile delinquency and crime also indicated a rejection of the earlier hypothesis that the Troubles would accelerate amoral or anti-social behaviour (Jardine 1989). In fact, Jardine (1989: 97) noted that Northern Ireland has a 'significantly lower rate of juvenile involvement in crime than elsewhere in the UK'. Two studies have also explored how approving Northern Irish children are of violence. In the first of these studies, Cairns (1983) examined the responses of 600 children to a series of situations in which another child received verbal or physical aggression. The 600 children were then asked how the child in the particular situation should respond. Cairns (1983) found that all children agreed on the correct levels of aggression that should be used for each situation, irrespective of whether they lived in a high or low violence area in Northern Ireland or an area in the Republic of Ireland. Thus exposure to the violent society of Northern Ireland had not altered their views of what was acceptable behaviour in classroom and playground situations. Further, Lorenc and Branthwaite (1986) approached this same issue by comparing Northern Irish primary school children from Londonderry with a comparison group from England. Lorenc and Branthwaite (1986) employed short stories depicting a violent event to examine how right or wrong the children thought the violent acts to be. The study also investigated the idea that Northern Ireland's apparently amoral, violent environment would lead the children to generalize their support for violence towards the security forces to other authority figures, such as parents and teachers. Lorenc and Branthwaite's (1986) findings suggested that Northern Irish children were growing up with a sense of right and wrong which has not been affected by the violent environment in which they live. Furthermore, they found no evidence to support Fraser's (1973) hypothesis that the children would develop new moral 'norms' and generalize the anti-authority feelings.

A number of studies employing Kohlberg's theory of moral reasoning (Kohlberg 1984) in Northern Ireland have produced a changing picture of the relationship between exposure to political violence and moral development among children (Fields 1976; Breslin 1982; Cairns and Conlon 1985; Ferguson and Cairns 2002). Research from the early years of this period of conflict described the children as morally truncated and predicted that this situation would become more profound, while research from the 1980s and 1990s depicted the children as morally mature in relation to their peers in the Republic of Ireland and Scotland. A similar trend has been found more widely in research focusing on child psychological well-being in Northern Ireland (Muldoon and Trew 2000; Muldoon et al. 2000).

The interpretation of conflict: ideological and religious commitment

Research indicates that an active engagement with the violence or ideological commitment to the political agenda can also increase resilience in children (Muldoon and Wilson 2001; Punamaki 1996). Punamaki's research with Israeli and Palestinian children demonstrated a negative correlation between ideological commitment and psychological problems but a positive correlation between the amount of violent exposure and this commitment. Muldoon and Wilson replicated Punamaki's research with Northern Irish adolescents and found a complex relationship between experience of conflict and psychological well-being. In general, their findings propose that those who showed most ideological commitment to their community and who were involved or exposed to the most violence had the best mental health. McWhirter (1990) supports these findings and suggests that commitment to political ideology can help young people resist the psychological damage of being exposed to political violence. As McWhirter continues, displaying some commitment to the political cause and becoming actively involved in the political struggle often have a very positive influence on a young person's level of self-esteem, and therefore this patriotic connection may mediate the psychological impact of the exposure to political violence.

Other work by Punamaki and Suleiman (1990) proposes that the perception and interpretation of the traumatic event are affected by the political context and that this is important in determining the impact that the event has on mental health. Straker et al. (1996) further researched this area and determined that political violence was not always viewed as being problematic. They indicated that the context was important in deciding whether the violence is a problem and what this violence actually means. Jones (2002: 1352) concludes that the 'subjective understanding and political context do mediate the impact of political violence'. Although there are many factors which could contribute to the apparent resilience of children and adolescents in countries such as Northern Ireland, one major factor may be that of religion. Research in this area (Park et al. 1990) has indicated that religion may influence not only a child's understanding of an event, but also the method chosen by the child in order to deal with that event. Research in this area conducted in Northern Ireland has suggested that the Christian Church has a highly positive effect on children's abilities to cope with the political violence in the province (McWhirter 1983). However, similar research by Roe (1993) has indicated that although commitment to religious ideology can assist in positive development, such as that described by McWhirter (1983), attempts at community development can be truncated by this religious commitment and, in some cases, this religious ideology can actually serve to exacerbate the conflict. This point finds resonance with Muldoon and Wilson's (2001: 121) research on ideological commitment, in which it is suggested that 'increased experience of conflict may result in more socially polarized views, greater intransigence, and a decreased willingness to accommodate the other side'.

Coping strategies: denial, dissociation and habituation

Cairns and Wilson (1989) suggest that people in Northern Ireland use coping mechanisms such as denial and distancing, in addition to a tendency to seek high levels of social support, to deal with the violence. This proposal by Cairns and Wilson is in line with suggestions made by Folkman and Lazarus (1988) who indicate that in situations that are irresolvable, coping strategies are often employed. In addition, there is evidence to suggest that children's well-being is increased with social support (Cauce et al. 1990). Fraser (1973) emphasized this point and believed one of the main mediating factors between exposure to violence and mental health among children was the vulnerability of the child's parents, either because of a lack of adequate emotional support or because they communicated their anxieties to the child.

Although denial and distancing are coping mechanisms which are actively employed by individuals after exposure to trauma in Northern Ireland, direct and indirect exposure to political violence can also elicit dissociative states. However, unlike denial and distancing, dissociation is a psychological response which is elicited both during (peri-) and after (post-) trauma rather than just after the event (Spiegel 1986). Consequently, dissociation is an immediate psychological response to trauma that is not dependent upon active cognitive processes (Counts 1990). In addition to this, although direct and indirect exposure to political violence can elicit dissociative states, there are other indirect factors which might lead to dissociation in the Northern Ireland population (Dorahy and Lewis 1998). Irwin (1994a) has suggested that dissociation levels are often increased in individuals who experienced the death or long-term loss of a parent as a child and also that dissociation is enhanced by feelings of unresolved grief (Irwin 1994b). Although dissociation research is ongoing in Northern Ireland, there is a need for this research area to expand to include dissociation in children and adolescents.

One key factor not to be overlooked when discussing Northern Irish children's resilience to their exposure to political violence is that of habituation. With specific regard to Northern Ireland, McWhirter

(1988) concluded that because the state of political violence and societal instability had become so characteristic of life in the province, the abnormal (i.e. that state of unease) had become the norm and children were therefore less likely to make unprompted references to the violence and on-going conflict because it was as much a part of their lives as anything else. However, if this is the case and McWhirter's suggestions about habituation are correct, then it may be, as Cairns (1996) suggests, that habituation should only be prevalent in societies characterized by prolonged political violence, such as Northern Ireland. This, Cairns (1996) suggests, goes hand in hand with Breznitz's (1983) immunization model which suggests that survival of a traumatic stressor will leave an individual better equipped to deal with subsequent stressors. This model, proposed by Breznitz, infers that in situations of repeated or prolonged stress, accurate preparatory information about the imminent crisis provides the individual with the opportunity to mobilize their defence mechanisms and coping strategies: they can foresee any loss which might be incurred, manage their anxiety, develop more adequate coping mechanisms and develop models which might prevent them becoming beleaguered by the stressful events (Janis 1971; Meichenbaum and Turk 1976; Girodo 1977; Meichenbaum 1977). This increased predictability results in reduced stress and a reduction in fear (Weiss 1970).

Due to this resilience, research in Northern Ireland has tended to present an argument that 'only a small proportion of children exposed to political violence require specialist treatment. Such children, however, tend to show a wide variety of symptoms' (Cairns 1996: 32), including signs of PTSD.

Post-Traumatic Stress Disorder among children in Northern Ireland

The majority of research into the impact of exposure to political violence and child mental health has focused heavily upon PTSD and its development as a consequence of exposure to trauma. The *Diagnostic and Statistical Manual of Mental Disorders* (*DSM-IV-R*) (APA 2000) indicates that although prevention of natural disasters is impossible and prediction of them is often difficult with any degree of accuracy, these events are still less psychologically disabling than those which are manmade or perpetrated by humans against other humans because these man-made events can all be either reduced or prevented. Although research has shown that psychological symptomatology is prevalent in children that have been exposed to organized violence (e.g. Adjukovic and Adjukovic 1993; Hjern et al. 1991; Thien and Malapert 1988), other researchers (e.g. Almqvist and Brandell-Forsberg 1997) have questioned the veracity of employing a PTSD diagnosis in children. Research has shown, however, that PTSD does occur in school age children and adolescents (e.g. Famularo et al. 1990) and further research by investigators such as Saigh (1989) have supported the *DSM-IV-R* proposal that PTSD can actually occur at any age, including childhood (APA 2000).

Joseph et al. (1993), however, determined that there was no significant difference between Northern Irish children from high violence areas and those from low violence areas on PTSD symptomatology, while McWhirter (1983) also found this to be the case. Cairns and Dawes (1996) further indicated that children exposed to this violence can remain free of adjustment problems and clinical disorders and further research by Perrin et al. (2000) confirms that the majority of children and adolescents who are exposed to traumatic stressors do not go on to develop full blown PTSD. Although research such as that conducted by Foy et al. (1996) reported that there is a direct relationship between the level of violence the child is exposed to and PTSD manifestations, other researchers would suggest that the meaning of the violence is far more important than the level of exposure to life threatening events (e.g. Ziv and Israel 1973; Malmquist 1986).

Implications for the peace process

The Northern Ireland peace process, which began with the signing of the Downing Street Declaration in December 2003, witnessed the paramilitary ceasefires in 1994, and led to the positive 'yes' vote for the Good Friday Agreement in the 22 May Referendum. Parallel to these events Northern Ireland has observed a reduction in paramilitary activity, but not a disappearance, with paramilitaries still involved in murder and vigilante-style punishment attacks. Post-1998 Northern Ireland also still suffers an annual cycle of dispute and civil disorder surrounding controversial Orange Order demonstrations and increasing residential segregation (McKittrick et al. 2004; Police Service of Northern Ireland 2005; Shirlow 2003). A reason for this slow progress and inability to leave the past behind could be in some way due to strong ideological/religious commitments – suggested coping strategies employed to reduce the impact of the conflict. Researchers (Muldoon and Wilson 2001; Roe 1993) have warned that religious and/or ideological commitments may protect from trauma, but exacerbate and perpetuate the conflict, while Ferguson and Cairns (1996) have illustrated that short-term coping strategies, such as avoiding the conflict, will only maintain that conflict in the long term. Therefore the peace process offers new challenges for the psychological well-being of Northern Irish children as they try to adjust to the challenges ahead and leave the culture of violence behind.

Concluding remarks

Although research has attempted to illustrate that the political violence in Northern Ireland has had a negative impact on psychological well-being, few of these studies have provided evidence to support the theory that children and young people in Northern Ireland have become psychiatric casualties of the political violence (Cairns and Wilson 1991). Instead most evidence would seem to suggest that the majority of children living in violent societies appear to be coping and well adjusted. Cairns (1996) questions whether the lack of psychological symptomatology in these children is an indicator of well-being or, rather, an indicator of severe traumatization, and other research in this area (Dawes et al. 1989) warns that the expectation that children are resilient may have led to a situation where the psychological distress encountered by children in societies such as Northern Ireland is under-estimated. Indeed, it may be the case that the low prevalence of mental health problems in children in Northern Ireland is the result of the changes in referral criteria by the responsible agencies (Cairns 1987) and therefore as the criteria change so do the number of children being referred – although the actual number of children being psychologically affected by the violence does not decrease/increase. Secondly, it is true to say that family support and cohesion in Northern Ireland are par-ticularly strong. Further explanation of this low prevalence of mental health problems may be explained by family and social support: Cairns (1996) has suggested that stable parents act as a protective factor and, in addition, that when the stress of living with political violence is chronic, rather than acute, it serves to strengthen family ties. Further, it may be suggested that the anti-social behaviour that is exhibited by some children and adolescents in Northern Ireland is an externalization of the psychological impact of exposure to trauma and political vio-lence. However, researchers such as Muldoon and Trew (2000) caution against making this connection as this anti-social behaviour is also related to socio-economic disadvantage, and Muldoon et al. (2000) indi-cate that although psychometric profiles would suggest that there is evi-dence of acting-out behaviour, this is not always the case when the actual behaviour is examined. However, it must also be remembered that although research suggests that exposure to political violence does not have an increasingly detrimental effect on children and their behaviour, there are a minority of children who are severely affected when violence harms themselves or their families.

References

Adjukovic, M. and Adjukovic, D. (1993) 'Psychological well-being of refugee children'. *Child Abuse and Neglect*, 17: 843–54.

Almqvist, K. and Brandell-Forsberg, M. (1997) 'Refugee children in Sweden: posttraumatic stress disorder in Iranian preschool children exposed to organised violence'. *Child Abuse and Neglect*, 21(4): 351–66.

American Psychiatric Association (2000) *Diagnostic and Statistical Manual of Mental Disorders* (Revised 4th edition) Washington DC: American Psychiatric Association.

Barenbaum, J., Ruchkin, V. and Schwab-Stone, M. (2004) 'The psychosocial aspects of children exposed to war: practice and policy initiatives'. *Journal of Child Psychology and Psychiatry*, 45(1): 41–62.

Boal, F. W. (1978) 'Ethnic residential segregation'. In D. Herbert and R. Johnston (eds), *Social Areas in Cities: Processes, Patterns and Problems*. London: John Wiley, pp. 57–95.

Breslin, A. (1982) 'Tolerance and moral reasoning among adolescents in Ireland'. *Journal of Moral Education*, 11(2): 112–27.

Breznitz, S. (ed.) (1983) *The Denial of Stress*. New York: International Universities Press.

Cairns, E. (1983) 'Children's perceptions of normative and prescriptive interpersonal aggression in high and low areas of violence in Northern Ireland'. Unpublished paper.

Cairns, E. (1987) *Caught in the Crossfire: Children and the Northern Ireland Conflict*. Belfast and New York: Appletree Press and Syracuse University Press.

Cairns, E. (1990) 'Impact of television news exposure on children's perceptions of violence in Northern Ireland'. *Journal of Social Psychology*, 130(4): 447–52.

Cairns, E. (1996) *Children and Political Violence*. Oxford: Blackwell.

Cairns, E. and Conlon, L. (1985) 'Children's moral reasoning and the Northern Irish violence'. Unpublished paper.

Cairns, E. and Darby, J. (1998) 'The conflict in Northern Ireland: causes, consequences and controls'. *American Psychologist*, 53(7): 754–60.

Cairns, E. and Dawes, A. (1996) 'Children: ethnic and political violence: a commentary'. *Child Development*, 67: 129–39.

Cairns, E., Hunter, D. and Herring, L. (1980) 'Young children's awareness of violence in Northern Ireland: the influence of television'. *British Journal of Social and Clinical Psychology*, 19: 3–6.

Cairns, E. and Wilson, R. (1989) 'Mental health aspects of political violence in Northern Ireland'. *International Journal of Mental Health*, 18: 38–56.

Cairns, E. and Wilson, R. (1991) 'Nothern Ireland: political violence and self-reported physical symptoms in a community sample'. *Journal of Psychosomatic Research*, 35: 707–11.

Cairns, E. and Wilson, R. (1993) 'Stress, coping and political violence in Northern Ireland'. In J. P. Wilson and B. Raphael (eds), *International Handbook of Traumatic Stress Syndromes*. New York: Plenum Press.

Cairns, E., Wilson, R., Gallagher, T. and Trew, K. (1995) 'Psychology's contribution to understanding conflict in Northern Ireland'. *Peace and Conflict: Journal of Peace Psychology*, 1(2): 131–48.

Cauce, A. M., Reid, M., Landesman, S. and Gonzales, N. (1990) 'Social support in young children: measurement, structure and behavioural impact'. In B. R. Sarason, I. G. Sarason and G. R. Pierce (eds) *Social Support: an Interactional View*. New York: Wiley.

Cohen, J. A. (1998) 'Practice parameters for the assessment of treatment of children and adolescents with posttraumatic stress disorder'. *Journal of the American Academy of Child and Adolescent Psychiatry*, 37: 4–26.

Connolly, P. and Healy, J. (2004) 'The development of children's attitudes towards "the Troubles" in Northern Ireland'. In O. Hargie and D. Dickson (eds), *Researching the Troubles: Social Science Perspectives on the Northern Ireland Conflict*. UK: Mainstream Publishing Ltd, pp. 37–57.

Counts, R. M. (1990) 'The concept of dissociation'. *Journal of the American Academy of Psychoanalysis*, 18: 460–79.

Dawes, A., Tredoux, C. and Feinstein, A. (1989) 'Political violence in South Africa: some effects on children of the violent destruction of their community'. *International Journal of Mental Health*, 18(2): 16–43.

Donnelly, M. (1995) 'Depression among adolescents in Northern Ireland'. *Adolescence*, 30: 339–50.

Dorahy, M. J. and Lewis, C. A. (1998) 'Trauma induced dissociation and the psychological effects of the "Troubles" in Northern Ireland: an overview and integration'. *Irish Journal of Psychology*, 19(2–3): 332–44.

Elbedour, S., Baker, A. M. and Charlesworth, W. R. (1997) 'The impact of political violence on moral reasoning in children'. *Child Abuse and Neglect*, 21(11): 1053–66.

Famularo, R., Kinscherff, R. and Fenton, T. (1990) 'Symptom differences in acute and chronic presentation of childhood Post-Traumatic Stress Disorder'. *Child Abuse and Neglect*, 14: 439–44.

Fee, F. (1980) 'Responses to a behavioural questionnaire of a group of Belfast children'. In J. Harbison and J. Harbison (eds), *A Society Under Stress: Children and Young People in Northern Ireland*. Somerset, England: Open Books, pp. 31–42.

Fee, F. (1983) 'Educational change in Belfast school children 1975–81'. In J. Harbison (ed.), *Children of the Troubles: Children in Northern Ireland*. Belfast, Northern Ireland: Stranmillis College Leaning Resources Unit, pp. 44–58.

Ferguson, N. and Cairns, E. (1996) 'Political violence and moral maturity in Northern Ireland'. *Political Psychology*, 17(4): 713–25.

Ferguson, N. and Cairns, E. (2002) 'The impact of political conflict on moral maturity: a cross-national perspective'. *Journal of Adolescence*, 25: 441–51.

Fields, R. M. (1976) *Society under Siege: a Psychology of Northern Ireland*. Philadelphia: Temple University Press.

Folkman, S. and Lazarus, R. S. (1988) 'The relationship between coping and emotion: implications for theory and research'. *Social Science and Medicine*, 26(3): 309–17.

Foy, D. W., Madvig, B. T., Pynoos, R. S. and Camilleri, A. J. (1996) 'Etiological factors in the development of post traumatic stress disorder in children and adolescents'. *Journal of School Psychology*, 34: 133–45.

Fraser, M. (1972) 'At school during a guerrilla war'. *Special Education*, 61: 6–8.

Fraser, M. (1973) *Children in Conflict*. London: Secker and Warburg.

Girodo, M. (1977) 'Self-talk: mechanisms in anxiety and stress management'. In C.D. Spielberger, I. G. Sarason, *Stress and Anxiety*, Volume 4. New York: Wiley and Sons.

Hjern, A., Angel, B. and Höjer, B. (1991) 'Persecution and behaviour: a report of refugee children from Chile'. *Child Abuse and Neglect*, 15: 945–51.

Irwin, H. J. (1994a) 'Proneness to dissociation and traumatic childhood events'. *Journal of Nervous and Mental Disease*, 182: 456–60.

Irwin, H. J. (1994b) 'Affective predictors of dissociation I: the case of unresolved grief'. *Dissociation*, 7: 86–91.

Janis, I. L. (1971) *Stress and Frustration*. New York: Harcourt Brace Jovanovich.

Jardine, E. (1989) 'Trends in juvenile crime'. In J. Harbison (ed.), *Growing Up in Northern Ireland*. Belfast: Stramillis College.

Jarman, N. and O'Halloran, C. (2001) 'Recreational rioting, young people, interface areas and violence'. *Child Care in Practice*, 7(1): 2–16.

Jones, L. (2002) 'Adolescent understandings of political violence and psychological well-being: a qualitative study from Bosnia Herzegovina'. *Social Science and Medicine*, 55: 1351–71.

Joseph, S., Cairns, E. and McCollam, P. (1993) 'Political violence, coping, and depressive symptomatology in Northern Irish children'. *Personality and Individual Differences*, 15(4): 471–3.

Kohlberg, L. (1984) *Essays in Moral Development: Vol. II. The Psychology of Moral Development: Moral Stages, their Nature and Validity*. San Francisco: Harper and Row.

Liddell, C., Kemp, J. and Moema, M. (1993) 'The young lions – South African children and youth in political struggle'. In L. Leavitt and N. Fox (eds), *The Psychological Effects of War and Violence on Children*. Hillsdale, NJ: Lawrence Erlbaum.

Lorenc, L. and Branthwaite, A. (1986) 'Evaluations of political violence by English and Northern Irish schoolchildren'. *British Journal of Social Psychology*, 25: 349–52.

Lyons, H. A. (1973) 'The psychological effects of the civil disturbances on children'. *The Northern Teacher*, Winter: 19–30.

Malmquist, C. (1986) 'Children who witness parental murder: posttraumatic aspects'. *Journal of the American Academy of Child Psychiatry*, 25: 320–5.

McAuley, P. and Kremmer, J. (1990) 'On the fringes of society: adults and children in a West Belfast community'. *New Community*, 16(2): 247–59.

McAuley, R. and Troy, M. (1983) 'The impact of urban conflict and violence on children referred to a child guidance clinic'. In J. Harbison (ed.), *Children of the Troubles: Children in Northern Ireland*. Belfast: Stanmillis College Learning Resources Unit.

McGrath, A. and Wilson, R. (1985) 'Factors which influence the prevalence and variation of psychological problems in children in Northern Ireland'. Paper presented at the annual conference of the Developmental Section of the British Psychological Society, Belfast, Northern Ireland, September.

McKeown, J. (1973) 'Civil unrest: secondary schools survey'. *The Northern Teacher*, Winter: 39–42.

McKittrick, D., Kelters, S., Feeney B. and Thornton, C. (2004) *Lost Lives: the Stories of the Men, Women and Children Who Died as a Result of the Northern Ireland Troubles* (2nd edn.). Edinburgh: Mainstream Publishing.

McWhirter, L. (1983) 'Growing up in Northern Ireland: from aggression to the troubles'. In A. P. Goldstein and M. H. Segall (eds), *Aggression in a Global Perspective*. New York: Pergamon, pp. 367–400.

McWhirter, L. (1988) 'Psychological impact of violence in Northern Ireland: recent research findings and issues'. In N. Eisenberg and D. Glasgow (eds), *Recent Advances in Clinical Psychology*. London: Gower.

McWhirter, L. (1990) 'How do children cope with the chronic troubles of Northern Ireland?' Paper presented at the Conference on Children in War, Jerusalem, June.

Meichenbaum, D. (1977) *Cognitive-Behaviour Modifications: an Integrated Approach*. New York: Plenum.

Meichenbaum, D. and Turk, D. C. (1976) 'The cognitive-behavioural management of anxiety, anger, and pain'. In P. O. Davidson (ed.), *The Behavioural Management of Anxiety, Depression and Pain*. New York: Brunner/Mazel.

Mercer, G. W. and Bunting, B. (1980) 'Some motivations of adolescent demonstrators in Northern Ireland civil disturbances'. In J. Harbison and J. Harbison (eds), *A Society Under Stress: Children and Young People in Northern Ireland*. Somerset, England: Open Books, pp. 153–66.

Muldoon, O. T. and Trew, K. (2000) 'Children's experience and adjustment to political conflict in Northern Ireland'. *Peace and Conflict: Journal of Peace Psychology*, 6(2): 157–76.

Muldoon, O., Trew, K. and Kilpatrick, R. (2000) 'The legacy of the troubles on the young people's psychological and social development and their school life'. *Youth and Society*, 32(1): 6–28.

Muldoon, O. and Wilson, R. (2001) 'Ideological commitment, experience of conflict and adjustment in Northern Irish adolescents'. *Medicine, Conflict and Survival*, 17: 112–24.

Murray, H. B. M. (1982) 'Prospect for psychology'. In G. S. Neilsen (ed.), *Psychology and International Affairs: Can We Contribute?* Copenhagen: Munksgaard.

Park, C., Cohen, L. H. and Herb, L. (1990) 'Intrinsic religiousness and religious coping as life stress moderators for Catholic versus Protestants'. *Journal of Personality and Social Psychology*, 5(3): 562–74.

Perrin, S., Smith, P. and Yule, W. (2000) 'Practitioner review: the assessment and treatment of posttraumatic stress disorder in children and adolescents'. *Journal of Child Psychology and Psychiatry*, 41(3): 277–89.

Persistent School Absenteeism in Northern Ireland (1977, 1982) Belfast: Department of Education for Northern Ireland.

Police Service of Northern Ireland (2005) *Casualties as a Result of Paramilitary-Style Attacks 1990/91–2004/05*. Retrieved 22 May 2005 from http://www.psni.police.uk/

Punamaki, R.-L. (1996) 'Can ideological commitment protect children's psychological well-being in situations of political violence?' *Child Development*, 67(1): 55–69.

Punamaki, R-L. and Suleiman, R. (1990) 'Predictors and effectiveness of coping with political violence among Palestinian children'. *British Journal of Social Psychology*, 29(1): 67–77.

Roe, M. D. (1993) 'Psychological and social resilience to political violence: role of faith communities'. Paper presented to the 101st Annual Convention of the American Psychological Association. Toronto, Canada, August.

Rutter, M., Cox, A., Tupling, C., Berger, M. and Yule, W. (1975) 'Attainment and adjustment in two geographical areas: 1. The prevalence of psychiatric disorder'. *British Journal of Psychiatry*, 126: 520–33.

Saigh, P. (1989) 'The validity of the DSM-III Post-Traumatic Stress Disorder classification as applied to children'. *Journal of Abnormal Psychology*, 98: 189–92.

Shirlow, P. (2003) '"Who fears to speak": fear, mobility and ethno-sectarianism in the two "Ardoynes"'. *The Global Review of Ethnopolitics*, 3(1): 76–91.

Smith, D. J. (1987) *Equality and Inequality in Northern Ireland, Part 3: Perceptions and Views*. London: Policy Studies Institute.

Smyth, M. and Hamilton, J. (2004) 'The human cost of the troubles'. In O. Hargie and D. Dickson (eds), *Researching the Troubles: Social Science Perspectives on the Northern Ireland Conflict*. UK: Mainstream Publishing Ltd, pp. 15–36.

Spiegel, D. (1986) 'Dissociating damage'. *American Journal of Clinical Hypnosis*, 29: 123–31.

Straker, G., Mendelshon, M., Tudin, P. and Mooza, F. (1996) 'Violent political contexts and the emotional concerns of township youth'. *Child Development*, 67(1): 46–54.

Stroufe, L. A. and Rutter, M. (1984) 'The domain of developmental psychology'. *Child Development*, 55: 17–29.

Thein, N. and Malapert, B. (1988) 'The psychological consequences for children of war traumata and migration'. In D. Miserez (ed.) *Refugees: the Trauma of Exile*. League of Red Cross and Red Crescent Societies, Geneva, Switzerland: Martinus Nijhoff Publishers, pp. 248–86.

Weiss, J. M. (1970) 'Somatic effects of predictable and unpredictable shock'. *Psychosomatic Medicine*, 32: 397–409.

Wilson, R. and Cairns, E. (1992) 'Troubles, stress and psychological disorder in Northern Ireland'. *The Psychologist*, 5(8) 347–50.

Wilson, R. and Cairns, E. (1996) 'Coping processes and emotions in relation to political violence in Northern Ireland'. In G. Mulhearn and S. Joseph (eds), *Psychological Perspectives on Stress and Trauma: From Disaster to Political Violence*. Leicester: British Psychological Society, pp. 19–28.

Yule, W., Bolton, D., Udwin, O., Boyle, S., O'Ryan, D. and Nurrish, J. (2000) 'The long-term psychological effects of a disaster experienced in adolescence: I: the incidence and course of PTSD'. *Journal of Child Psychology and Psychiatry*, 41(4): 503–11.

Ziv, A. and Israeli, R. (1973) 'Effects of bombardment on the manifest anxiety level of children living in kibbutzim'. *Journal of Counselling and Clinical Psychology*, 40: 287–91.

13
Adjustment of Both Parents and Children of Exiled and Traumatized Refugees in the Host Country

Amer Hosin

Introduction

This chapter aims to examine the adjustment processes among both parents and children of traumatized and exiled refugees who live in a host culture. It is also hoped that the work will help to answer a few important questions on how children react to the refugee experience, how they adjust to and cope in the host culture, and what their mental health problems are. The answers provided to these questions are important to a number of professionals and individuals, e.g. policy-makers, researchers and many practitioners such as psychiatrists, psychologists, social workers, mental health nurses, etc. As well as identifying factors that contribute to traumatization in a refugee population, parental health and variables such as the duration and number of years spent in the host country, the group's background, current level of social contact and support, numbers of family members sharing the household, and the nature of the traumatic experience prior to their flight are also investigated.

A considerable amount of research literature on ethnic minority groups has been published so far (e.g. Fernando 1995, 2002; Karami 1990; King 1994; Littlewood and Lipsedge 1989; Pilgrim and Rogers 1994) on culture, race, ethnicity and mental health. Indeed, this amount of literature has promoted knowledge and increased professional understanding in this specific area. However, apart from some very recent publications (Aldous et al. 1999; Hosin 2000, 2001; Black et al. 1997; Woodhead 2000; Burnett and Peel 2001a, 2001b, 2001c; Smith et al. 2001; Westermeyer 1988, 1989; Turner et al. 2003) very little attention has been paid to the links between children's adjustment and that of adult family members of traumatized refugees living together in a host culture. In other words, published research which links both children's adjustment and parental problems (particularly among those refugees who have escaped civil strife, wars, suffered multiple traumas or displacement) is very limited. A recent study by Jafar (2000), which was funded by the King's Fund (UK) on the Health Needs' Assessment of the Iraqi community in London, suggested that 53 per cent of the adult population studied (n = 420 adult refugees) had a wide range of mental health problems, 49 per cent had heart diseases and 24 per cent suffered from various type of cancers. These findings confirm the reported result by Gorst-Unsworth and Goldenberg (1998) and Lavik et al. (1996). The former examined the importance of social factors in exile among 84 Iraqi refugees and found depression in 44 per cent of the sample. This study suggests that many of the most important factors in continuing morbidity can be modified in the country of exile. It has also highlighted the importance of family reunion where the survivor is separated from close relatives (wife and children). Lavik et al. (1996) meanwhile found that 46.6 per cent of the patients included in their study had a Post-Traumatic Stress Disorder (PTSD) according to the *DSM-IV* criteria (1994). However, age, gender, unemployment and torture emerged as important predictors of emotional withdrawal in this study. Both of the above-mentioned studies seem to place more emphasis on the multifactorial nature of risk factors in the psychological health of refugees and the need for integrated rehabilitation efforts as well as professional help to improve the social environment, and the need to provide appropriate social activities and support to the refugee population.

Refugees' experience, post-migration and adjustment

Focusing further on the traumatized children of war regions, parental adjustment and children's reactions, Smith et al. (2001) cited several studies and reported that children's reactions to direct exposure and living through war conditions may contribute to producing negative outcomes, including high levels of PTSD symptoms among children who have survived conflict in war regions. This study further added that traumatic stressors in war are commonly multiple, diverse, chronic and repeated. Other researchers in this area such as Bryce et al. (1989) and Dawes et al. (1989), have focused on parental adjustment and children's reactions to traumatic events. In fact, all these studies (including Smith et al.'s study) which were conducted in former conflict regions such as Lebanon, South Africa and Bosnia have found that parental mental health, particularly that of mothers in times of conflict, was a significant predictor of children's adjustment and morbidity. Baker (1992) supports the above-mentioned findings and added, 'tortured individuals are less likely to function as parents, spouses or employees. Tortured survivors can have difficulty in establishing relationship and trust with their spouse and children and are therefore more likely to transmit their problem to their offspring' (see also Basoğlu 1992).

Furthermore, Almqvist and Broberg (1999) investigated the relative importance of various risk and protective factors for mental health and social adjustment in 50 young Iranian pre-school refugee children after arriving in Sweden. The results of this study indicated that although exposure to war and political violence were important risk factors for long-lasting post-traumatic stress symptoms in children, their mothers' emotional well-being predicted strong emotional well-being in children. This study also noted that, overall, children's adaptation in the host culture is the result of a complex process involving several interacting risk and protective factors. These may include peer relationships, current life circumstances in the receiving host countries, and exposure to bullying, all of which are of equal or greater importance than previous exposure to organized violence.

Likewise, Hjern and Angel (2000) and Montgomery and Foldspang (2001) reported a family history of violence (parental exposure to torture) as well as a distressed present family situation were the strongest predictors of sleep disturbance among recently arrived refugee children. Sourander (1998) looked at the extent of damage on the separated refugee minors waiting for placement in an asylum centre in Finland and reported that about half of the minors were functioning within clinical or borderline range when evaluated with the Child Behaviour Checklist. This study also claimed that very young and unaccompanied refugee minors are more vulnerable to emotional distress than older children. Hauff and Vaglum (1995) studied 145 Vietnamese boat refugees aged 15 and above. The population of this community sample were interviewed on their arrival in Norway and again three years later. Major findings of this investigation unexpectedly suggested three years later that there was no decline in self-rated emotional and psychological distress, almost one in four suffered from a psychiatric disorder, and the depression rate in this research was prevalent in both men and women. Female gender, negative life events, a lack of a close confidante and chronic family separation were identified as predictors for psychopathology. This suggests that the availability of a close confidante (spouse, children, or close relatives) in periods of psychosocial transition has a protective effect against psychiatric disorders. This research also noted that married refugees separated from their spouses by the flight were more emotionally distressed than other refugees on arrival in Norway. Focusing further on children of exiled and tortured survivors living in Denmark, Cohn et al. (1980, 1985) found that more than one-third of the children were anxious and hypersensitive to noise, suffered from insomnia and frequent nightmares, and 23 per cent had a regular nocturnal enuresis. Allodi (1989) indicated that emotional distress in children was related to previous traumatization of the parents and the current coping styles of the latter. These conclusions are in agreement with Acuna's (1989) findings which noted that withdrawal, depression, irritability, aggressiveness, generalized fear, and excessive clinging were common characteristics of the children of torture survivors. An interesting commentary concerning the above-mentioned features was illustrated by Weile et al. (1990) who stated that children of traumatized families were fragile, vulnerable, and had more psychosomatic problems than age-matched native school children.

Making sense of attachment theory and applying research to practice

This section could be regarded as an extension to Felicity de Zulueta's earlier discussion of the treatment of psychological trauma from the perspective of attachment theory (see Chapter 5 above).

Attachment theory, as indicated earlier, was developed by John Bowlby (1908–90). Bowlby (1971, 1975, 1980) described attachment, especially to the mother, as an adaptive, biological process serving the needs of the child for protection and nurturing. So what is the part of the adult's relation that influences the life of the developing child? Indeed, family functioning and quality of parental care and affection are crucial in development. According to Mary Ainsworth and her co-workers (Ainsworth et al. 1978) there are three main patterns of attachment that can be characterized by observation of the toddler's behaviour with the mother. It has been suggested that emotionally warm, sensitive care and a high quality parent–child relationship result in the young child developing a whole range of adaptive forms of behaviour including confident exploration of the environment. Emphasis has been placed on the importance of early child contact particularly over the first three years of the child's life (Klaus and Kennl 1976; Herbert et al. 1982). Likewise, Mills and colleagues (1984) found that that mental ill-health makes both parents unavailable to the child and impairs the quality of care. For example, a depressed mother is likely to be less responsive to the needs of the child, less able to provide consistent discipline and less likely to stimulate or initiate interaction (Weissman and Paykel 1974). Further, a morbidly anxious mother often transmits her anxieties through identification, imitation and example. Further a mother who is frightened of lifts or flying will communicate fear of flying to her children (Graham 1994: 37; Freud and Burlingham 1943). Similarly, Spence et al. (2002) recently reported in their longitudinal and community-based study (n = 4434 families followed up from infancy to adolescence) that symptoms of anxiety and depression in young children are found to be associated with early childhood experience of maternal anxiety and depression. This study also indicates that the effect would be much greater with prolonged, persistent or repeated exposure to high maternal anxiety and depression. It was also noted that family adversity such as poverty, distressed marital relationship and break-up during the child's first five years produced a small but significant increase in the risk of high anxiety and depression in young children. Furthermore, this study also claimed that such internalized emotional problems during childhood and adolescence could be regarded as significant mental health issues that are not only more stable than traditionally thought but also result in long-term consequences if left untreated. Other conclusions reached in this study which looked at the link between children's mental health and parental psychopathology suggested again that anxious and depressed children are more likely to have parents who have experienced some form of psychological difficulties including anxiety, depression or substance abuse. Overall, this investigation seems to confirm earlier findings (Biederman et al. 1991; Weissman et al. 1984) which reported that depressed and/or anxious parents are more likely to have children who manifest emotional and behavioural difficulties such as anxiety, depression, attention deficit and behavioural problems. Spence and colleagues (2002) who cited Whaley et al. (1999) also did not rule out genetic factors but suggested that parenting styles and communication can provide some explanation for this complex interaction. However, the explanation offered in the literature suggested anxious and/or depressed refugee mothers are more likely to provide little autonomy, display less warmth and engage in more criticism. Hence, such mothers consequently provide inadequate care and tend less to discharge parental responsibilities (Westermeyer 1991: 137; Howe et al. 1999).

Clearly some of the above-cited literature gives a clear association between the attachment styles of the care provider and the predicted behaviour of the infant. Still within the attachment framework, Cairns (2002: 60–89) stated that infants who were cared for by adults who are emotionally available and responsive (simply enjoyed the benefit of secure attachment) are likely to be curious, playful, sociable, confident and more cooperative than those children who experience an unmet attachment needs pattern and who are described as 'insecure'. This study also reported that insecure attachments lead to inhibition, fear, anxiety, irritability and inadequate toleration or regulation of stress, as well as difficulties in forming relationships with people and the wider environment. Further, it was also indicated that children with an unmet attachment will struggle more in the recovery from losses and are less able to draw on the comfort of substitute carers. These children may also find it difficult to think and construct narratives and could struggle more than their peers when it comes to learning. Hence the education system must provide for the educational needs of all children, and perhaps recognize the needs of traumatized children as totally different from those of non-traumatized children. Cairns (2002), before ending her various book chapters on attachment, trauma and resilience, noted that children can survive and thrive even in terrible conditions, and should be given the opportunity to develop the resilience they need. She further added that unattached children and refugees need to develop social resilience, new interest, new activities, hobbies and sports, and to be taken on group adventure trips and be given opportunities which may help them to learn the art of planning for their own lives (see also Wolin and Wolin 1993).

Extent of trauma exposure, vulnerabilities and legacies of displacement

It is worth noting here that the extent of vulnerability depends on the impact of violence and migration on the child's family and community. This may include witnessing the death and injury of a parent or sibling and perhaps persistent exposure to death, destruction and ultimately separation from parents. Researchers (e.g. Freud and Burlingham 1943) regard separation from family support, siblings and friends as more stressful than exposure to bombing and injury. However, the most vulnerable time appears to be the pre-school years and early adolescence (Bowlby 1980; Rutter 1966; Black 1974). Other risk factors may include sudden (unanticipated) death of parents or siblings, radical change in family circumstances and roles, poor access to family support and an unstable, inconsistent environment. It would be fair to suggest here that rapidly changing environments with little stability as well as parental psychopathology and lack of security or protection have implications for the physical health and mental well-being of the refugee population. As indicated above, children who live under the threat of adversity and who cope well have been referred to as 'resilient children' (Cairns 2002; Masten 2001; see also Chapter 8, this volume, on trauma, resilience and growth in children).

However, Rutter (1985), Garmezy (1987) and Werner (1989) have looked at the factors which help children to cope with severe and stress-ful life events. Their research indicated that lack of immediate support (e.g. disintegration of family) and the more risk factors a child is exposed to are more likely to make children vulnerable to psychiatric or mental health problems. In sum, and as Ahearn and Athey (1991) stated, expo-sure to multiple traumas (stressors), both chronic and acute, greatly decrease a child's ability to cope successfully. Indeed, much needs to be learned about coping in children. Masten (2001: 227) stated that 'resilience appears to be a common phenomenon that results in most cases from the operation of basic human adaptation systems. If those systems are protected and in good working order, development is robust even in the face of severe adversity; if these major systems are impaired then the risks for developmental hazard are prolonged.'

Masten (2001) also defined resilience as a class of phenomena charac-terized by good outcomes in spite of serious threat to adaptation or devel-opment. So far, an important message has emerged from research on resilience which suggests that psychology has neglected important phe-nomena in human adjustment and development in the last few decades (see also Bonanno 2004; Linley and Joseph 2005). Hence, it has focused mainly on risks, pathology and treatment. Williamson (1988) and Ahearn and Athey (1991) have summarized the plight of refugees, and empha-sized the extent of their vulnerability. Williamson suggested: 'at any point in time, half of the refugees in the world are children. Most large-scale flights involve children, young adults and women. These children often experience malnutrition, lack of a balanced diet for normal growth, infectious diseases during the flights, exposure to crowded conditions, and poor sanitation. Many children also may lose siblings due to infec-tious diseases, experience separation, death of parents, become victims of violence, be beaten and suffer injuries, and are more likely to assume an adult role when the family structure changes through the death of parents and during illness' (Williamson 1988: 16).

Further, and while writing on the legacies of war, atrocities and refu-gees, Summerfield (1997: 360) noted that there have been an estimated 160 wars and armed conflicts in the developing world since 1945, with 22 million deaths and three times as many injured. He quoted UNICEF figures for 1986 and suggested that 'in the First World War, 5% of all casualties were civilians, 50% in the Second World War, over 80% in the US war in Vietnam and in present conflicts over 90%.' He went further to add that 80 per cent of all war refugees are in developing countries, many among the poorest on earth. In parts of Central America, he claimed, 50 per cent of households are headed by a woman and these are much more likely to be poor. Mortality rates during the acute phase of displacement by war are up to 60 times those of expected rates. Those at extra risk are households headed by an unprotected woman (often widowed), those without a community or marginalized in an alien cul-ture, those at serious socio-economic disadvantage or in severe poverty, and those with poor physical health or a disability. The emotional well-being of children remains reasonably intact for as long as their parents, or other significant figures, can absorb the continuing pressure of the situ-ation. Once parents can no longer cope with day-to-day living, child well-being deteriorates rapidly and infant mortality rates rise. Summerfield is one of the few professionals who regards the Western diagnostic classi-fications of PTSD as somewhat problematic when applied to diverse non-Western survivor populations. He stresses that a checklist of mental state features cannot provide a rigorous distinction between subjective distress and objective disorder. Much of the distress experienced and communi-cated by victims of extreme trauma is normal and adaptive. He argues that despite a PTSD prevalence of 14–50 per cent found in various studies of survivor populations in both third world and Western settings, the suf-ferers are often active and have good social as well as work function. That is to say there has been a tendency to rely on an ethnocentric interpreta-tion of disorder, based upon Western medical theories of traumatization, adjustment problems and psychiatric treatments. Thus, Summerfield regards a diagnosis of PTSD as poorly predictive and an unreliable indica-tor of a need for psychological treatment.

Assessment of refugees, integration and therapeutic approaches

Westermeyer (1991: 127–62), in a comprehensive review, suggested that assessment and treatment should take into consideration a wider range of past experience and current life situations as well as medical history, family illnesses and social background. This should include physical examination, developmental data, pre-natal and post-natal problems, social and emotional development, pre-flight stressors, losses, length of stay in refugee camps, and early resettlement experience. That is to say pre-migration, transmigration and post-migration experiences are frequently traumatic and must be assessed. Treatment, however, should resemble that offered to indigenous populations (see also Chapter 2 of this book) and should include counselling, cognitive and behavioural therapy, as well as pharmacotherapy if necessary. Compliance problems and complaints regarding side-effects may occur more often among refugees who are not familiar with long-term medications. These can be reduced through education and re-education of the parents and the child. In sum, refugee problems are too complex to rely on medication to solve mental health and psychiatric problems. Doctors and therapists therefore should direct patients to counselling, social activities, play, group work, stress management, education and recommendation of other psychotherapies available to deal with stressful and long-term problems. Jones (1998) worked with adolescent refugees in Bosnia who experienced uprooting and various losses – i.e. losses of family, home, school, town, friends and relatives – and suggested that greater flexibility over boundaries is required, particularly regarding time and setting. In addition, therapists working in a human rights/refugee camps context should be prepared to acknowledge their own impartiality and subjectivity and allow the discussion of political and social issues within the group. It is also suggested that such support can be of use through providing a space for expressing feelings, problem-solving and rebuilding of social ties. Eisenbruch (1990) uses the term *cultural bereavement* to describe the losses, and sees this as a condition that can affect both physical and mental health. Jones (1998) and Eisenbruch (1990) both agreed on the fundamental task of rebuilding first the social networks, engaging in community support, facilitating the development of problem-solving skills and addressing the collective experience of loss rather than focusing entirely on the psychopathological impact of trauma on the individual. It has been claimed that the most important task to accomplish during debriefing is to educate the victims and survivors about the psychological sequel frequently experienced by most refugees. This normalization of stress through debriefing can reduce people's responses to the inevitable symptoms of stress, depression, guilt, sleep disturbance, etc. The socio-cultural background of the survivor may be an important consideration in the screening process. Some survivors may be from certain cultures or from certain parts of a particular country where psychotherapy is not recognized as a form of treatment. In such cases an offer of psychotherapy may be rejected by the client, or even when accepted, premature termination of treatment is always a possibility.

In refugee camps and on arrival, physical needs such as food, water, clothes, shelter, sanitation, immunization and care for infectious diseases should be a priority. Psychological and social needs should follow and must include reduction in uncertainty, improving education and links with religious groups, expatriate groups and other social agencies. Moreover, screening for problems of mental health and social adjustment should occur in school, through the social services and perhaps through primary care clinics and hospitals. Staff in these locations should be sensitive to the special needs and problems of refugees. Woodhead (2000) summarized the needs of refugees as follows:

> Refugees arrive from different countries – with different historical, age, gender and cultural backgrounds – seeking safety, accommodation and security. Some arrive in considerable distress, are victims of war and torture and may have complex physical and mental health needs. However, food and a safe environment (home) is likely to be their first priority. Those who arrive from war-torn regions tend to show signs of post-traumatic stress disorder alongside other psychiatric and health problems such as anxiety, depression, insomnia, malnutrition, intestinal problems, skin complaints, stigma, poor self esteem.

Overall, refugee assessments demand special sensitivity to anxiety, fear and shyness, and should show reassurance, clarity and understanding. Refugees are individuals with a well-founded fear arising from one of a number of causes from witnessing malicious violence and losses, to being subject to interrogation, imprisonment and oppression. Hence, research instruments used with the refugee population should be unintrusive, unprovocative and sensitive to the participant's culture and values. In a recent article on refugees' health and instruments used, Turner et al. (2003: 444) stated that 'despite the resilience of many refugees coming to the UK, there was a substantial proportion who have evidence of serious psychological difficulties. Newly arrived refugees not only need community support but also many will have significant mental health problems and will need access to effective mental health treatment. Therefore, screening questionnaires are likely to be helpful with the refugee population but the threshold needs careful clinical validation. That is cut-off scores from these measures should never be used rigidly or by themselves in making a diagnosis.' Further details on the needs assessment of refugees can be found in Westermeyer (1991).

In general, contemporary data on PTSD prevalence (for a complete review see Meichenbaum 1994; Yule 1999, Yule et al. 2000; Fairbank et al. 1995; Koopman 1997; Resick 2001; Deivedi 2000; Thomas 1995) has revealed that approximately 25–30 per cent of individuals who witness a traumatic event may develop chronic PTSD and other forms of mental disorders, e.g. depression, etc. Pre-existing psychopathology, degree of horror, duration, frequency and level of exposure, gender, age, suddenness, controllability, inflicted damage and intensity of the disaster, perceived threat at the time, early separation from family and availability of support would all be risk factors which determine PTSD development in both children and adults (see Chapters 1 and 2 of this book for further details). In summary, the prevalence of symptoms is related to a variety of factors including the nature of trauma, the child's own experience, age, sex, past psychiatric illnesses and the degree of social support received from parents at home. It is worth noting, however, that a high prevalence of some forms of mental health problems is a characteristic of studies of refugee communities. For example Brent and Harrow's (1995) survey indicated that self-reported mental health problems were over five times higher in a refugee sample than in the general population sample. Levin (1999: 345) also reported that around 30 per cent of refugee children are in a severe state of mental discomfort and are in urgent need of child psychiatric or psychosocial rehabilitation.

Finally Stimpson et al. (2003) confirmed the above findings and indicate that psychiatric disorder is common, disabling and burdensome after war. Treatment approaches and rehabilitation of trauma must include the whole family, i.e. spouses, children and the whole social network of the victims. However, working with refugee families and their children who may have witnessed displacement, exile, torture, atrocity or separation is at best difficult. The stress levels suffered by such traumatized patients are chronic and sometimes severe. It is advisable to use a combination of approaches, e.g. counselling, cognitive therapy, drugs and other psychotherapeutic approaches to treat the problems of decrease of social interest, isolation, chronic depression, nightmares, poor concentration, irrational behaviour and avoidance behaviour (see Part I of this book). Dedicated professionals with the necessary energy and expertise may be able to provide specialized treatment, recognize the role of current stresses, relieve some symptoms by medication and also help traumatized individuals to get the social, emotional and financial support that they require. Jumaian et al. (1997) touched on this issue by suggesting that the treatment approach for survivors of traumatic events often begins with debriefing. Yule and Udwin (1991) and Stallard and Law (1993) compared debriefed and non-debriefed individuals and found that the debriefed samples showed lower levels of distress particularly in relation to intrusive thoughts. Other studies (Yule 1991, 1992; Saigh 1991; Joseph et al. 1991; Basoğlu 1992) suggested that there is a wide range of effective strategies including group therapy, behaviour and cognitive approaches, desensitization, flooding techniques as well as relaxation training used for tension, anxiety and intrusive thoughts. Most of these techniques can help sufferers to enhance their coping skills. Sleep problems and nightmares are other aspects of PTSD symptoms among children who have witnessed disasters. Halliday (1987) and Palace and Johnson (1989) found that relaxation and music before bedtime could be useful techniques for alleviating the recurrence of nightmares. Other reactions, which need careful intervention and therapy, include depression, guilt feelings, pessimism, irritability and anger.

In any event, Yule and Canterbury (1994) suggested that treatment approaches need flexibility and both clinicians and therapists should be prepared to draw upon a wide range of available techniques. Priority should be given to those at risk. Furthermore, whatever approach is used, establishing a supportive, trusted relationship and being in a safe environment are essential elements in therapy. Joseph et al. (1992) supported this by suggesting that social support can contribute to the reduction of the probability of the individual developing full-blown PTSD, and may also help speed up the adjustment required before recovery can occur (see also Yule et al. 2000). Finally, Levin (1999) indicated that professionals should consider the following aspects while assessing or offering rehabilitation programmes to traumatized refugees: (a) the type of trauma; (b) difficult life events before the flight; (c) experience in refugee camps; (d) cultural and ethnic background; (e) gender perspectives; (f) language difficulties and life in exile

Unaccompanied children, women and refugee families

Every year a few thousand children arrive in the UK without a parent or guardian to look after them. According to Home Office statistics, the UK received 2733 asylum applications from unaccompanied children in 2000. Some of these children arrived completely alone while others were with relatives or non-governmental organizations. Their parents could be dead, ill, imprisoned or simply did not have the money to flee as well. The reasons for leaving a country can vary widely, and can include armed conflicts that target children to forced military service. Figures available in the UK suggested that in 1999, 45 per cent of unaccompanied child refugees came from Kosovo. The next highest proportion came from Afghanistan, followed by Somalia, China, Albania, Turkey, Sierra Leone, Sri Lanka, Romania, Eritrea, Ethiopia, Iraq, Nigeria, Angola and the Democratic Republic of Congo (mainly from war regions). Studies show that refugee women and their children are extremely vulnerable, as are the elderly. Rape is a common element in the pattern of persecution, terror and ethnic cleansing that uproot refugee families from their homes and communities. The UNHCR in their worldwide web page reported that from Somalia to Bosnia refugee families frequently cite rape or the fear of rape as a key factor in their decision to leave (UNHCR 2000).

It has also been estimated that no less than 20–30 per cent of refugees up to 1990 have been tortured. Domovitch et al. (1984), in a study of 104 torture survivors, observed the following mental symptoms in descending order of frequency: anxiety, insomnia, nightmares, depression, withdrawal, irritability, loss of concentration, sexual dysfunction, memory disturbance, fatigue, aggressiveness, impulsiveness, and hypersensitivity to noise. Similarly, Somnier and Genefke (1986) reported that the most common symptoms were sleep disturbances, nightmares, headaches, impaired memory, poor concentration, fatigue, fear/anxiety and social withdrawal. It should be emphasized here that refugee populations cannot be regarded as a homogeneous group. Although they share the experience of forced uprooting, their reactions to trauma are not necessarily similar or totally predictable. Some refugees have highly developed occupational skills, while others are educated and have various abilities which enable them to resettle and perhaps make a useful contribution to the new host country. Some become depressed or lack the skills to adapt quickly to a new culture. Due to their near-death experiences and exposure to violence either before or during the flight, many adults (see earlier accounts above) are unable to function adequately as parents, spouses, employees or citizens, and they are likely to experience a series of strained relationships as a result. In addition, their mental health problem is significantly higher when compared with the general non-refugee population.

A recent research study (Hosin et al. 2006) which studied adjustment of 61 traumatized Iraqi families and their 162 children in London again found a wide range of mental health problems among both parents and their offspring. The main aim of this study was to investigate the relationship between the parental well-being of Iraqi refugees and the psychological adjustment of their offspring, using both the General Health Questionnaire (GHQ-30 item version, Goldberg and Hillier 1979; Goldberg and Williams 1988) and a short and modified version of the Children Behavioural Checklist questionnaire (CBCL, Achenbach et al. 1991; Achenbach 1991, 1993). Both of the above-mentioned measures (i.e. the GHQ and CBCL) have been translated and used in different cultures with success (see El-Rufaie and Daradkeh 1996; Ormel et al. 1989; Kitamure et al. 1994; Henderson et al. 1981; Visser et al. 2003; Crijnen et al. 1997).

All parents (n = 61parents) included in this community-based study were asked to complete both the GHQ questionnaire and a very short, modified version of CBCL. In the latter, parents were asked to reflect on any problems (including psychosocial and behavioural symptoms of ill-health) which may have manifested themselves in the recent past among their children. Good psychological adjustment amongst refugee children was expected to be associated or more likely to manifest itself when parents are psychologically healthy and less distressed. As well as parental health, variables such as the duration and number of years spent in the host country, the group's background, current level of social contact and support, numbers of family members sharing the household, and the nature of the traumatic experience prior to their flight were investigated. As expected, this study seems to confirm many earlier findings reported in previous literature (see Jafar 2000). For example, the main result of this study appears to indicate that the estimated level of distress (caseness) among parents who completed the GHQ was very high, with 52.46 per cent of the sample reaching the threshold level (the threshold level chosen for this study was adjusted to 8 negative items). It was also suggested that adult refugees in this study manifested poor mental health, and this in turn was found to be associated positively with children's poor adjustment in the host culture. Overall results (using independent t-tests) revealed that there were no significant differences between male and female scores on the GHQ. Surprisingly, other findings of this study indicated that educational background (i.e. secondary school, high school or university qualifications) was not a significant factor in determining the adjustment and/or level of distress amongst the population of this study. Rather, large family size and refugee parents who have more than one child at home appear to be more vulnerable to distress than those who have smaller families. Further, newly arrived refugees (recently exposed to the host culture, i.e. one year or less) seem to score higher on the GHQ than their counterparts who have been in the host culture for longer periods of time.

The above-mentioned outcomes (particularly high scores on the GHQ and high self-reported distress levels) were expected and discussed within the frameworks of culture learning theory, U-curve theory and the multi-dimensional model on acculturation. It was claimed (see Hosin et al. 2006) that such problems can be attributed to problems prior to displacement, the new demands of the host culture, daily stresses, unmet expectations, isolation and perhaps lack of skills and social support in the new and unfamiliar culture. On the other hand, the manifestation of social, emotional and behavioural problems among children were related to their home surroundings, isolation, and lack of care provided by the suffering and traumatized parents. This research has also suggested that emotional and adjustment problems manifested among children in this study will not disappear without proper intervention programmes, and proper consideration of all risk factors, including family circumstances and previous parental psychopathology

Is it possible to suggest that children's adjustment here was influenced by their parents' history of unpleasant interactions with the environment? Probably yes if we adopt attachment theory highlighted above, that is, the internal models and early social relationships with the mother as outlined in the 'maternal responsiveness/sensitivity hypothesis' suggested by Ainsworth's original research (Ainsworth et al. 1978), and subsequently by a number of studies (Kochanska 2001; Oppenheim et al. 1988; Lewis et al. 1984; Cairns 2002: 57). These studies reported that the quality and sensitivity of mother–child interactions from as early as a few months and through early childhood predicted secure attachment, curiosity, problem solving, social confidence, interest in the world around them and perhaps independence and lack of behaviour problems. Indeed, in some cases, a parent's depression can contribute directly to the child's difficulties and poor adjustment among children (Graham 1994: 37; Mills et al. 1984; Hewison and Tizard 1980). Further, a young person must also be understood in the context of the family, peers, and the school system and therefore aspects of this whole system must be addressed too. No doubt, such a broad perspective (using multi-methods or triangulation measures to test assumptions or hypotheses) will certainly inject further rigour and validity assurance to any study on children. In brief, assessing child and adolescent problems is a complex process that most often involves evaluating multiple aspects of functioning. Thus a broad range of behavioural, affective, cognitive and physical components must be considered. Knowledge of age-related changes and the impact of problems on the developing child at school, with peers and at home is also required. Finally, if assessment demands contact with young person and refugee families, then such assessment measures require special sensitivity to anxiety, fear, shyness, safety, reassurance, clarity and understanding. Indeed, research instruments used with refugee populations should also be unintrusive, unprovocative and sensitive to the participants culture and values.

Learning a new language, internalizing different social norms and finding new employment are great challenges for even the most able and creative refugees. Westermeyer (1989, 1991), Westermeyer et al. (1983) and Hauff and Vaglum (1995) confirmed this and pointed out that upon assessment it is important to take into account the conditions during exile and pre-migration experience, the traumatization in the host country (i.e. the acculturation stress and the pressure of assimilation during the first years of resettlement) and other predisposing factors which are not related to their experience. In other words, research on the mental health of refugees should take into account the complexity of their holistic situation. That is to say, the quality of life and the health situation of the refugee population demand considerable attention, including the delivery of services which should be available, effective and aimed at reducing stress. However, lack of social support and isolation appear to be much stronger predictor of poor mental health and depression in the long term than severity of trauma. Indeed, an early period of adjustment to a new environment and coming to terms with post-traumatic experiences need a much more sensitive approach, particularly for the most vulnerable refugees such as victims of torture and rape and for unaccompanied children (Clinton-Davis and Fassil 1992). It should also be remembered that while refugee experiences can generate a number of mental health problems, some refugees are reluctant to seek help, and their tendency to somatize emotional problems is particularly common because they come from societies that stigmatize mental illnesses.

Almqvist and Hwang (1999: 169) addressed the importance of parental coping and parental functioning and stated that young children will continue to cope with difficult environments as long as their parents are not pushed beyond the stress threshold level capacity. It was suggested that once that point is exceeded, the development of young children deteriorates rapidly and markedly. This research also added that parents who are hopeful and optimistic are more likely to influence children's adjustment in the host culture. Freud and Burlingham (1943) identified the importance of the family as a buffer for stress, and separation from the family as a major stress crisis period. Ahearn and Athey (1991: 4–7) stated that children cannot be understood independently of their environments. Thus, an ecological framework in which the child is viewed as a part of a family system and of a larger social system should be considered.

Various writers, however, seem to place emphasis on different variables to help refugees to make the transition and adjust to the host and unfamiliar culture. Ward et al. (2001) for example, claimed that successful adjustment in the unfamiliar culture is greatly dependent on not only individual but on other situational factors and the reasons for the exposure to the host culture (i.e. reasons for the contact), the length of the stay as well as culture norms and policies. Furthermore, Ward and Kennedy (1994) and Berry et al. (1992) maintained that both assimilation policies and integration are facilitative strategies for adjusting into the new culture as compared to separation. Furnham and Bochner (1986) and Lysgaard (1955) meanwhile argue that the least stress occurs during the early stage of contact with the host culture, while the most stress occurs during the intermediate phase of acculturation processes. The latter relates adjustment to the duration and stages of time spent in a host culture. It involves (the U-curve hypothesis, see below) an initial stage of optimism, which Lysgaard (1955) describes as the honeymoon period, followed by a culture shock and the process of improvement of adjustment in the host society. In fact others (Noels et al. 1996) associate an individual's reactions to the nature of the displacement to complex factors such as personality, temperament, the extent of social support, cultural similarity, prior knowledge of the language, reasons for contact, and perceived cognitive control over the experience. Using a stress model, Williams and Berry (1991) and Lazarus and Folkman (1984) suggested that any move to a new place creates stressful demands, and a major task confronting individuals in stressful situations is a cognitive one. This implies that the interpretation of the situation and the activation of the coping response could maximize a sense of control over the situation. Similarly, Ward et al. (2001) and Berry et al. (1992) claimed that an individual who possesses positive cognitive control and views the changes resulting from the acculturating experience as being constructive, adapts better to the host culture. Ward and Change (1997), who develop the culture fit hypothesis, see adjustment from a different angle and claim that acculturating individuals whose own culture is very different from the host culture are more likely to suffer poor adjustment and high levels of stress than others whose culture is similar to their new surroundings (cited in Hosin et al. 2006). Bochner (1999) meanwhile found that the level of tolerance within the host culture is an important factor, which helps adjustment in the host environment. In their article on refugees and adjustment, Hosin et al. (2006) added: 'there is a somewhat complex interplay amongst a variety of factors, which influence the extent to which successful adjustment can be made in the host culture'. Having discussed all possible factors which may contribute to the poor psychological well-being of the refugee population, a good understanding of this complexity and the relationship between migration and mental health is essential for any assessment or rehabilitation programme.

Being in an unfamiliar, unknown host culture: an acculturative perspective

Cross-cultural transition is a significant life event involving un-accustomed changes and new forms of intercultural contact (Ward et al. 2001: 43). Early perspectives on the intercultural contact were influenced by research on migration and mental health (Murphy 1973, 1977; Fernando 2002). Much of the previous research was not only epidemiological in its orientation but relied heavily on a medical model, case study and sample of convenience (Brislin and Baum-gardner 1971). However, during the 1980s this area of research began to shift its database from hospital archive records to community surveys. One aspect of this new research wave started to question why migrants have a higher rate of psychological disorders than the domi-nant groups. In sum, early theories applied to the study of inter-cultural contact were clinically oriented and strongly related to a medical model of adjustment (Ward et al. 2001). A different view of adjustment research emerged during the late 1970s and early 1980s (Furnham and Bochner 1982) and it was mainly driven by the core proposition that learning about the host culture influences adjust-ment. This shift of emphasis has certainly laid the foundation for a culture learning approach. This approach, alongside the multi-dimensional model of social support network, life events and stress model, was offered as a competing theoretical framework for the analysis of intercultural contact and adjustment processes (Ward et al. 2001: 19–46).

At the individual level, Berry (1997) and Hsiao-Ying (1995) consider acculturation and adjustment to the new and unfamiliar host culture as a psychosocial process by which the individual should achieve harmony with the new surroundings through interaction, changes in knowledge, attitudes and in cognitions. Meanwhile Bochner (1982, 1986) relates successful adjustment to culture learning which embraces the acquisition of appropriate social skills and behaviours necessary to conduct successful daily activities and negotiate the cultural milieu. This of course includes general knowledge about the specific culture, length of residence in the host culture, language and communication competence, quantity and quality of contact with the host nationals. Other factors which are relatively important for adjustment are pre-migration stress, cognitive reappraisal of change, personality, loneliness and quality of social relationships. Adjustment here is discussed in terms of skills deficit and acculturative stress and a range of mediating variables which can either increase or decrease the deficit and the psychosocial stress that refugees may face. In general, these influential variables can be related to the individual, cultural knowledge, self-efficacy, the available resources, social support, and host cultural relations.

Furthermore, an early theoretical perspective in this area was the U-curve model developed by Lysgaard (1955). The U-curve theory describes the three stages of emotional adjustment one often experiences in a host culture. The initial stage is the honeymoon period, which may be characterized by high levels of positive adjustment due to enthusiasm, excitement and a positive expectation of being in the host culture. This is followed by decreased adjustment, frustration and distress due to lack of interaction, culture shock, lack of understanding of the native language and the sharp disparities between the dominant and the original culture (Oberg 1960; Vaughan 1962). The third stage, however, is characterized by a gradual learning, acquisition of necessary skills, social interaction and possible integration with the new culture, and above all else, familiarity with the customs and value system of the host culture which may promote positive and successful adjustment. Critics of the U-curve theory (e.g. Bochner 1986) claimed that since there are many variations within the process of adjustment so it is difficult to see a universal pattern emerging across various situations and individuals. On the other hand, cultural maintenance theory (Berry et al. 1989) links the individual's adjustment and coping to the process of assimilation and/or integration within the host culture, and to the efforts that may be made by individuals to maintain their own cultural identity alongside the host culture. That is to say attitudes that are adopted towards the host culture are fundamental factors which determine the path of adjustment among the sojourners. Finally, in their attempt to establish a distinct model for both psychological and socio-cultural adjustment Ward and Kennedy (1992) and Church (1982) found the following variables predict successful adjustment in the host culture: prior contact with host cultures, language capability, attitudes, personal relationships and duration of stay and cultural distance. Ward and Kennedy also suggested that strategies which could lead to a more positive adjustment include assimilation or integration. Thus the newcomers are required to be open and integrate with the host culture values and oppose the alternative strategies of alienation or marginalization which are more likely to lead to poor adjustment and high levels of acculturative stress.

National and international policies on refugees

Although Helen O'Nions (in Chapter 14) will address this issue and provides more depth and focus on 'the legal framework' and both national and international policies on refugees, here are a few summarized accounts to orient our readers to legislation and policies that may exacerbate the trauma among such vulnerable groups in a host culture.

Woodhead (2000) has conducted a recent study for the King's Fund and was concerned about the effect of the changes brought by the Immigration and Asylum Act 1999 on the health of asylum seekers and refugees in the UK. The two changes which the act brought in were the introduction of the dispersal system – authorities are able to disperse asylum seekers and refugees to a number of designated sites across the country – and the use of vouchers instead of cash benefits. The latter system was in place for a short period of time and allowed all refugees and asylum seekers to purchase their food in designated shops and supermarkets. This study indicates that health services are generally not geared up to cope with the needs of asylum seekers and refugees. Woodhead's report further states that the quality of health services for asylum seekers and refugees around the country is inconsistent. London, for example, remains better than other parts of the country where there is little history of incoming asylum seekers or refugee communities. This critical report also suggested that communication between health professionals and asylum seekers and refugees who do not speak English is often difficult and leads to misdiagnosis. The report also criticized the short-lived vouchers system and described it as divisive, excluding and inequitable. Woodhead, in his report, further added that the dispersal system places individuals away from their community, area of worship and friends, confronts them with loneliness and isolation and perhaps keeps them from links which are vital for their well-being. Overall, most asylum seekers in Britain are single men under the age of 40 (Burnett and Peel 2001a, 2001b, 2001c). However, worldwide most refugees are women. Refugees arrive with a wide range of experiences including massacres and threats of massacres, detention, beatings, torture, rape, sexual assault, witnessing death and torture of others as well as destruction of homes and property and forcible eviction, etc. Unfortunately, and despite the guidelines of the 1951 Geneva Convention which aim to protect and care for refugees, most Western countries are now seeking to implement new deterrent policies characterized by indefinite detention of all refugees (children, women and young adult men who arrive at their shores and ports of entry). This is very much the case in Australia, the Netherlands, Germany and Britain. Britain detains illegal immigrants awaiting deportation. Furthermore, Home Office statistics for 2002 revealed that there were 1440 asylum seekers held in detention camps in the UK at the end of June 2002, including 300 held at the 'fast-track' Oakington reception centre near Cambridge, and the remainder in immigration service removal centres.

With regard to targets and the current movement's pledge of removal of failed asylum seekers or unsuccessful applications which were running at around 1000 a month, the latest Home Office figures show that 9630 asylum seekers were removed in the financial year 2001–2. Immigration officials also confirmed recently that a more 'achievable' deportation target is to be set later this year, as the target of 30 000 set some time ago was not achievable.

The Home Office Statistics Report (2002) suggested that asylum seekers arriving in Britain rose by 4 per cent to 20 400 between April and June of that year. The report also showed that most asylum seekers are genuine, and more than 50 per cent were given permission to stay. The largest group, 3420, came from Iraq with numbers up by a fifth, followed by Afghanistan (2130), Somalia (1455) and Zimbabwe (1345) and a few other countries going through political upheaval. On the other hand, the proportion of asylum seekers who have not been given full refugee status but have been given exceptional leave to stay in Britain has also risen over the last two years. In 2000 only 12 per cent were given exceptional leave to remain compared to 17 per cent during 2001 and 26 per cent in the current year.

Internationally, the number of refugees who try to enter Australia is far smaller than the 71 000 asylum seekers who applied to come to Britain in 1999–2000. Since it was first introduced in 1994 by Australia's Labor government, Australia's refugee policy not only isolates refugees from the real world but offers refugees indefinite detention. That is, it detains indefinitely all men, women and children until the authorities decide whether or not they deserve refugee status (Barkham 2002). Overall, this large country is only offering 12 000 permanent places each year taken from a UNHCR campus. Former staff who worked in some of these oppressive, remote detention camps in Australia (for example in Woomera) described the psychological well-being of detainees as very poor. Many suffered high level anxiety and were on anti-depressant drugs. It must be mentioned here that a total of 139 countries have signed the 1951 Geneva Refugee Convention. However, international protection of refugees comprises more than physical safety. That is, refugees should at least receive the same rights and basic help as any other foreigner who is a legal resident, including certain fundamental entitlements of every individual. That is, refugees should have basic civil rights including freedom of movement, thought, and freedom from torture and degrading treatment. Thus as a general rule, detention of asylum seekers is not acceptable by international law. It is particularly undesirable, the UNHCR claimed, when those detained include the very vulnerable, children, single women and people with special medical and psychological needs.

Many countries are aware that the 1951 Geneva Convention specifically bars countries from punishing people who have arrived directly from a country of persecution provided that they present themselves speedily to the authorities and show good cause for their illegal entry. With regard to detention and repatriation policies of failed asylum, Germany, Denmark, the Netherlands, Austria, Switzerland and the United Kingdom have already sent refugees home. In the Netherlands, five Kurds from Northern Iraq went on hunger strike for more than 80 days protesting at the Dutch decision to deport them. The hunger strikers were aged between 25 and 36. According to *The Guardian* (26 April 2001), deportation is already deployed by the Home Office and has led to a dramatic increase in the refusal rate. Various other measures have been taken by the present Labour government in Britain to speed up the removal of illegal immigrant and asylum seekers whose appeals have been rejected. Furthermore, the UK government regulations on asylum indicate that asylum seekers can only get residency in Britain if they meet the 1951 UN Convention's definition of a refugee.

This means they must have a 'well-founded fear of persecution' on the grounds of race, religion, nationality, membership of a particular social group or political opinion. Asylum seekers can make a verbal application for residency at a British port and then have five days to collect evidence to substantiate their claim. The application is then sent to the Home Office's Immigration and Nationality Directorate for a decision. If it is turned down, the asylum seeker can appeal; if that appeal is turned down by the Immigration Appeals Tribunal the asylum seeker will be deported. Britain has already called for the modernization of the 1951 United Nations Convention on Refugees. In particular, Britain wants the right to automatically reject asylum seekers if they have passed through Europe to get to Britain instead of applying for asylum in the first safe country they reach.

In sum, it should be stated here that people who are seeking asylum are not a homogeneous population. However, previous studies (Burnett and Peel 2001b) have found that one in six refugees has a physical health problem severe enough to affect their life, and two-thirds have experienced anxiety or depression, sleep problems and poor memory. Social isolation and poverty have a compounding negative impact on mental health, as do hostility and racism. Reducing isolation and dependence, having suitable accommodation and spending time more creatively through education or work can often do much to help adjustment. Moreover, positive changes can be seen if immigrants are reunited with families and take up educational and employment opportunities. Refugee community organizations are invaluable in supporting refugees. They can provide information and orientation and reduce the isolation experienced by so many refugees. In a study of Iraqi asylum seekers, Gorst-Unsworth and Goldenberg (1998) have found depression was more closely linked with poor social support than with a history of torture. It is important for refugees to develop ongoing links and friendships with people in the host community. Indeed, the best mental health outcomes may be achieved in this way. Further details on the health and well-being of asylum seekers and refugees can be found in Burnett and Peel (2001a, 2001b, 2001c) and Keyes (2000).

References

Achenbach, T. M. (1991) *Manual for the Child Behaviour Checklist 4–18 and 1991 Profile.* Burlington: Department of Psychiatry, University of Vermont.

Achenbach, T. M. (1993) *Empirically Based Taxonomy: How to Use Syndromes and Profile Derived from the CBCL/4–18, TRF and YSR.* Burlington: Department of Psychiatry, University of Vermont.

Acehnbach, T. M., Howell, C. T., Quay, H. C. and Conner, C. K. (1991) 'National survey of problems and competencies among four to sixteen-year-olds: parents' reports for normative and clinical samples', *Monographs of the Society for Research and Child Development*, 56(3), Serial No. 225.

Acuna, J. E. (1989) *Children of the Storm*. Philippines: Children Rehabilitation Centre.

Ahearn, F. L. and Athey, J. L. (eds) (1991) *Refugee Children: Theory, Research and Services*. Baltimore: Johns Hopkins University Press.

Ainsworth, M., Blehar, M. C., Waters, E. and Wall, S. (1978) *Patterns of Attachment: a Psychological Study of Strange Situations*. Hillsdale, NJ: Lawrence Erlbaum.

Aldous, J., Bardsley, M. and Daniell, R. (1999) *Refugee Health in London: Key Issues in Public Health*. East London and City Health Authority: The Health of Londoners Project.

Allodi, E. (1989) 'The children of victims of political persecution and torture: a psychological study of a Latin American refugee community'. *International Journal of Mental Health*, 18: 3–15.

Almqvist, K. and Broberg, A. G. (1999) 'Mental health and social adjustment in young refugee children 3½ years after their arrival in Sweden'. *Journal of the American Academy of Child and Adolescent Psychiatry*, 38(6): 723–30.

Almqvist, K. and Hwang, P. (1999) 'Iranian refugees in Sweden: coping processes in children and their families'. *Childhood*, 6(2): 167–87.

Bahugra, D. and Bhui, K. (2001) *Cross-cultural Psychiatry: a Practical Guide*. London: Arnold.

Baker, R. (1992) 'Psychological consequences for tortured refugees seeking asylum and refugee status in Europe'. In M. Basoglu (ed.), *Torture and its Consequences: Current Treatment Approaches*. Cambridge: Cambridge University Press.

Barkham, P. (2002) 'No waltzing in Woomera'. *The Guardian Weekend*, 25 May.

Basoğlu, M. (ed.) (1992) *Torture and its Consequences: Current Treatment Approaches*. Cambridge: Cambridge University Press.

Berry, J. W. (1997) 'Immigration, acculturation and adpatation'. *Applied Psychology: an International Review*, 46: 5–34.

Berry, J. W., Kim, U., Power, S., Young, M. and Bujaki, M. (1989) 'Acculturation attitudes in plural societies'. *Applied Psychology*, 38: 185–206.

Berry, J. W., Poortinga, Y. H., Segall, M. H. and Dasen, P. R. (1992) *Cross-cultural Psychology: Research and Application*. Cambridg: Cambridge University Press.

Biederman, J., Rosenbaum, J. F., Hirshfeld, D. R. and Faronone, S. V. (1991) 'Psychiatric correlates of behavioural inhibition in young children of parents with or without psychiatric disorders'. *Annual Progress in Child Psychiatry and Child Development*: 269–4.

Black, D. (1974) 'What happens to bereaved children?' *Proceedings of the Royal Society of Medicine*, 69: 842–4.

Black, D., Newman, M., Harris-Hendriks, J. and Mezey, G. (eds) (1997) *Psychological Trauma: a Developmental Approach*. Gaskell and Royal College of Psychiatrists.

Bochner, S. (1982) 'The social psychology of cross-cultural relations'. In S. Bochner (ed.), *Cultures in Contact: Studies in Cross-Cultural Interaction*. Oxford: Pergamon.

Bochner, S. (1986) 'Coping with unfamiliar cultures: adjustment or culture learning?' *Australian Journal of Psychology*, 38: 347–58.

Bochner, S. (1999) 'Cultural diversity within and between societies: implication for a multicultural social system'. In P. B. Pedersen (ed.), *Multiculturalism as a Fourth Force*. Washington DC: Taylor & Francis, pp. 19–60.

Bonanno, G. (2004) 'Loss, trauma and human resilience'. *American Psychologist*, 59(1): 20–8.

Bowlby, J. (1971) *Attachment and Loss*. Vol. 1, *Attachment*. Harmondsworth: Penguin.

Bowlby, J. (1975) *Attachment and Loss*. Vol. 2, *Separation Anxiety and Anger*. Harmondsworth: Penguin.

Bowlby, J. (1980) *Attachment and Loss*, Vol. 3, *Loss*. New York: Basic Books.

Brent and Harrow Refugee Survey (1995) London Brent and Harrow Health Agency.

Brislin, R. and Baumgardner, S. (1971) 'Non-random sampling of individuals in cross-cultural psychology'. *Journal of Cross-cultural Psychology*, 2: 397–400.

Bryce, J., Walker, N., Ghorayeb, F. and Kanj, M. (1989) 'Life experience, response styles and mental health among mothers and children in Beirut, Lebanon'. *Social Science and Medicine*, 28: 685–95.

Burnett, Angela and Peel, Michael (2001a) 'Asylum seekers and refugees in Britain'. *British Medical Journal*, 24 February.

Burnett, Angela and Peel, Michael (2001b) 'Asylum seekers and refugees in Britain: health needs of asylum seekers and refugees'. *British Medical Journal*, 322: 544–7, 3 March.

Burnett, Angela and Peel, Michael (2001c) 'Asylum seekers and refugees in Britain: the health of survivors of torture and organized violence'. *British Medical Journal*, 322: 606–9, 10 March.

Burvill, P. W. and Knuiman, M. W. (1983) 'Which version of the GHQ should be used in community studies?' *Australian and New Zealand Journal of Psychiatry*, 17: 237–42.

Cairns, K. (2002) *Attachment, Trauma and Resilience*. London: British Association of Adopting and Fostering (BAAF).

Cheung, P. (1994) 'Reliability and validity of the Cambodian version of the 28-item General Health Questionnaire'. *Social Psychiatry and Psychiatric Epidemiology*, 29(2): 95–9.

Church, A. T. (1982) 'Sojourner adjustment'. *Psychological Bulletin*, 91: 540–72.

Clinton-Davis, Lord and Fassil, Yohannes (1992) 'Health and social problems of refugees'. *Social Science Medicine*, 35(4): 507–13.

Cohn, J., Danielsen, L., Koch, L. et al. (1985) 'A study of Chilean refugee children in Denmark'. *Lancet*, 2: 437–8.

Cohn, J., Holzer, K., Koch, L. and Severin, B. (1980) 'Children and torture: an investigation of Chilean immigrant children in Denmark'. *Danish Medical Bulletin*, 27: 238–9.

Crijnen, A. M., Achenbach, T. M. and Verhulst, F. C. (1997) 'Comparison of problems reported by parents of children in 12 cultures: total problems, externalising and internalising'. *Journal of the American Academy of Child and Adolescent Psychiatry*, 36: 1269–77.

Dawes, A., Tredoux, C. and Feinstein, A. (1989) 'Political violence in South Africa: some effects on children of the violent destruction of their community'. *International Journal of Mental Health*, 18: 16–43.

Deivedi, K. N. (ed.) (2000) *Post-Traumtic Stress Disorder in Children and Adolescents*. London: Whurr Publishers.

Domovitch, E., Berger, P. B., Wawe, M. J., Etlin, D. D. and Marshall, J. C. (1984) 'Human torture: description and sequal of 104 cases'. *Canadian Family Physician*, 30: 827–30.

Eisenbruch, M. (1990) 'Cultural bereavement and homesickness'. In S. Fisher and C. L. Cooper (eds), *On the Move: the Psychology of Change and Transition*. London: Wiley.

El-Rufaie, O. E. and Daradkeh, T. K. (1996) 'Validation of the Arabic versions of the thirty and twelve-item General Health Questionnaires in primary care patients'. *British Journal of Psychiatry*, 169(5): 662–4.

Fairbank, J. A., Schlenger, W. E., Saigh, P. A. and Davidson, J. R. T. (1995) 'An epidemiological profile of post-traumatic stress disorder: prevalence, co-morbidity, and risk factors'. In M. J. Friedman, D. S. Charney and A. Y. Deutch (eds), *Neurobiological and Clinical Consequences of Stress: From Normal Adaptation to PTSD*. Philadelphia: Lippincott-Raven.

Fernando, S. (1995) *Mental Health in a Multi-Ethnic Society*. London: Routledge.

Fernando, S. (2002) *Mental Health, Race and Culture*. New York and Basingstoke: Palgrave Macmillan.

Freud, A. and Burlingham, D. (1943) *Young Children in War Time*. London: George Allen & Unwin Ltd.

Furnham, A. and Bochner, S. (1982) 'Social diffculity in a foreign culture: an empirical analysis of culture schock'. In S. Bochner (ed.), *Cultures in Contact: Studies in Cross-cultural Interactions*. Oxford: Pergamon, pp. 161–98.

Furnham, A. and Bochner, S. (1986) *Culture Shock: Psychological Reactions to Unfamiliar Environments*. London: Methuen.

Garmezy, N. (1987) 'Stress, competence and development: continuities in the study of schizophrenic adults and children vulnerable to psychopathology, and the research for stress-resistant children'. *American Journal of Orthopsychiatry*, 57(2): 159–74.

Goldberg, D. P. and Hillier, V. F. (1979) 'A scaled version of the General Health Questionnaire'. *Psychological Medicine*, 9: 139–45.

Goldberg, D. P. and Williams, P. (1988) *A User's Guide to the General Health Questionnaire*. Windsor, UK: NFER-Neslon.

Gorst-Unsworth, C. and Goldenberg, E. (1998) 'Psychological sequel of torture and organised violence suffered by refugees from Iraq: trauma-related factors compared with social factors in exile'. *British Journal of Psychiatry*, 172: 90–4.

Graham, P. (1994) *Child Psychiatry*. Oxford: Oxford University Press.

Halliday, G. (1987) 'Direct psychological therapies for nightmares: a review'. *Clinical Psychology Review*, 7: 501–23.

Hauff, E. and Vaglum, P. (1995) 'Organised violence and the stress of exile: predictors of mental health in a community cohort of Vietnamese refugees three years after resettlement'. *British Journal of Psychiatry*, 166: 360–7.

Henderson, S. H., Byrne, D. G. and Duncan-Jones, L. (1981) *Neurosis and the Social Environment*. Sydney: Academic Press of Australia.

Herbert, M., Slukin, W. and Sluckin, A. (1982) 'Mother to infant "bonding"'. *Journal of Child Pycology and Pychaitry*, 23: 205–21.

Hewison, J. and Tizard, J. (1980) 'Parental involvement and reading attainment'. *British Journal of Educational Psychology*, 50: 209–15.

Hjern, A. and Angel, B. (2000) 'Organized violence and mental health of refugee children in exile: a six-year follow-up'. *Acta Paediatric*, 89(6): 722–7.

Hosin, A. (ed.) (2000) *Essays on Issues in Applied Developmental Psychology and Child Psychiatry*. New York: Edwin Mellen Press (see Ch. 5).

Hosin, A. (2001) 'Children of traumatised and exiled refugee families: resilience and vulnerability'. *Medicine, Conflict and Survival*, 17(2): 137–45.

Hosin, A., Moore, S. and Gaitanou, C. (2006) 'The relationship between psychological well-being and adjustment of both parents and children of exiled and traumatized Iraqi refugees'. *Journal of Muslim Mental Health*, 1(2) (October).

Howe, D., Brandon, M., Hinings, D. and Schofield, A. (1999) *Attachment Theory, Child Maltreatment and Family Support: a Practical and Assessment Model.* Basingstoke: Palgrave Macmillan.

Hsiao-Ying, T. (1995) 'Sojourner adjustment: the case of foreigners in Japan'. *Journal of Cross-cultural Psychology*, 26: 523–36.

Jafar, S. (2000) *Health Needs Assessment Study of the Iraqi Community in London.* London: Iraqi Community Association in cooperation with King's Fund.

Jones, L. (1998) 'Adolescent groups for encamped Bosnian refugees: some problems and solutions'. *Clinical Child Psychology and Psychiatry*, 3(4): 541–51.

Joseph, S. A., Berwin, C. R., Yule, W. and William, R. (1991) 'Causal attributions and psychiatric symptoms in survivors of the *Herald of Free Enterprise* disaster'. *British Journal of Psychiatry*, 159: 245–6.

Joseph, S. A., Williams, R., Yule, W. and Walker, A. (1992) 'Factor analysis of the impact of events scale with survivors of two disasters at sea'. *Personality and Individual Differences*, 13(6): 693–7.

Jumaian, A., Hosin, A. and Rahmatallh, A. (1997) 'Post-traumatic stress disorder in children: symptoms, assessment and treatment'. *Arab Journal of Psychiatry*, 8(2): 127–39.

Karami, G. (1990) *Ethnicity and Health*. North East Thames Regional Health Authority. The Health Report.

Keyes, E. (2000) 'Mental health status in refugees: an integrative review of current research'. *Issues in Mental Health Nursing*, 21: 397–410.

King, M. (1994) 'Incidence of psychotic illness in London: comparison of ethnic groups'. *British Medical Journal*, 309: 1115–19, 29 October.

Kitamure, T., Shima, S., Sugawara, M. and Toda, M. A. (1994) 'Temporal variation of validity of self-rating questionnaires – repeated use of the general health questionnaire and Zung's self-rating depression scale among women during antenatal and postnatal periods'. *Acta Psychiatrica Scandinavia*, 90: 446–50.

Klaus, M. and Kennell, J. (1976) *Maternal Infant Bonding: the Impact of Early Separation or Loss on Family Development.* St. Louis: Mosby.

Kochanska, G. (2001) 'Emotional development in children with different attachment histories: the first three years'. *Child Development*, 67: 474–90.

Koopman, C. (1997) 'Political psychology as a lens for viewing traumatic events'. *Journal of Political Psychology*, 18(4): 831–47.

Lancet (2003) 'Editorial', Vol. 361, No. 9367, 26 April.

Lavik, N., Hauff, E., Skrondal, A. and Oivind, Solberg (1996) 'Mental disorder among refugees and the impact of persecution and exile: some findings from an out-patient population'. *British Journal of Psychiatry*, 169: 726–32.

Lazarus, R. S. and Folkman, S. (1984) *Stress, Appraisal and Coping*. New York: Springer.

Levin, L. (1999) 'Traumatised refugee children: a challenge for mental rehabilitation'. *Medicine, Conflict and Survival*, 15(4): 342–51.

Lewis, M., Feiring, C., McGuffoy, C., and Jaskir, J. (1984) 'Predicting psychopathology in six year olds from early social relations'. *Child Development*, 55: 123–36.

Linley, P. A. and Joseph, S. (2005) 'The human capacity for growth through adversity'. *American Psychologist*, 60(3): 261–72.

Littlewood, R. and Lipsedge, M. (1989) *Aliens and Alienists: Ethnic Minorities and Psychiatry*. London: Unwin Hyman.

Lysgaard, S. (1955) 'Adjustment in a foreign society: Norwegian Fulbright grantees visiting the United States'. *International Social Science Bulletin*, 7: 45–51.

Masten, A. S. (2001) 'Ordinary magic: resilience processes in development'. *American Psychologist*, 56(3): 227–38 (special issue on Positive Psychology).

Meichenbaum, D. (1994) *A Clinical Handbook: Practical Therapist Manual for Assessing and Treating Adults with Post Traumatic Stresses Disorder*. Canada, Ontario: Institute Press.

Mills, M., Puckering, C., Pound, A. and Cox, A. (1984) 'What is it about depressed mothers that influences their children's functioning'. In J. Stevenson (ed.), *Recent Research in Developmental Psychology*. Oxford: Pergamon, pp. 11–17.

Montgomery, E. and Foldspang, A. (2001) 'Traumatic experience and sleep disturbance in refugee children from the Middle East'. *European Journal of Public Health*. 11(1): 18–22.

Murphy, H. B. (1973) 'Migration and major mental disorders: a reapprisal'. In C. Swingmann and M. Pfister-Ammende (eds), *Uprooting and After*, New York: Springer-Verlag, pp. 221–31.

Murphy, H. B. (1977) 'Migration, culture and mental health'. *Psychological Medicine*, 7: 677–84.

Noels, K. A., Pon, G. and Clement, R. (1996) 'Language, identity and adjustment: the role of linguistic self confidence in the acculturation process'. *Journal of Language and Social Psychology*, 15(3): 246–64.

Oberg, K. (1960) 'Culture shock: adjusting to new cultural environments'. *Practical Anthropology*, 7: 177–82.

Oppenhiem, D., Sagi, A. and Lamb, M. E. (1988) 'Infant–adult attachments on the kibbutz and their relation to socioemotional development four years later'. *Developmental Psychology*, 24: 427–33.

Ormel, J., Koeter, M. W. J. and van de Brink, W. (1989) 'Measuring change with the General Health Questionnaire: the problem of retest effects'. *Social Psychiatry and Psychiatric Epidemiology*, 24: 227–32.

Palace, E. M. and Johnson, C. (1989) 'Treatment of recurrent nightmares by the dream reorganisation approach'. *Journal of Behaviour, Therapy and Experimental Psychology*, 20: 219–26.

Pilgrim, D. and Rogers, A. (1994) *A Sociology of Mental Health and Illness*. Buckingham: Open University Press.

Resick, P. (2001) *Stress and Trauma*. Philadelphia: Taylor & Francis.

Rutter, M. (1966) *Children of Sick Parents*. London: Oxford University Press.

Rutter, M. (1985) 'Resilience in the face of adversity: protective factors and resistance to psychiatric disorder'. *British Journal of Psychiatry*, 147: 598–611.

Saigh, P. A. (1991) 'The development of posttraumatic stress disorder'. *Behaviour Therapy*, 2: 213–16.

Smith, P., Perrin, S., Yule, W. and Rabe-Hesketh, S. (2001) 'War exposure and maternal reactions in the psychological adjustment of children from Bosnia-Hercegovina'. *Journal of Child Psychology and Psychiatry*, 42(3): 395–404.

Somnier, F. E. and Genefke, I. K. (1986) 'Psychotherapy for victims of torture'. *British Journal of Psychiatry*, 149: 323–9.

Sourander, A. (1998) 'Behaviour problems and traumatic events of unaccompanied refugee minors'. *Child Abuse and Neglect*, 22(7): 719–27.

Spence, S., Najman, J., Bor, W., O'Callaghan, M. and Willimas, G. (2002) 'Maternal anxiety and depression, poverty and marital relationship factors during early childhood as predictors of anxiety and depressive symptoms in adolescence'. *Journal of Child Psychology and Psychiatry*, 43(4): 457–69.

Stallard, P. and Law, F. (1993) 'Screening and psychological debriefing of adolescent survivors of life threatening events'. *British Journal of Psychiatry*, 163: 660–5.

Stimpson, N., Thomas, H., Weightman, L., Dunstan, F. and Lewis, G. (2003) 'Psychiatric disorder in veterans of the Persian Gulf'. *British Journal of Psychiatry*, 182: 391–403

Summerfield, D. (1997) 'The impact of war and atrocity on civilian populations three years after resettlement'. *British Journal of Psychiatry*, 166: 360–67.

Thomas, T. N. (1995) 'Acculturative stress in the adjustment of immigrant families'. *Journal of Social Distress and the Homeless*, 4(2): 131–42.

Turner, S., Bowie, C., Dunn, G., Shapo, L. and Yule, W. (2003) 'Mental health of Kosovan refugees in the UK'. *British Journal of Psychiatry*, 182: 444–8.

UNHCR (United Nations High Commissioner Refugees) (2000 edition) *Refugees by Numbers*. Available at: http://www.unhcr/un&ref/number2000

Vaughan, G. M. (1962) 'The social distance attitudes of New Zealand students towards Maoris and fifteen other national groups'. *Journal of Social Psychology*, 57: 85–92.

Verhulst, F. C. and Koot, H. M. (1992) *Child Psychiatric Epidemiology – Concepts, Methods and Findings*. London: Sage Publications.

Visser, J. H., Van de Ende, J., Koot, H. M. and Verhulst, F. C. (2003) 'Predicting change in psychopathology in youth referred to mental health services in childhood and adolescence'. *Journal of Child Psychology and Psychiatry*, 44(4): 509–19.

Ward, C., Bochner, S. and Furnham, A. (2001) *The Psychology of Culture Shock*, 2nd edn. Philadelphia and Hove, East Sussex: Routledge.

Ward, C. and Change, W. C. (1997) 'Cultural fit: a new perspective on personality and sojourner adjustment'. *International Journal of Intercultural Relations*, 21: 525–33.

Ward, C. and Kennedy, A. (1992) 'Locus of control, mood disturbance, and social difficulty during cross-cultural transitions'. *International Journal of Intercultural Relations*, 16: 175–94.

Ward, C. and Kennedy, A. (1994) 'Acculturation strategies, psychological adjustment and sociocultural competence during cross–cultural transitions'. *International Journal of Intercultural Relations*, 18: 329–43.

Weile, B., Wingender, L. B., Bach-Mortensen, N. and Busch, P. (1990) 'Behavioural problems in children of torture victims: a sequel to cultural maladaptation or to parent torture?' *Journal of Development and Behavioural Paediatrics*, 11: 79–80.

Weissman, M. M., Leckman, J. F., Merikangas, K. R., Gammon, G. D. and Prusoff, B. A. (1984) 'Depression and anxiety disorders in parents and children: results from Yale family study'. *Archive of General Psychiatry*, 41: 845–52.

Weissman, M and Paykel, E. (1974) *The Depressed Women: a Study of Social Relationships*. Chicago: Chicago University Press.

Werner, E. E. (1989) 'High risk children in young adulthood: a longitudinal study from birth to 32 years'. *American Journal of Orthopsychiatry*, 59(1): 72–81.

Westermeyer, J. (1988) 'DSM-IV psychiatric disorders among Hmong refugees in the United States: a point of prevalence study'. *American Journal of Psychiatry*, 145: 197–202.

Westermeyer, J. (1989) *Psychiatric Care of Migrants*. Washington DC: American Psychiatric Press.

Westermeyer, J. (1991) 'Psychiatric service for refugee children: an overview'. In F. Ahearn and J. L. Athey (eds), *Refugee Children: Theory, Research and Services*. Baltimore: Johns Hopkins University Press.

Westermeyer, J., Vang, T. and Neider, J. (1983) 'Refugees who do and do not seek psychiatric care: an analysis of premigration and postmigration characteristics'. *Journal of Nervous and Mental Disease*, 171: 86–91.

Whaley, S. E., Pinton, A. and Sigman, M. (1999) 'Characterising interactions between anxious mothers and their children'. *Journal of Consulting and Clinical Psychology*, 67: 826–36.

Williams, C. L. and Berry, J. W. (1991) 'Primary prevention of acculturation stress among refugees: application of psychological theory and practice'. *American Psychologist*, 46(6): 632–41.

Williamson, J. (1988) 'Half the world's refugees'. *Refugees*, 54: 16–18.

Wolin, S. J. and Wolin, S. (1993) *The Reslient Self: How Survivors of Troubled Families Rise Above Adversity*. New York: Villard Books.

Woodhead, D. (2000) *The Health and Wellbeing of Asylum Seekers and Refugees*. London: King's Fund Report.

Yule, W. (1992) 'Post traumatic stress disorder in children'. *Current Opinion in Paediatrics*, 4: 623–9.

Yule, W. (ed.) (1999) *Post Traumatic Stress Disorders: Concepts and Therapy*. Chichester: Wiley.

Yule, W. and Canterbury, R. (1994) 'The treatment of posttraumatic stress disorder in children and adolescents'. *International Review of Psychiatry*, 6: 141–51.

Yule, W. and Udwin, O. (1991) 'Screening child survivors for posttraumatic stress disorder: experience from the *Jupiter* sinking'. *British Journal of Clinical Psychology*, 30: 131–8.

Yule, W., Bolton, D., Udwin, O., Boyle, S., O'Ryan, D. and Nurrish, J. (2000) 'The long-term psychological effects of a disaster experienced in adolescence: I: the incidence and course of PTSD'. *Journal of Child Psychology and Psychiatry*, 41(4): 503–11.

14
The Effects of Deterrence-Based Policies on Vulnerable, Traumatized Asylum Seekers and Refugees

Helen O'Nions

The scale of refugee movements in the world today is alarming, with around twenty million people across the globe considered to be 'of concern' to the UNHCR (UNHCR 2004). The reasons for large-scale refugee movements are numerous, including famine, civil war and ethnic violence.[1] On an individual level, the Medical Foundation for the Care of Victims of Torture documents hundreds of cases involving human rights abuses, torture, sexual exploitation, domestic violence and slavery. In 2003, the organization dealt with over 2000 individual cases (Medical Foundation 2004). Some of these applications will result in a grant of refugee status, but many more will not.

The aim of this chapter is to explore the way that refugee law, now rooted in a policy of deterrence, can intensify the suffering and distress experienced by vulnerable asylum seekers. It will be shown that in attempting to deter illegitimate asylum seekers or 'economic migrants' the current policy is failing to protect those most at risk. It is now almost impossible for those fleeing persecution to find safe and legal means of travel (Hayter 2000; Hathaway 1991). Across Europe there has been a convergence of approaches based on preventing entry and restricting welfare provisions (Schuster 2000). The harmonization of asylum policies across Europe is almost complete (Joly 1996). The same deterrence-based strategy, discussed below in the context of the UK, is found across Europe and the same tragic consequences result.

The law in the United Kingdom and Europe has its origins in the 1951 Convention on the Status of Refugees and its protocol of 1967 (hereafter Geneva Convention 1951). However, the interpretation of these legal provisions varies widely between signatory states. In recent years, the British government has discussed the possibility of repealing the international framework, which forms a minimum level of protection for those defined as refugees. In such a discussion it is often suggested that the Convention obligations place too great a financial burden on the affluent states of the West. This debate ignores the evidence that the vast majority of refugees live in countries outside of Europe (UNHCR 2004). In fact, the burden of providing and supporting these people rests largely on a handful of African and Asian states. Before examining the effects of the current policy, this chapter will first identify the key elements which an applicant must demonstrate in order to claim refugee status.

Minimum legal standards

In order for an asylum seeker to be recognized as a 'refugee' and consequently to be afforded the protection that the Geneva Convention requires, he or she will have to demonstrate a well-founded fear of persecution. The applicant will also need to establish that the persecutory treatment arises due to one of the five trigger factors: race, religion, national origins, political opinion or membership of a particular social group (see UNHCR 1992). If the applicant has experienced persecution for reasons other than those listed he/she will not be able to demand protection as a Convention refugee. In addition, if a person has acted in a purposeful way to fall within the definition once in the UK, the courts will tend to regard them cynically.

These categories are largely self-explanatory and should be given a purposive, broad definition in keeping with the spirit of the Convention. However, as the category most open to interpretation, 'membership of a particular social group' requires further attention. The UNHCR handbook states that it covers persons with 'similar habits, background or social status' (UNHCR 1992). Similarly, the EU joint position refers to people from the same background or with the same customs or same social status. It can be attributed by the persecutor rather than existing in fact (Council Joint Position 96/196/JHA).

Conscientious objectors may fall within this provision, although it appears from the case of *Sepet and Bulbul v SSHD and UNHCR* ([2003] 3 All ER 304) that the consequence of refusal to perform military service must be more than mere imprisonment in order to amount to persecution. It also appears that a person forced into serving in an internationally condemned military action or an abhorrent campaign which is considered to be outside the normal rules of military conduct, such as the Russian military campaign in Chechnya, could suffice to demonstrate persecution (*Krotov v SSHD* [2004] EWCA Civ 69). However, this subjective assessment will vary depending on the particular receiving state's view about what is or is not a legitimate military campaign.

Persecution on the basis of homosexuality could also fall within this provision. In the past the courts have required that the applicant alleging persecution on the grounds of homosexuality must demonstrate that he or she is an 'active' homosexual. However the case of *Jain v SSHD* ([2000] Imm AR 76) provides judicial recognition that homosexuals do form a social group under the Convention due to the presence of certain immutable characteristics, which a person cannot change without undermining their identity. This approach reflects the House of Lords decision in the case of *R v IAT and SSHD exp Shah and Islam* ([1999] 2 AC 629), in which women who were accused of adultery and faced a punishment of stoning to death, were considered to constitute a social group within Pakistan. Given the wording of the Convention, the Shah decision involves a certain amount of creativity and is certainly welcome from the perspective of justice. However, legalistically the decision is questionable as it appears at odds with a series of decisions in which a person can be denied protection because their social group is constituted primarily from the persecution directed at it. These are complex legal technicalities, which are beyond the scope of this chapter. However, they serve to remind us of the wide margin of discretion given to all levels of decision-makers in refugee determinations.

The meaning of well-founded persecution

Persecution is not defined in the Convention but is clearly interpreted to be more serious than simple discrimination (*R v SSHD exp Gashi and Nikshiqi* [1997] INLR 96). Indeed, it is best understood as a persistent pattern of 'serious harm' (Berkowitz and Jarvis 2000). The requirement that the fear of persecution is 'well-founded' requires decision-makers to consider both the applicant's state of mind (subjective test) and also information pertaining to the likelihood of persecution should they be returned (objective test). It is clear from the case of *R v SSHD exp Adan* ([1998] Imm AR 338) that the fear needs to be present rather than being constituted from past events.

Significantly, the court held in *Karanakaran* ([2000] Imm AR 271) that the decision-maker should consider each case on its facts and evaluate all the evidence whilst contemplating the consequences of their decision should it be incorrect. Typically, the objective assessment is based largely on Home Office documentation concerning the political situation in the country of origin and it can be difficult for the applicant to disprove these assessments. This is particularly disconcerting given research by the Immigration Advisory Service which found the information contained in these 'objective reports' to be 'dangerously inaccurate and misleading' (IAS 2003). The Home Office's own Advisory Panel on Country Information established in the face of such criticisms has endorsed these concerns (Advisory Panel on Country Information 2004).

The Convention categories: an overview

If a person's claim does not fit within one of these categories, there will prima facie be no legal obligation on a state to recognize them as a refugee. In many cases, across Europe, such people are afforded a temporary status, such that when the conflict in their homeland is over they will be returned. In the UK this has traditionally been exceptional leave to remain, which was initially given for a four-year period after which time the case would be reviewed. This has now been replaced with humanitarian leave (initially for three years) or discretionary leave. Both afford the Home Office a large degree of discretion and the opportunities for an applicant to challenge an adverse decision are strictly limited. Some of the more obvious cases of vulnerable individuals who do not fit neatly within the Convention criteria include women persecuted specifically because of their gender, persons fleeing a civil war or situation of conflict and those who have experienced prolonged discrimination falling short of persecution (see Crawley 2001; Refugee Women's Resource Project 2004).

There is no requirement that the state or its agents must have perpetrated the persecution. If the particular state is unable or unwilling to prevent persecutory actions perpetrated by others within its jurisdiction this will satisfy the Convention criteria. This fact could certainly be relevant in the decision by a government to condemn a particular regime, and it may go some way to explaining the reluctance of many European nations to acknowledge the full extent of the conflict and humanitarian crisis in Sudan. However, in France and Germany there has been a reluctance to recognize persecution in cases where non-state agents have perpetrated the actions (Phuong 2002); controversially, the EU has now endorsed their restrictive interpretation (Joly 1996: 71). This has had a knock-on effect in the British courts as a decision to remove an applicant to these countries has the potential to threaten the principle of non-refoulement. Indeed, the Court of Appeal in *Adan, Subaskaran and Aitsegur* ([1999] 3 WLR 1274) ruled that the Home Secretary had an obligation to ensure that the 'safe' country applied the correct Convention interpretation irrespective of the EU joint position.

The principle of non-refoulement

The principle of non-refoulement (from the French word meaning 'to expel') is the key to refugee protection under the Convention. Article 33(1) establishes that a person cannot be returned *in any manner* to the frontiers of territories where their life or freedom would be threatened on account of one of the Convention grounds. Furthermore, the UNHCR has clarified that this obligation extends beyond those formally recognized as refugees. The use of temporary protection was endorsed by the UNHCR in response to the crisis in the former Yugoslavia, where a strict application of the Convention was not made out – for example, in cases of serious injury requiring treatment, or sexual assault.

The non-refoulement obligation must be viewed in the light of Article 3 of the Convention Against Torture and other Cruel, Inhuman or Degrading Treatment or Punishment 1984, which establishes, inter alia, that no state shall return a person where there are substantial grounds for believing that she/he would be in danger of being subjected to torture (Gorlick 1999). The Committee Against Torture has received some individual complaints on this issue and established in the case of *Elmi v Australia* ([1999] INLR 341) that the non-refoulement obligation is wider than that afforded to those formally defined as 'refugees' under the 1951 Convention, such as those who are fleeing clan violence. In this sense it could be applied to many people presently caught up in the rebel violence in Sudan. It would also apply in circumstances where a person would otherwise be excluded from protection under the 1951 Convention, such as those suspected of terrorist activities. However, the 1984 Convention is not a legally binding instrument, as it has not been incorporated into domestic law. Of more contemporary significance therefore, is the obligation contained in Article 3 of the European Convention on Human Rights and Fundamental Freedoms incorporated via the Human Rights Act 1998. Signatories to the European Convention on Human Rights 1950 have found it difficult to remove a person in such circumstances because of the absolute prohibition on torture and inhuman and degrading treatment contained in Article 3. The latter is an absolute right (i.e. it permits no restrictions or limitations by the state) and applies to everyone irrespective of nationality. It is possibly the most useful tool in improving the treatment of those claiming asylum across Europe and recent case law in the UK has indicated that it may be deployed in cases ranging from detention to withdrawal of state support (discussed below). However, the fact that Article 3 is increasingly being raised in legal argument is extremely alarming as it indicates that many asylum seekers and refugees are experiencing degrees of hardship such that inhuman and degrading treatment may be alleged.

European cooperation

The issue of immigration and asylum has gradually moved up the European agenda and cooperation between European states has developed dramatically. Since the Treaty of Amsterdam (1997) cooperation on asylum policy is now in the first pillar of the Union. The Dublin Convention 1990 requires that asylum seekers' applications be processed and determined in the first European state of arrival. The Convention was strengthened by EU Regulation 343/2003 which provides that they will not be permitted to make an application elsewhere unless there are significant family ties. In practice, this means that those seeking refugee status in Europe will be returned to the first European state of arrival, typically following a period of detention whilst their removal is facilitated. This obviously places a disproportionate burden on the poorer countries of southern Europe and may mean that applicants spend a great deal of time in transit (Blake 2001: 116).

More recently, the UK has signed up to EU Directive 2003/9/EC establishing minimum standards for the reception of asylum seekers. The directive includes a variety of significant principles, including access to education and health care as well as recognition of the specific needs of vulnerable groups. However, member states retain a wide margin of discretion as to the way they administer asylum control. A proposed directive 'On Minimum Standards for Granting and Withdrawing Refugee Status' (14203/04) adopts the lowest common denominator approach and supports controversial domestic policies including the recognition of certain countries as safe and a restricted right of appeal in such cases (ECRE et al. 2004).

The Resolution on Unaccompanied Children (1997), which established common standards for the reception and treatment of this vulnerable group, has yet to have the force of European law. The new Procedures Directive makes the child's welfare a 'primary' but not the paramount consideration and there is a presumption that, on reaching the age of 16, the child can be treated as an adult and denied specialist legal representation (Article 17).

Protecting the most vulnerable

Unaccompanied children seeking asylum are the most vulnerable of this vulnerable diaspora. According to the Refugee Council, unaccompanied children are marginalized in two ways: 'as children, to whom societies tend to ascribe fewer rights, and as refugees or migrants, who are invariably denied, usually by legislation, the same rights as host community nationals' (Refugee Council 2003: Part 9).

The term 'unaccompanied' refers to children who arrive without any parent or guardian. It can be misleading given that many children who appear accompanied may in fact be 'unaccompanied' by a person who has their welfare at heart. In some cases they will be 'accompanied' by traffickers or relatives who intend to sell them as forced labour – a fact that will rarely be detected by immigration officers.

The number of those officially defined as 'unaccompanied' has risen dramatically from 192 cases in 1992 to over 6000 in 2002, with the consequence that the government now targets special procedures and services to assist them. In the autumn quarter of 2003, 565 asylum applications were submitted by unaccompanied children (Kundnani 2003). Home Office statistics do not distinguish between adults and children who are granted refugee status, but it is apparent that the majority of unaccompanied children will be granted temporary leave to stay rather than refugee status (Ayotte and Williamson 2001: 4). The law provides that they may not be removed whilst they remain a child unless a suitable and willing carer emerges in the country of origin (Home Office Policy DP 4/96). However, there are several case studies that demonstrate that children have been refused admission without a suitable carer to return to. In two cases documented by Russell (1999: 139–40), boys as young as 13 were expected to return to countries in the midst of civil war without any family to turn to.

The reasonable degree of likelihood test established by the House of Lords in *SSHD v Sivakumaran* ([1988] Imm AR 147) is used to determine whether a person is at risk of persecution on their return. The standard of proof is lower than the typical civil standard of balance of probabilities and incorporates both subjective and objective elements. This test is applied equally to children, although it is often more difficult to assess in a child's case as information can often be confused and conflicting as a result of trauma and stress. According to the immigration rules, credibility will then become a key issue and may justify an application being refused. There has been some judicial recognition of the need to modify the strict decision-making process when dealing with children but the immigration rules do not specifically address this issue.

The degree of stress and trauma experienced by these children cannot be understated. A recent comparative study in Oxford found that 'more than a quarter of refugee children had significant psychological disturbance – greater than in both control groups and three times the national average' (Fazal and Stein 2003). Evidence also suggests that children may experience Post-Traumatic Stress Disorder (PTSD) following the violent death of family members and symptoms tend to manifest themselves at times of acute stress, such as waiting for a refugee determination (Hosin 2001). In 2001, Save the Children studied the experiences of unaccompanied child asylum seekers and found that this background of trauma and possible PTSD was being exacerbated by chaotic and frenetic social care provision on arrival in the UK (Stanley 2001). Many of the children experienced lengthy delays in their asylum hearing and some received little or no support on their arrival.

Perhaps the biggest concern from a human rights law perspective is that the government has entered a reservation against Article 22 of the Convention on the Rights of the Child 1989 (hereafter CRC), an international treaty that has received widespread international support. Article 22 recognizes the vulnerability of child refugees and obliges states to afford them appropriate protection and humanitarian assistance. The reservation states that the UK retains the right to administer immigration law, irrespective of this right, when it is deemed necessary. The effect of the reservation is that Article 22 cannot be relied upon in domestic legal proceedings. It has become apparent that the welfare of the child is not the paramount consideration in immigration cases, contradicting the obligation in Article 3 of the CRC and the founding principle of the Children Act 1989. The Refugee Council have argued in their response to the government's Green Paper *Every Child Matters*: 'Whilst the reservation remains in force we have a two-tier system, one tier of children for whom their best interests are the paramount consideration, and another for those whose best interests are a secondary consideration' (Refugee Council 2003).

It has been contended that the reservation undermines the whole object and purpose of the Convention and therefore that it is invalid under international law (Russell 1999: 131). Indeed, the UN committee charged with overseeing the Convention has been critical of the UK's stance (UNCRC 1999). However, the government has repeatedly argued that the reservation does not undermine the Convention per se and has stressed that its purpose is to prevent a claim for asylum solely on the basis of Convention rights. Recent research undertaken by Save the Children has found that the UK's approach is reflected in most other European countries. The importance of the child's best interests in immigration and asylum decisions is not emphasized in the EU harmonization context and the child's interests are seldom prioritized in decision-making (Ruxton 2000).

Identifying a child

The immigration rules define a child as someone who, in the absence of documentary evidence, appears to be under the age of 18 (HC 395 para. 349). There are numerous accounts of child asylum seekers struggling to convince immigration officers of their age. The child may be required to undergo an intimate medical examination, which, in the context of the experience and the trauma which the child may have already experienced, may be distressing and damaging to the child. The consequence of an error may be extreme. Russell documents an incident of a 13-year-old girl detained for several months despite evidence from a paediatrician and social worker confirming her age, and in another case, a 14-year-old boy was admitted temporarily into the UK with nowhere to stay and no money only to suffer abuse at the hands of other, adult asylum seekers (Russell 1999: 136). Given the difficulties created by the imposition of visas, many asylum-seeking children will not have correct documentation to prove their age. Indeed in some cases, children do not actually know their age – this could be due to custom (there may be no formal recognition of births in the country of origin), to confusion on arrival in an alien environment or to trauma that they have experienced. It is therefore regrettable that detention is used in order to determine the age of any young person. In a report to the National Audit Office, the Refugee Legal Centre stated: 'In our experience such disputes often become protracted and take a significant amount of effort and resources to resolve. Leaving aside the cost of such disputes, we are particularly concerned that Home Office intransigence leaves minors in a vulnerable position, often in detention' (Refugee Legal Centre 2003). Judicial decisions have been critical of the Home Office approach. It is clear from the case of *B, R (on the application of) v London Borough of Merton* ([2003] EWHC 1689 (Admin)) that the onus of proof should not be placed on the applicant and that the Home Office needs to consider factors beyond the applicant's immediate appearance such as family circumstances and history, educational background and wider cultural factors.

Recent research on a small sample of cases by the Refugee Council indicated that, as well as being distressing and unpleasant for the applicant, detention for the purpose of age verification is commonly found to have been unnecessary. In their survey of 23 cases in which age was disputed, the overwhelming majority were either conceded by the Home Office or ruled in the applicant's favour by the court (Refugee Council 2003). The Guidelines for Paediatricians published in November 1999 by the Royal College of Paediatrics and Child Health state:

> In practice, age determination is extremely difficult to do with certainty, and no single approach to this can be relied on. Moreover, for young people aged 15–18, it is even less possible to be certain about age ... Age determination is an inexact science and the margin of error can sometimes be a much as 5 years either side. (Stanley 2001: 30)

A further consequence of the tightening of borders across Europe is the need for asylum seekers to obtain false documents in order to travel. This may undermine the applicant's credibility and potentially lead to disputed minors being imprisoned for entering with false documentation (Lumley 2003; Tuitt 1996). The consequences of detaining minors were raised in the recent report by Her Majesty's Inspector of Prisons in relation to Dungavel prison: 'It remains our view that, however conscientiously and humanely children in detention are dealt with, it is not possible to meet the full range of their developmental needs. We therefore remain of the view that the detention of children should be an exceptional course, and only for a very short period – no more than a matter of days' (HMIP 2003a: 45). Despite these concerns Dungavel is still being used to detain children, in some cases for as long as nine months (BBC News 2005c; Crawley and Lester 2005). A Save the Children study found that half the children surveyed had been detained for more than one month with detrimental consequences for their emotional, psychological and physical welfare (Crawley and Lester 2005: 9). The detention of children potentially violates international legal provisions requiring states to promote rehabilitation and recovery of such children. As Russell argues, 'the UK authorities compound the trauma they have suffered through arbitrary detention, before any decision has been made on the asylum claim' (Russell 1999: 153).

Care and support for child asylum seekers

Until an asylum seeker turns 16 they are entitled to the same level of support from local authorities as other vulnerable children, including foster care and a social worker. However, the suitability of this accommodation varies and is often inadequate with a significant number of minors placed in single adult accommodation (Audit Commission 2000). In the past there have been reports of unaccompanied female asylum seekers simply disappearing from local authority care, the most likely explanation being recruitment into child prostitution (UNICEF 2001).

Between the ages of 16 and 18, there is discretionary support provided and consequently there is often a variation between local authorities. Once they turn 18 many find that they are cast out of the support system and left to fend for themselves. Many children surveyed by the Children's Refugee Consortium expressed anxiety at turning 18 and uncertainty about their future (Dennis 2002). Recently, in *R on app of Helen Berhe and others v LB Hillingdon* ([2003] EWHC 2075 (Admin)), the High Court interpreted the Children Leaving Care Act as providing the same level as support for young adult vulnerable asylum seekers as British children of the same age. This could include an aftercare package up to the age of 25. Children with families may find that they experience destitution by virtue of a recent legislative change. Section 9 of the Asylum and Immigration (treatment of claimants etc.) 2004 Act withdraws support for families with children who have failed in their final asylum appeal. Support will not be withdrawn unless the Secretary of State certifies that the family without reasonable excuse, failed to take reasonable steps to leave the UK voluntarily. Any dependent child of the asylum seeker would be liable to be taken into the care of the local authority, which would continue to have responsibility for providing accommodation for the child under Section 20 of the Children Act 1989 if the adult claimant were to be unable to provide it. As it would not be possible for social services to offer help to the adult on whom the child is dependent, there are likely to be a significant number of cases in which the authority could only discharge its responsibility towards the child by taking the child into its care.

During the passage of the Bill, the multi-party Joint Committee on Human Rights expressed reservations about the operation of Section 9, noting that violations of the Convention on the Rights of the Child and the European Convention on Human Rights could 'all too easily follow in practice' (JCHR 2003–4: para 45). In a recent report by the charity Barnados, Section 9 was strongly criticized by 33 Local Authorities who found that it was 'wholly incompatible' with their obligations under the Children Act 1989 (Kelly and Meldgaard 2005: 24). The government pilot study of Section 9 covered 116 families; so far none have been reported to have been returned and at least 35 families have disappeared into the margins of society. The consequences of this policy for the children of failed asylum seekers is extremely worrying. The presumption of depriving families of support and forcing them into destitution and homelessness is, like so many Home Office policies, flawed. Even on the disputed assumption that return is a realistic proposition, children risk being exposed to extreme deprivation through its policy and Local Authorities are unclear as to how it should be implemented.

Education of child asylum seekers

In the face of overwhelming criticism from educationalists, refugee groups and MPs, government plans to use accommodation centres to provide separate education for asylum-seeking children, were recently shelved. However, it remains apparent that access to education is a big problem for all children awaiting a refugee determination. The 1996 Education Act places a duty on Local Education Authorities in England to provide a school place for all children of compulsory school age (5–16 years) in their area. It is apparent that this duty is simply not being realized in the case of child asylum applicants. This may be a result of the dispersal policy in which access to schools and language support is rendered problematic. It could also be a consequence of a policy which detains children of an uncertain age. In addition, attitudes of education authorities and schools as well as the attitudes and experiences of the children themselves may undermine access. Many unaccompanied children are given discretionary leave as an alternative to refugee status and the temporary nature of this status causes insecurity and uncertainty and can obviously undermine educational success (OFSTED 2003: 5; Rutter 2003: 4; Dummett 2001). In a recent report by the Children's Refugee Consortium, which monitored the experience of a group of 118 child asylum seekers, almost half were not attending school and some had been waiting for a place for over six months (Dennis 2002). This is notwithstanding the duty laid down in Article 10 of the recent EC Directive 2003/9/EC requiring asylum seekers to be given access to education under similar conditions as nationals of the host state. The same study also found that a significant number had no access to health care and were not registered with a GP (Dennis 2002).

The focus on deterrence

Adults and children are suffering as a result of an asylum policy based on deterrence and prevention. The focus of this policy is flawed. It is flawed from a humanitarian perspective because it is directly responsible for additional deprivation and trauma that many genuine refugees experience when trying to exercise their rights as guaranteed in the UN Declaration on Human Rights. It is also flawed because it simply does not succeed in the stated objective of preventing bogus applications. The only people benefiting from these restrictive measures are traffickers. Their clients may be economic migrants or they may be genuine, there is simply no way of knowing the true figures. The only data we do have suggest that the number of asylum applications is falling (BBC News 2004b); we certainly cannot say that the new measures assist the genuine refugee and deter the bogus. Home Office research has found that across Europe, it is impossible to show that a reduction in the number of asylum seekers is simply attributable to particular policy initiatives. Furthermore, there was no evidence that conclusively demonstrated a reduction in the number of bogus applications as a result of more restrictive policy changes (Zetter et al. 2003). Dallal Stevens advises that we take a lesson from history and recognize that 'when human beings feel impelled to migrate, there is little that states can do to prevent it' (Stevens 2004: 436). However, since the increasing number of persons coming to the UK to seek asylum in the 1990s (Harding 2000; Harvey 2000) and the media frenzy which continues to drive anti-refugee rhetoric, successive governments have changed their focus from ending primary immigration to deterring asylum seekers. The international legal right to seek asylum guaranteed in Article 14 of the Universal Declaration of Human Rights (1948) has been substantially eroded by these initiatives.

Criminalizing illegal entry

A statement attached to the latest legislation on the Immigration and Nationality Directorate website makes it clear that those who arrive in the UK without correct documentation may not expect favourable treatment:

> Those claiming to be escaping death and torture must be honest with us – if they cannot explain how they got here without travel documents they should not expect to benefit from our protection and will face criminal prosecution if they deliberately seek to mislead the authorities by disposing of or destroying their documents before making their claim. (http://www.ind.homeoffice.gov.uk/ind/en/home/laws_policy/legislation/main_provisions.html)

Under Section 14A (1) Immigration Act 1971, a person who enters the UK by deception is now guilty of an offence and is liable to up to two years' imprisonment. This offence is broadly worded to encompass destroying travel documents, possession of false documents and entering under false pretences. There is also an offence committed under Section 25(1) by anyone who assists the unlawful entry of an asylum seeker. The asylum applicant has the opportunity to rebut the presumption of guilt by demonstrating reasonable excuse. The Joint Committee on Human Rights have expressed concern at the criminalization of illegal entry in the light of the Geneva Convention obligations as well as the right to fair trial guaranteed by the Human Rights Act 1998 (Joint Committee on Human Rights 2004). The provision fails to recognize the inevitability of illegal entry. There is no doubt that it is almost impossible for an asylum seeker to board an airplane and apply for entry legally in this capacity. If they come from a visa national country, as most do, the consequence of applying for a visa based on the desire to seek asylum in the destination state would, at best, lead to a refusal, and at worst, lead to imprisonment and possibly torture or death. This provision has nothing to do with protecting the interests of legitimate claimants. Rather it is entirely focused on prevention and deterrence that does not discriminate between the deserving and the undeserving applicant (see Immigration Advisory Service 2003).

There has clearly been a tendency to introduce visa requirements for people travelling from countries, which have generated a high number of asylum claims. Tony Blair's 2003 promise to reduce the number of people claiming asylum in the UK has seen asylum applications fall by roughly half: from 22 030 in the third quarter of 2002, to 11 955 in the third quarter of 2003 (excluding any accompanying spouses and children). In its press release announcing the figures, the government claimed that the reduction in numbers was caused by its policy of deterring those making 'abusive' claims (Kundnani 2003). However, the difficulty of substantiating this claim has already been noted with reference to the Home Office's own research (Zetter et al. 2003). The simple reduction cannot accurately differentiate between genuine and bogus. To illustrate this point one can refer to Zimbabwe. The number of refugee applicants from Zimbabwe fell by three-quarters, from 2750 in the last quarter of 2002 to 710 in the third quarter of 2003, since the introduction of a visa regime at the end of that year. Yet the British government has continued to criticize the Mugabe regime and has lobbied the European Union for sanctions to be applied (Black and Meldrum 2002).

Carriers liability provisions first introduced in 1987 combine with visa restrictions to prevent asylum seekers from taking legitimate routes to enter the West. In addition, the government has been stationing Immigration officials at ports to prevent people who are suspected of being asylum seekers from travelling to the UK (O'Nions 2002). Such a practice appears to undermine the international right to 'seek' asylum and was recently ruled unlawful by the House of Lords in *R (on the app of European Roma Rights Centre) v SSHD* ([2005] 1 All ER 527) in respect of Roma travellers prevented from boarding aeroplanes at Prague airport (Travis 2004). The decision highlighted the subjective and discriminatory nature of these actions.

The Home Office operates a safe country list, which was originally confined to EU accession states. The presumption is that people who come from countries on this list are unlikely to be legitimate asylum seekers. In most cases, people will then be detained pending removal. The safe country list has recently been extended to include countries such as Jamaica, Ukraine, Albania and Sri Lanka (Home Office 2003). Home Office instructions indicate that most asylum seekers from these countries will be presumed to be 'clearly unfounded' and will thus be detained at Oakington reception centre pending removal (see Nicholson and Twomey 1998 1999; Shah 2000 for further information on UK law and refugee policies).

The absence of an in-country right of appeal deprives many asylum seekers from the opportunity of presenting their case before an independent adjudicator. The quality of initial decision-making has been an issue attracting major criticism and has seen many decisions, primarily those based on adverse credibility findings, being overturned on appeal (Amnesty International 2004; Asylum Aid 2003). In 2003, Amnesty International examined 170 refusal letters and claimed that the Home Office was responsible for approximately 14 000 incorrect asylum decisions, which were subsequently overturned on appeal. The director of Amnesty, Kate Allen, commented: 'The appeals system is presently the only thing keeping thousands of people each year from persecution. When initial decision-making is so frequently wrong, reducing appeal rights against these decisions could mean returning people to face torture or execution' (Amnesty International 2004b). However, an out-of-country appeal does not enable credibility findings to be adequately challenged as the applicant will not be physically present to respond to such questions (Baldaccini 2004). The presumption that these countries are safe is not borne out by legitimate, detailed research. On the contrary, a detailed report on the persecution of women by the Refugee Women's Resource Project documents cases where women from Albania are sold to traffickers, lesbians in Jamaica are persecuted by vigilantes, and Ukrainian domestic violence legislation fails to protect the interests of female victims (Refugee Women's Resource Project 2004).

Denial of support

The 1999 Immigration and Asylum Act repealed the disastrous voucher system and instead introduced a regime whereby support would only be provided to those deemed 'destitute' through the National Asylum Support Service (NASS). Since January 2003, 'destitute' adult, childless asylum seekers whose claims were not submitted 'as soon as reasonably practicable' after arriving in Britain have been denied any kind of housing or subsistence, as a result of Section 55 of the Nationality, Immigration and Asylum Act 2002. When deciding whether a claim has been made 'as soon as reasonably practicable' case-workers must consider any physical or practical impediments to applying and the mental state of the applicant In 2004, the Refugee Council estimate that 9000 people were refused support for this reason alone, although many applied within hours of arrival (Refugee Council 2004). Their *Hungry and Homeless* study found that three-quarters of the voluntary organizations interviewed had experienced people sleeping rough as a consequence of Section 55. The justification of this move was in keeping with the government's attempts to deter people from entering the UK in order to take advantage of the welfare system.

The deterrent effect of Section 55 can be questioned as the number of in-country applications actually increased by 7 per cent in 2003 (HL debates. Col. 658, 26 April 2004). In addition, research suggests that the time that a person applies for asylum has little to do with the legitimacy of their claim. Indeed, statistically those that claim 'late' are more likely to be successful than those who apply immediately upon arrival. There is certainly no evidence to suggest that late claimants are always bogus. An unsuccessful attempt to repeal Section 55 was mounted in the legislative division of the House of Lords in 2003. It was noted that 81 per cent of successful claimants in the first three terms of 2003 were in-country applicants (HL debates. Col. 657, 26 April 2004). Furthermore, in London half those denied support under this provision are women and around 29 per cent end up sleeping rough. Having lost a high-profile legal challenge the government introduced a concession in December 2003 to enable people to apply for support if they make an application within three days of arrival A person is exempt from Section 55 if denial of such support would breach the prohibition on inhuman and degrading treatment contained in Article 3 of the Human Rights Act 1998 following the Court of Appeal decision in *R on application of Q v SSHD* ([2003] EWCA Civ 364). It is clear, however, from this case and the Home Office guidance that destitution in itself will not amount to inhuman or degrading treatment and the courts will look to see whether such support can be gained through a charitable organization. If a person is destitute but is able to get some food and shelter from a charity or friends, the Home Office is under no additional obligation to support them. Lord Phillips cited the definition of inhuman and degrading treatment in *R (on the app of Pretty) v DPP* ([2001] UKHL 61):

> Where treatment humiliates or debases an individual showing lack of respect for, or diminishing, his or her human dignity or arouses feelings of fear, anguish or inferiority capable of breaking an individual's moral and physical resistance, it may be characterized as degrading and also fall within the prohibition of Article 3 ... (para.119).

It is therefore apparent that inhuman and degrading treatment could indeed include 'sleeping rough, begging for food or money with which to buy it, and the fear, humiliation and mental suffering which soon ensue'. In December 2005, the House of Lords issued a major blow to the new support policy by deciding that the Pretty threshold was reached and there was a breach of Article 3 where asylum applicants struggled to find basic food and were forced to sleep rough as a consequence of Section 55 (*R v SSHD exp Adam, Limbuela and Tesema* ([2005] UKHL 66)). Nevertheless, the Section 55 approach has been implicitly endorsed by the EU and will not contravene the new directive on minimum standards. The UK lobbied the EU for the late inclusion of Article 16(2) which mirrors the wording of Section 55 allowing benefits to be refused if an asylum seeker has not made an application as soon as reasonably practicable.

Those who are refused asylum and may not be able to return, for example because of ill health or the condition of the country to which they will be returned, will normally be refused benefits and are prohibited from working. However, there is discretion to provide hard-case support when such persons are destitute and have no other means of support. In the case of *Ibraheem Mohammed Tajir Salih* ([2003] EWHC 2273 (Admin)) it was revealed that the Home Office had a policy not to inform rejected applicants of the existence of this provision. The court found this approach to be irrational and also criticized the five-day delay in finding accommodation for the homeless applicants. Hard-case support cases are now required to engage in 'voluntary' community work in order to receive support. It is also evident that many asylum seekers who are receiving support are living in conditions of extreme poverty (BBC News 2005b). Support is set at 70 per cent below the national subsistence level provided to those receiving state benefits. In addition, the dispersal system throws up many problems which impact negatively on the health of asylum seekers. There is ample evidence from across Europe of alienation, victimization and heightened vulnerability as a result of this system, which separates people from their communities and places them in deprived, hostile environments (Save the Children 2000; Institute of Race Relations 2000). Other recent findings from research into the asylum system in Leeds also found that many people who are accepted as refugees become homeless after transferring from accommodation under the NASS scheme (BBC News 2005c; Cholewinski 1998). It is clear that this complex and divisive system is failing to provide basic support for the most vulnerable.

Detention

The practice of detaining asylum seekers can be seen as another example of a restriction aimed at deterring asylum seekers and it represents one of the greatest threats to their well-being (see Hughes and Liebaut 1998: 199–209; Fabbricotti 1998). Persons may be detained in specialized immigration centres or in the prison system. The provision of specialized detention centres is common throughout Europe with approximately 100 000 asylum seekers detained at any one time (Jesuit Refugee Service 2004). Detention is considered to fall within the basic standards of support to be given to asylum seekers as laid down in the recent EU Directive 2003/9. The reasons for detention vary between states and there is little reliable statistical information available on the number of persons detained (HMIP 2003a).

The British government detain more asylum applicants than any other European state and the arbitrary nature of this detention policy has prompted criticism from a variety of sources including the UNHCR (see interview with Hope Hanlan 2000; HMIP 2003b). The number of persons detained is rising at a steady and alarming rate (Lumley 2003). In Northern Ireland there has been a doubling of the number of asylum seekers imprisoned, including infants and children, and a fivefold increase in the number of women applicants detained in mainstream prisons (Wiesener and Corrigan 2004).

Until 2002, detention in the UK was only used pending an order for deportation. However, this has now been extended by Section 62 of the 2002 Nationality Immigration and Asylum Act to enable detention pending examination or a decision whether to remove or removal itself. As the government has publicly committed itself to removing more failed asylum seekers the number of persons in detention will continue to increase. Home Office statistics listed 1105 asylum seekers detained solely under immigration law provisions on 25 September 2004 (Home Office 2004: 9). Despite constructing many new detention establishments, a significant number are placed in mainstream prisons and 22 per cent of asylum detainees had been held in detention for more than four months (Home Office 2004: 9). Many fast-tracked applicants whose cases are considered to be 'clearly unfounded' will be detained at Oakington Reception Centre pending removal (Home Office 2004). The conditions of this detention have very recently been illustrated in an undercover BBC investigation that documented acts of violence and abuse in a culture of insensitivity and racism (BBC1 2005a). Detention is also used in cases where removal is not imminent. Indeed, the extent of arbitrariness surrounding detention appears to conflict with international legal provisions. The UNHCR guidelines establish that detention should not be used unless absolutely necessary and specify the exceptional reasons which may justify confinement (UNHCR 1999). They also state that unaccompanied minors, pregnant and nursing mothers should not be detained under any circumstances. In the case of unaccompanied elderly persons, those with disabilities or who have experienced torture or trauma, alternatives should be sought and detention should only be considered when medical evidence confirms that there would be no adverse effect to health or well-being (UNHCR 1999; UNHCR 1997; Clayton 2004: 432).

In 2002, the Chief Inspector of Prisons conducted the most comprehensive report to be issued on the detention of asylum seekers in the UK. Her findings give grave cause for concern. In particular she noted that the psychological well-being of detainees worsened over time and that many detainees experienced frustration, abuse and humiliation by centre staff (HMIP 2003b; BBC News 2003). More recent reports suggest that these criticisms have not been addressed consistently (BBC News 2004; BBC1 2005a). The findings are supported by several other studies and are clearly hard to reconcile with UNHCR guidelines (Dell and Salinsky 2001; McLeish et al. 2002).

Article 51(f) of the European Convention on Human Rights, now incorporated in the Human Rights Act 1998, establishes that immigration detention can be justified very specifically to prevent unauthorized entry and to detain a person against whom action is being taken with a view to deportation or extradition. In order to comply with the rule of law, one would expect any deprivation of liberty to be clearly enunciated with reference to these two exceptions and to be proportionate to the given need. However, the House of Lords have adopted a narrow interpretation of this provision by interpreting unauthorized entry to constitute any entry that has not been specifically authorized by the Home Office (*R v SSHD exp Saadi and Others* ([2002] 1 WLR 3131)). In addition, Home Office policy allows for the detention of families and unaccompanied minors despite UNHCR guidance (Cole 2003: 96–113). At any one time it is estimated that between 30 and 40 families are detained in specific family units (Home Office 2004: 9). In the case of unaccompanied minors, the justification for confinement is one of credibility. The *Operational Enforcement Manual* says that unaccompanied minors should be treated as adults where their appearance 'strongly suggests' that they are over 18. Given the difficulties in establishing age, discussed above, this inevitably means that many vulnerable minors will be placed in detention (see Crawley and Lester 2005). The policy on detention has become progressively more restrictive with increasing numbers of people, including families and unaccompanied children, being detained. The right to an automatic bail hearing, which had been introduced but never implemented in 1999, has now been repealed. It must be remembered that, discounting unauthorized entry, these asylum detainees have not committed any criminal offence. The House of Lords' interpretation of unauthorized entry in this context is lamentable given the obstacles designed to prevent legitimate entry.

The future of European refugee protection

In 2003, Labour proposed a 'new vision for Refugees', which would see refugee claims processed externally (Fekete 2003). The EU Commission has adopted the UK's proposals, the effect of which is that migrants will have to make asylum claims as close to their country of origin as possible (European Commission 2004). The justification for this action is twofold – the assumed increase in applications from economic migrants and the unprecedented rise in the use of human traffickers. As the human rights monitoring group, Statewatch, has argued, these assumptions are not questioned and the EU appears incapable of understanding that human traffickers are a product of exclusionary immigration rules which prevent asylum seekers and migrants alike from getting legitimate access to the West (Statewatch 2004; Fekete 2003). It appears from UNHCR proposals that this scheme would primarily target arrivals from countries deemed to be 'safe' and that such applicants would be housed in closed reception centres in poorer countries bordering Europe. Obviously, there will be no guarantee that such initiatives will not eventually be applied to all asylum seekers. States such as Turkey have been proposed as processing centres, conveniently forgetting that a large number of asylum applications in the West come from Turkish Kurds. It is also worth remembering that many countries are designated as safe in the absence of evidence to the contrary. For example Afghanistan was considered safe for refugee repatriations in 2003 despite NGO evidence to the contrary. The welfare of asylum seekers will not be a priority if these recommendations are accepted and accountability will further be diminished. Raekha Prasad, writing for the *Guardian* comments: 'In all but name, Britain is proposing a new network of refugee camps – designated areas where those inside have different rights from those outside. To envisage such a plan is to imagine ghettoes created by the world's most peaceful and richest countries in some of the world poorest and most unstable regions' (quoted in Statewatch 2004). There is no doubt that an honest debate on asylum is required. European media and governments must be held accountable for the perception that all asylum seekers are bogus (Mollard 2001). Refugee organizations should be given the opportunity to lead and inform this debate (Goodwin-Gill 1996).

Conclusion

In 1997, a 12-year-old Kenyan boy was found crushed to death after stowing in the landing gear of a plane bound for Gatwick (Ayotte and Williamson 2001: 54). In December 2004, a Zimbabwean citizen beaten and tortured by agents of Mugabe's Zanu PF party had his application for asylum rejected by the Home Office on the basis that he could have expected nothing less given his opposition to the regime (Johnston and Breslin 2004; Ayotte 2000).

As the numbers of refugees continue to rise and the opportunities for legal travel diminish, the traffickers profit at the expense of the vulnerable (Morrison 2000). Asylum seekers have no choice but to resort to increasingly dangerous and devious methods of travel. On arrival, most are considered to be 'bogus' and many face detention, repatriation, poverty or homelessness. The particular vulnerability of children is seldom recognized by a system operating in a culture of disbelief and denial. This culture of disbelief pervades Home Office decision-making as people with traumatic experiences and mental illness are detained pending decisions and removals. The constant change in immigration and asylum law and policy, evidenced by a new piece of legislation every 18 months, demonstrates the climate of confusion and misinformation. It has been shown that the current obsession with deterrence is flawed on many levels. On a humanitarian level, it undermines the right of every person to seek asylum. On a practical level, it leaves people with no option but to resort to clandestine, illicit and dangerous means of travel. Finally, on an economic level, global economists have now recognized that Europe needs immigration in order to stabilize the retirement age (UN Study 2000). It is sadly an unsurprising paradox that the immigration controls of the West serve the interests of the strong, determined and wealthy whilst working to deprive the vulnerable of the protection they desperately need.

Note

1   Stevens notes that one of the greatest refugee movements of all may be about to happen as a result of global climate change. The fall-out from the Asian tsunami of December 2004 may indeed see this prediction becoming a reality (Stevens 2004).

References

Advisory Panel on Country Information (2004) 'Commentary on October 2003 CIPU report on Somalia', 2nd meeting, 2 March 2004. Available at: www.ind.homeoffice.co.uk/filestore/APCI2.2.doc

Amnesty International (2004a) 'Get it right: how Home Office decision making fails refugees'. Amnesty International, London.

Amnesty International (2004b) 'UK asylum – new report exposes Home Office failures causing nearly 14,000 wrong asylum decisions in one year'. Press briefing, 9 February 2004. Amnesty International.

Asylum Aid (2003) *Safe for Whom?* Available at: www.asylumaid.org

Audit Commission Briefing (2000) 'A new city: supporting asylum seekers and refugees in London'. July.

Ayotte, W. (2000) *Separated Children Coming to Western Europe: Why they Travel and How they Arrive.* Save the Children.

Ayotte, W. and Williamson, L. (2001) *Separated Children in the UK.* Refugee Council and Save the Children.

Baldaccini, A. (2004) 'Providing protection in the 21st century: refugee rights at the heart of UK asylum policy'. Asylum Rights Campaign, London.

BBC News (2003) 'Asylum detention needs reform'.

BBC News (2004a) '"Prison culture" at asylum centre'. 16 June.

BBC News (2004b) 'Asylum applications fall sharply'. 24 February.

BBC News (2005a) 'Asylum undercover'. 3 March.

BBC News (2005b) 'Benefits fail city asylum seekers'. 10 January.

BBC News (2005c) 'Child detention regulation urged'. 28 February.

Berkowitz, N. and Jarvis, C. (2000) *Asylum Gender Guidelines*. Immigration Appellate Authority.

Black, I. and Meldrum, A. (2002) 'EU agonizes over Mugabe sanctions'. Guardian Unlimited (www.guardianunlimited.co.uk), 18 February.

Blake, N. (2001) 'The Dublin Convention and rights of asylum seekers in the European Union'. In E. Guild and C. Harlow (eds), *Implementing Amsterdam: Immigration and Asylum Rights in EC Law*. Oxford: Hart Publishers.

Blake, N. and Husain, R. (2003) *Immigration, Asylum and Human Rights*. Oxford: Oxford University Press.

British Medical Association (2002) *Report on Asylum Seekers and Health*. BMA.

Cholewinski, R. (1998) 'Enforced destitution of asylum seekers in the UK'. *International Journal of Refugee Law*, 10(3): 462.

Clayton, G. (2004) *Textbook on Immigration and Asylum Law*. Oxford: Oxford University Press.

Cole, D. (2003) 'The detention of asylum-seeking families in the UK'. *Immigration, Asylum and Nationality Law*, 17(2): 96–113.

Crawley, H. (2001) *Refugees and Gender: Law and Process*. Bristol: Jordan.

Crawley, H. and Lester, T. (2005) *No Place for a Child*. February. Save the Children.

Dell, M. and Salinsky, S. (2001) *Protection not Prison: Torture Survivors Detained in the UK*. September, Medical Foundation for the Care of Victims of Torture.

Dennis, J. (2002) *A Case of Change: How Refugee Children in England are Missing Out*. Refugee Council.

Dummett, M. (2001) *On Immigration and Refugees*. London: Routledge.

European Commission Communication to the European Parliament (2004) 'Improving access to durable solutions' 4 June. COM (2004) 410.

European Council on Refugees and Exiles, Amnesty International and Others (2004) 'Call for withdrawal of asylum procedures directive'. Letter to Mr Vittorino, 22 March 2004. Available at: http://www.statewatch.org/news/2004/mar/ngo-asylum-leter.pdf.

Fabbricotti, A. (1998) 'The concept of inhuman or degrading treatment in international law and its application in asylum cases'. *International Journal of Refugee Law*, 10(4): 637.

Fazal, M. and Stein, A. (2003) *Mental Health of Refugee Children: Comparative Study*. May 2003 Section of Child and Adolescent Psychiatry, University Department of Psychiatry, Warneford Hospital, Oxford.

Fekete, L. (2003) 'The EU's new border control programme'. Independent Race and Refugee News Network, 27 March.

Goodwin-Gill, G. (1996) *The Refugee in International Law*. Oxford: Clarendon Press.

Gorlick, B (1999) 'The Convention and the Committee Against Torture: a complementary protection regime for refugees'. *International Journal of Refugee Law*, 11(3): 479–95.

Harding, J. (2000) *The Uninvited: Refugees at the Rich Man's Gate*. London: Profile Books.

Harvey, C. (2000) *Seeking Asylum in the UK: Problems and Prospects*. London: LexisNexis.

Hathaway, J. (1991) *The Law of Refugee Status*. London: Butterworths.

Hayter, T. (2000) *Open Borders*. London: Pluto.

HMIP (2003a) Her Majesty's Inspectorate of Prisons. *Report on Dungavel*. August. HMI 042/2003.

HMIP (2003b) 'Introduction and summary of findings: inspection of five immigration service custodial establishments'. April. HMIP, Home Office. A summary of the report is available at: http://www.medact.org/content/refugees/ dungavel_14aug2003.pdf

Home Office (2003a) '"Safe country list" expanded to cut asylum abuse'. 17 June. Available at: www.ind.homeoffice.gov.uk/news.asp?NewsID=283

Home Office (2003b) 'Asylum statistics: 3rd quarter 2003'. September.

Home Office. (2004) 'Asylum statistics: 3rd quarter 2004'. September.

Hope Hanlan Interview October 2000. *In Exile*. Refugee Council.

Hosin, A. (2001) 'Children of traumatized and exiled refugee families: resilience and vulnerability'. *Medicine, Conflict and Survival*, 17: 137–45.

Hughes, F. and Liebaut, J. (eds) (1998) *Detention of Asylum Seekers in Europe: Analysis and Perspectives*. Netherlands: Kluwer.

Immigration Advisory Service (2003) *Home Office Country Assessment: an Analysis*. Available at: www.iasuk.org

Institute of Race Relations (2000) 'The dispersal of xenophobia'. *European Race Bulletin*, 33/34, 2000. www.irr.org.uk

Jesuit Refugee Service (2004) *Detention in Europe*. JRS Europe.

Johnston, J. and Breslin, J. P. (2004) 'Home office tells "foolhardy" asylum seekers: "It's your own fault you've been persecuted"'. *Sunday Herald*, 26 December.

Joint Committee on Human Rights (2004) 5th Report 2003–4. 10 February.

Joly, D. (1996) *Haven or Hell: Asylum Policies and Refugees in Europe*. Basingstoke: Macmillan.

Kelly, N. and Meldgaard, L. (2005) *The End of the Road*. Barnados.

Kundnani, A. (2003) 'Analysis: the quarterly asylum statistic'. Independent Race and Refugee News Network. 1 December. www.irr.org.uk

Lumley, R. (2003) *Children in Detention*. Refugee Council Policy Paper. Refugee Council.

McLeish, J., Culter, S. and Stancer, C. (2002) 'A crying shame: pregnant asylum seekers and their babies in detention'. Maternity Alliance. www.maternity-alliance.org.uk

Medical Foundation for the Care of Victims of Torture (2004a) *Opening Doors: Annual Review 2003–4* www.torturecare.org.uk. See also (2004b) *Implementation of Reception Directive*. Medical Foundation Response. December 2004.

Mollard, C. (2001) *Asylum: the Truth Behind the Headlines*. Oxfam.

Morrison, J. (2000) *The Trafficking and Smuggling of Refugees: the End Game of European Asylum Policy?* UNHCR.

Nicholson, F. and Twomey, P. (eds) (1998) *Current Issues of UK Asylum Law and Policy*. Aldershot: Ashgate.

Nicholson, F. and Twomey, P. (eds) (1999) *Refugee Rights and Realities*. Cambridge: Cambridge University Press.

OFSTED (2003) *The Education of Asylum-seeker Pupils*. HMI 453, October.

O'Nions, H. (2002) 'A litmus test for civil society'. *The Guardian Unlimited*, 31 July.

Phuong, C. (2002) 'Persecution by non-state agents: comparative judicial interpretations of the 1951 Refugee Convention'. *European Journal of Migration and Law*, 4(4): 521.

Refugee Council (2003) *Response to the Government's Green Paper: 'Every Child Matters'*. November. www.refugeecouncil.org.uk

Refugee Council (2004) *Hungry and Homeless: the Impact of the Withdrawal of State Support on Asylum Seekers, Refugee Communities and the Voluntary Sector*. April. www.refugeecouncil.org.uk

Refugee Legal Centre (2003) 'Response to national audit office study on asylum: deciding applications for asylum'. Available at: www.refugee-legal-centre. org.uk/NAO010703.doc

Refugee Women's Resource Project. (2004) *Safe for Whom? Women's Human Rights Abuses and Protection in 'Safe List' Countries: Albania, Jamaica and Ukraine*. Asylum Aid.

Russell, S. (1999) 'Unaccompanied refugee children in the UK'. *International Journal of Refugee Law*, 11(1).

Rutter, J. (2003) *Working with Refugee Children*. Joseph Rowntree Foundation.

Ruxton, S. (2000) *Separated Children in Europe: a programme for Action*. Save the Children and UNHCR.

Save the Children and the Scottish Refugee Council (2000) *I Didn't Come Here for Fun*. Save the Children.

Schuster, L. (2000) 'A comparative analysis of the asylum policy of seven European governments'. *Journal of Refugee Studies*, 13(1): 118–32.

Shah, P. (2000) *Refugees, Race and the Legal Concept of Asylum in Britain*. London: Cavendish.

Stanley, K. (2001) *Cold Comfort: Young Separated Refugees in England*. Save the Children.

Statewatch Press Release (2004) 'Analysis: "Killing me softly? Improving durable solutions": doublespeak and the dismantling of refugee protection in the EU'. Statewatch.

Stevens, D. (2004) *UK Asylum Law and Policy*. London: Sweet and Maxell.

Travis, A. (2004) 'Asylum operation racist say law lords'. *The Guardian Unlimited*, 10 December.

Tuitt, P. (1996) *False Images: the Law's Construction of the Refugee*. Pluto

UNCRC Committee on the Rights of the Child: consideration of report submitted by the UK. UN Doc CRC/C/15/add.34 (8th session 1995) and 2nd report to the UN Committee on the Rights of the Child by the UK. HMSO 1999.

UN Study (2000) *Replacement Migration: Is it a Solution to Declining and Ageing Populations?* Population Division of the Department of Social and Economic Affairs, New York.

UNHCR (1992) *Handbook on Procedures and Criteria for Determining Refugee Status*. UNHCR.

UNHCR (1997) *Guidelines on Policies and Procedures Dealing with Unaccompanied Children Asylum Seeking*. UNHCR.

UNHCR (1999) *Guidelines on Applicable Criteria and Standards Relating to the Detention of Asylum Seekers*. Februry. UNHCR.

UNHCR (2000) *The State of the World's Refugees: Fifty Years of Humanitarian Action*. Oxford: Oxford University Press.
UNHCR (2002) http://www.unhcr.org/cgi-bin/texis/vtx/home
UNHCR (2004) 'Refugees by number 2003'. UNHCR. http://www.unhcr.org/cgi-bin/texis/vtx/home
UNICEF (2001) 'Refugee and asylum seeking children'. May. Briefing. UNICEF. www.unicef.org.uk
Wiesener, C. and Corrigan, P. (2004) 'Measuring misery – detention of asylum seekers in Northern Ireland: a statistical analysis 2002–2004'. 17 June. Refugee Action Group, Belfast. Available at: http://www.amnesty.org.uk/images/ul/M/Measuring_Misery.pdf
Zetter, R., Griffiths, D., Ferretti, S. and Pearl, M. (2003) *An Assessment of the Impact of Asylum Policies in Europe 1990–2000*. Home Office Research Study 259.

Index

DATE DUE